Synaptic Plasticity

Synaptic Plasticity

Molecular, Cellular, and Functional Aspects

edited by Michel Baudry, Richard F. Thompson, and Joel L. Davis

A Bradford Book
The MIT Press
Cambridge, Massachusetts
London, England

This book was set in Palatino by Asco Trade Typesetting Ltd., Hong Kong and was printed and bound in the United States of America.

Library of Congress Cataloging-in-Publication Data

Synaptic plasticity : molecular, cellular, and functional aspects / edited by Michel Baudry, Richard F. Thompson, and Joel L. Davis.
  p.   cm.
"A Bradford book."
Includes bibliographical references and index.
ISBN 0-262-02359-8
  1. Neuroplasticity.   I. Baudry, M.   II. Thompson, Richard F.   III. Davis, Joel L., 1942–   .
QP363.3.S964   1993   76287   93–19699
612.8—dc20   CIP

Contents

Contributors

Alain Artola
Max-Planck Institute for
Brain Research
Frankfurt, Germany

German Barrionuevo
Department of Behavioral
Neuroscience
University of Pittsburgh
Pittsburgh, Pennsylvania

Michel Baudry
Department of Biological Sciences
University of Southern California
Los Angeles, California

Mark F. Bear
Neuroscience Department
Brown University
Providence, Rhode Island

Theodore W. Berger
Department of Biomedical
Engineering
University of Southern California
Los Angeles, California

Gilbert Chauvet
Institute for Theoretical Biology
University of Angers
Angers, France

Chong Chen
Neuroscience Program
University of Southern California
Los Angeles, California

Leon N. Cooper
Neuroscience and
Physics Department
Institute for Brain and
Neural Systems
Brown University
Providence, Rhode Island

Caleb E. Finch
Neurogerontology Division,
Andrus Gerontology Center and
Department of Biological Sciences
University of Southern California
Los Angeles, California

Leslie Grover
Neurobiology Department
Northeastern Ohio College of
Medicine
Rootstown, Ohio

Susan Hockfield
Section of Neurobiology
Yale University
New Haven, Connecticut

Nathan Intrator
Computer Science Department
Tel-Aviv University
Tel-Aviv, Israel

Masao Ito
Frontier Research Program, RIKEM
Wako, Saitama, Japan

Jeansok J. Kim
Neuroscience Program
University of Southern California
Los Angeles, California

Donald N. Krieger
Department of Neurological Surgery
University of Pittsburgh
Pittsburgh, Pennsylvania

David J. Krupa
Neuroscience Program
University of Southern California
Los Angeles, California

Gary Lynch
Center for the Neurobiology of
Learning and Memory
University of California, Irvine
Irvine, California

Thomas H. McNeill
Neurogerontology Division,
Andrus Gerontology Center
University of Southern California
Los Angeles, California

Alan F. Nordholm
Neuroscience Program
University of Southern California
Los Angeles, California

Michael A. Paradiso
Institute for Brain and
Neural Systems
Brown University
Providence, Rhode Island

Steven P. R. Rose
Brain and Behaviour Research Group
Open University
Milton Keynes, England

Robert J. Sclabassi
Department of Electrical Engineering
University of Pittsburgh
Pittsburgh, Pennsylvania

Wolf Singer
Max-Planck Institute for
Brain Research
Frankfurt, Germany

Oswald Steward
Departments of Neuroscience and
Neurosurgery
University of Virginia Health
Sciences Center
Charlottesville, Virginia

Timothy Teyler
Neurobiology Department
Northeastern Ohio College of
Medicine
Rootstown, Ohio

Judith K. Thompson
Neural, Informational and
Behavioral Sciences
University of Southern California
Los Angeles, California

Richard F. Thompson
Neural, Informational and
Behavioral Sciences
University of Southern California
Los Angeles, California

Introduction

What is synaptic plasticity, or rather, what do neurobiologists mean when they talk about synaptic plasticity? There are probably as many definitions of this expression as there are neuroscientists, and this may simply indicate that synaptic plasticity is an intrinsic property of the nervous system which neuroscientists, at whatever levels of analysis they operate, are compelled to integrate in their scientific approach. If such is the case, is there a molecular or cellular characteristic of nerve cells that could account for such an ubiquitous and predominant property? Or rather, is there a multitude of mechanisms that provide adaptive properties for a wide variety of phenomena?

This book represents an attempt to answer these questions. First, it reflects the diversity of phenomena included under the broad concept of synaptic plasticity and presents a number of illustrations of the different approaches used to both define and study synaptic plasticity. It also addresses the question of the mechanisms that participate in different forms of synaptic plasticity. Finally, and perhaps more importantly, it attempts to develop some of the ideas related to the functional consequences of synaptic plasticity in regard to brain development, recovery from injury, and learning and memory.

The first two chapters deal with brain development and synapse formation and describe mechanisms that are involved in activity-dependent modifications of synapse formation. Many neuroanatomists working on a variety of neural systems have demonstrated that synapses in the mature nervous system are a product of a competitive process in which some early-formed synaptic connections fail to develop, while others mature and become functional gates of relevant circuits. An important criterion for survival of a synapse and the resultant changes in plasticity that occur is the extent to which the synapse is active during development. A nervous system starts with a surplus of possible connections and evolves by synaptic elimination and selective stabilization as proposed by J.P. Changeux as well as by G. Edelman several years ago. In chapter 1, Susan Hockfield examines the role of the extracellular matrix in stabilizing mature synaptic structures and reviews several processes that could explain the loss of synaptic plasticity as development proceeds. In chapter 2, Oswald Steward tackles the very difficult problem of molecular targeting and develops the thesis that some synaptic constituents are locally synthesized. Such a mechanism would offer a possible candidate for producing local regulation of synaptic properties, something that neuro-scientists have long searched for.

Indeed, whether plasticity involves structural changes in synapses, new synapses, or changes in the composition of existing synapses, these modifications require new molecular constituents to be delivered and incorporated into the appropriate sites. Unfortunately, until recently, very little was known about the mechanisms involved in the process of synapse formation. Starting with the recent discoveries about how mRNAs are differentially distributed within neurons, Oswald Steward discusses three possible mechanisms. The first involves a sorting mechanism which determines whether particular mRNAs remain in the cell body or are transported to the dendrites. The second is a mechanism for transporting mRNAs into dendrites. The third suggestion is for a mechanism that connects the mRNAs with the ribosomes and the protein synthesis machinery which is involved in producing the required local structural changes.

Finch and McNeill (chapter 3) have approached the study of plasticity through that of the natural process of aging and the pathological processes that mimic (albeit with exceptions) the decreases in neuroplasticity that occur past maturation. They analyze some of the important molecular events that are taking place following lesions and which have been identified from the studies of two widely used models, the hippocampal response to entorhinal cortex lesion and the striatal response to decortication. Furthermore, this chapter also explores the links between these models of neuronal degeneration with the neuropathological manifestations associated with aging and neurodegenerative diseases, both pathologies resulting in decreased behavioral plasticity. In particular, this chapter describes the possible roles of a host of signaling molecules that have previously been shown to participate in immune responses in the organism, in neuronal and glial responses to deafferentation.

The next four chapters are devoted to a review of the properties and mechanisms of two forms of synaptic plasticity that have become extremely popular as potential candidates for memory storage devices, long-term potentiation and long-term depression of synaptic efficacy. Long-term potentiation (LTP) was discovered at the end of the 1960s but has only recently generated considerable excitement (as well as controversy) among neuroscientists as its mechanisms and properties are being unraveled. Long-term depression (LTD) was discovered more recently and has generated as much debate as long-term potentiation. These reviews address two major issues in this field: (1) are there different forms of LTP and LTD?, and (2) what are the functional roles of LTP and LTD in terms of information processing and storage?

Teyler and Grover (chapter 4) provide evidence for another LTP mechanism that may not be dependent on the glutamate NMDA receptor. The brief history of LTP has provided for a continuous expansion of conditions, time courses, and "rules" that produce the plasticity known as "potentiation." A mechanism for inducing potentiation based on activation of calcium channels greatly expands the universality of LTP. If all neuronal tissue is capable of plasticity to some degree, mechanisms must exist for potentiation to occur in the absence of NMDA receptors. Mechanisms should also exist to account for different kinetics and timing constraints in order to generate plasticity at different synapses. Michel Baudry and Gary Lynch begin their chapter (chapter 5) with a review of glutamatergic synapses with an emphasis on the properties of glutamate receptors which are likely to play critical roles for both LTP induction and maintenance. Numerous reviews have discussed the development and expression of LTP, and Lynch and Baudry critically consider the problem of long-term maintenance. Human memory can exist for many decades. What models of plasticity can account for this incredibly long (in biological terms) information storage period? The answers may be found in changes in gene expression and resultant protein synthesis and structural changes, but cell-adhesion mechanisms may also provide a key. All these chapters thus make a strong case that synaptic plasticity in nerve cells emerges from numerous cell biological mechanisms which are also used in a variety of other cells to produce long-lasting modifications of structures and functions and suggest that there might exist a small number of cellular principles underlying synaptic plasticity.

Masao Ito's contribution (chapter 6) examines a mechanism for plasticity in motor learning. Cerebellar Purkinje cells exhibit a long-term depression (LTD) of their responses to parallel fiber stimulation, which is thought to be important for describing mechanisms required for learning a motor task. Ito also suggests an analogy between movement and thought which, if carried to its logical conclusion, also implicates LTD in higher cognitive functions. In chapter 7, Artola and Singer move from plasticity in the hippocampus and cerebellum to the neocortex. They concentrate on describing heterosynaptic neocortical LTD, a depression of nonstimulated input systems that might possibly influence a variety of afferent pathways simultaneously.

Appropriately, these four chapters are followed by four others that directly address the question of the relationships between synaptic plasticity and information processing and learning and memory. The first, by Cooper and collaborators, (chapter 8) reviews the theory of Bienenstock, Cooper, and Munro (commonly known as the BCM theory of synaptic plasticity) that has been developed to account for the effects of the environment on the organization of the visual cortex. The chapter presents new experimental observations that verify certain key assumptions of the theory and compares the BCM theory with other theories of visual cortical plasticity. This chapter and the following one, by Ted Berger and collaborators, (chapter 9) represent a more theoretical, computational approach to the study of neural plasticity. While the BCM theory aims to provide a physiologically plausible account of synaptic plasticity in the kitten visual cortex, it does not suggest a biological mechanism for the decrease of plasticity at the end of the critical period. Both Cooper's and Berger's modeling depends on nonlinear characteristics of neurons. New mathematical approaches have made these efforts to model plasticity in biological systems very exciting.

Berger and his collaborators present an extensive review of their original interactive approach, which combines nonlinear mathematical analysis of input/output functions, computer simulations of network models, and experimental analyses of the processing of neural information by the hippocampal formation. This approach has the appealing property that it incorporates the interactions between all elements of the system, those known as well as those unknown. The chapter also describes preliminary attempts at incorporating synaptic plasticity in the system and the resulting effects on signal processing. Steven Rose then reviews the evidence that learning of simple tasks involves modulation of synaptic connectivity—in other words, a form of synaptic plasticity. His review also addresses the difficult issue of the time dimension in learning and attempts to present possible mechanisms that could be involved in generating stable, long-lasting modifications of synaptic efficacy.

Rose also raises the question of how information retrieval and synaptic plasticity are related. It is clearly not sufficient to provide an adequate description of the role of plasticity in an information storage process. That information is useless without a retrieval mechanism. The last two chapters (10 and 11) make a successful effort to relate synaptic plasticity to behavioral changes—the ultimate goal of all the work described in this volume. It is therefore appropriate that the last chapter, by Richard Thompson and collaborators, reviews synaptic plasticity from the behaviorist point of view and provides closure to many issues raised in this introduction. Furthermore, it attempts to give the readers who choose to proceed through this book in serial fashion an integrative summary of all the preceding chapters. Thompson and colleagues offer a comprehensive review of the properties and mechanisms of various forms of associative learning and link several mechanisms of synaptic plasticity discussed in the previous chapters (i.e., LTP and LTD) to associative learning. In addition, they make the point that different circuitries express different forms of synaptic plasticity and thus participate in different types of learning and memory.

The book thus reveals a surprising convergence of both experimental and theoretical concepts and does indeed suggest that a small number of molecular and cellular properties might well account for the various forms of synaptic plasticity observed in different physiological or pathological conditions. Overall, we believe that this book will be extremely useful for those scientists interested in the mechanisms and functional significance of synaptic plasticity during development, learning, and trauma.

Synaptic Plasticity

1 Molecular Correlates of Activity-dependent Development and Synaptic Plasticity

Susan Hockfield

1 INTRODUCTION

The acquisition of mature, differentiated neuronal properties takes place over an extended developmental period, through a number of different mechanisms. Some of the very last events in neuronal development occur late in the postnatal period when the mature set of synapses between neurons is selected and the adult anatomical and physiological properties of neurons are acquired. Experiments in many different systems have shown that the mature set of synapses is selected from an initial set by selective stabilization of some synapses and elimination of others (for review, see Purves and Lichtman, 1985). The process of synapse selection is governed, at least in part, by neuronal activity. External stimuli (such as visual or auditory signals) can be extremely effective in evoking the neuronal activity that mediates synapse selection and the acquisition of mature neuronal properties.

The visual system of vertebrates has provided some of the most compelling demonstrations of activity-dependent development (Hockfield and Kalb, 1993; Sherman and Spear, 1982). Visually evoked neuronal activity in the early postnatal period has profound effects on the anatomy and physiology of neurons in the visual system of mammals and amphibia. Visually evoked neuronal activity controls the segregation of geniculocortical input representing right and left eyes into ocular dominance columns in the primary visual cortex of cats and primates (for reviews, see Shatz, 1990; Shemman and Spear, 1982). Neuronal activity in the visual pathway during the prenatal period controls the segregation of retinal afferents into eye-specific layers in the cat lateral geniculate nucleus (LGN) (Shatz and Stryker, 1988). In the postnatal period visually evoked activity regulates the final size and distribution of retinogeniculate arbors (Garraghty et al., 1989; Sur et al., 1982). In amphibia, visually evoked activity drives the retinotopic mapping of afferents from the nucleus isthmi onto the tectum in two-eyed frogs (Udin and Keating, 1981) and the segregation of retinal afferents into ocular dominance stripes in the tectum of three-eyed frogs (Reh and Constantine-Paton, 1985).

Neuronal activity most dramatically influences mature neuronal phenotype during a circumscribed period in postnatal development called the critical or sensitive period. During the critical period a neuron exists in an immature, relatively plastic state. After the end of the critical period a neuron exists in a mature, relatively nonplastic state. Synapse stabilization is likely to be a key element in the transition from the immature, plastic to the mature, nonplastic state. The mechanisms by which the mature set of synapses is selected and stabilized are little understood.

Several lines of experimentation have led to the postulate that coincident activation of presynaptic and postsynaptic elements leads to the strengthening and stabilization of a subset of developing connections. A model put forth by Hebb (1949) forms the basis of one of the more popular postulated mechanisms for increased synapse efficacy and for synapse stabilization. In this model, concurrent activity of presynaptic and postsynaptic elements acts to increase synaptic strength. The cellular mechanisms underlying synapse potentiation and the postulated increase in dwell-time (that is, stabilization) of synapses during development have been active areas of research over the last several years.

2   ROLE OF RECEPTORS IN SYNAPTIC STABILIZATION

Potentiation and stabilization of synapses requires the participation of both the presynaptic and postsynaptic elements. The biophysical properties of the N-methyl-D-aspartate subclass of glutamate receptors suggest that it may play a postsynaptic role in activity-dependent increase in synaptic strength and in synapse stabilization. A review of this literature is well beyond the scope of the present chapter, but a number of excellent reviews have been published (Brown et al. 1990; Kennedy, 1989). As described further below, the distribution and temporal regulation of expression of the NMDA receptor in the cat visual cortex (Bode-Greuel and Singer, 1989; Fox et al., 1989) and rodent spinal cord (Hockfield et al., 1990a; Kalb and Hockfield, 1990a; Kalb et al., 1992 and Kalb and Hochfield, 1992) further suggest a role in developmental synaptic plasticity. More recently, nitric oxide has been suggested to be a retrograde signal released by the postsynaptic cell onto the presynaptic element to mediate changes in the efficacy and dwell-time of the synapse (Bredt and Snyder, 1992).

The kinds of processes that might be involved in the potentiation and stabilization of a group of synapses described above might operate over a relatively short period of time (seconds to weeks). The synapses in some areas of the mammalian CNS (for example, the thalamocortical synapses in primary visual cortex of cat and primate) that are established during the critical period remain stabilized for the life of the animal. During the sensitive or critical period in cortical development synaptic patterns can be continually modified by neuronal activity. After the close of the critical period, however, neuronal activity has no demonstrable effect on the pattern of thalamocortical synapses. This nonplastic period lasts the lifetime of the animal, suggesting that another mechanism might be involved in the long-term stabilization of synapses.

3 ROLE OF EXTRACELLULAR MATRIX

We have been exploring the possibility that the change in neuronal pheno-type from an immature, plastic state to a mature, less plastic state, might be reflected by changes in the molecular properties of neurons. Identification of proteins that are expressed at the close of the critical period could advance our understanding of the biological processes underlying the loss of synaptic plasticity in development.

The elements of the extracellular matrix (ECM) may play a role in stabiliz-ing mature synaptic structure. In many tissues, the ECM serves to stabilize intercellular interactions and helps to maintain tissue integrity (for reviews, see Hockfield, 1990; Ruoslahti, 1989). Extracellular matrices are often rich in proteoglycans, glycoproteins that are extensively modified by long, un-branched carbohydrate chains, called glycosaminoglycans, comprising repeat-ing disaccharide units. Recent studies have shown that the mature mammalian CNS contains a diverse population of surface-associated proteoglycans. The properties of some of these proteoglycans are very similar to those of proteo-glycans in nonneural extracellular matrices.

Early studies with the electron microscope showed that the mammalian CNS does not contain a clearly defined, electron-dense ECM (Peters et al., 1976). This led to the conclusion that the CNS was lacking a standard ECM. The application of a variety of staining techniques showed that ECM did indeed exist, and furthermore, indicated that molecules found in intercellular spaces in the CNS corresponded in many cases to components of ECM iden-tified in other tissues (Atoji et al., 1989; Castejon, 1970; Luft, 1966; Nakanishi, 1983).

4 EXTRACELLULAR PROTEOGLYCANS AND SYNAPTIC PLASTICITY

More contemporary approaches, using antibody probes, specific enzymes, and chromatographic techniques, have unequivocally demonstrated surface-associated or extracellular proteoglycans in the mature CNS (Atoji et al., 1990; Fryer et al., 1992; Naegele et al., 1988; Hockfield and McKey, 1983; Watanabe et al. 1989; Zaremba et al., 1989). A number of distinct proteo-glycans are expressed by distinct subsets of neurons (Hockfield et al., 1983, 1990a; Watanabe et al., 1989; Zaremba et al., 1989, 1990a, b). In almost all cases, surface-associated proteoglycans are expressed late in postnatal devel-opment, long after neurons have achieved their mature position in the CNS and have established initial dendritic and axonal arborizations (Hockfield et al., 1983, 1990a; Kalb and Hockfield, 1988; Sur et al., 1988; Watanabe et al., 1989; Zaremba et al., 1990a, 1992).

The subcellular localization of surface-associated CNS proteoglycans is consistent with a role in maintaining synaptic structure. Examination at the ultrastructural level has shown that several proteoglycans are distributed over the surface of neuronal cell bodies and proximal dendrites but are excluded from the synaptic cleft (Hockfield and McKay, 1983; Watanabe et al., 1989; Zaremba et al., 1989). Antibody labeling of live neurons has shown unequivocally that some of these surface-associated proteoglycans have extracellular epitopes (Zaremba et al., 1989, 1990a). Detergent extraction and partitioning experiments (Hockfield et al., 1990a) indicate that some chondroitin sulfate proteoglycans lack a transmembrane domain and, therefore, maybe entirely extracellular. This extrasynaptic distribution is reminiscent of the distribution of components of the ECM at the neuromuscular junction (for discussion, see Hockfield and McKay, 1983).

4.1 Regulation of Cat-301 Proteoglycan Expression in the Visual System

Several properties of the Cat-301 proteoglycan suggest a role in the acquisition of mature neuronal properties. First, as described above, surface-associated Cat-301 immunoreactivity is initially detected relatively late in neuronal development. In every case examined to date, neurons do not demonstrate Cat-301 surface staining until well into postnatal life. In the cat LGN, for example, surface-associated Cat-301 immunoreactivity is first seen around postnatal day 30 and adult levels are not reached until after postnatal day 90 (Sur et al., 1988). We have demonstrated by many different criteria that Cat-301 selectively recognizes LGN Y-cells (Hockfield and Sur, 1990; Sur et al., 1988). The time course of antigen expression parallels the previously described maturation of the electrophysiological properties of Y-cells (Daniels et al, 1978; Mangel et al., 1983).

The second property of the Cat-301 proteoglycan that suggests a role in neuronal maturation is the regulation of expression of the proteoglycan by manipulations that alter the acquisition of normal anatomical and physiological characteristics of neurons. For example, the acquisition of mature Y-cell electrophysiological properties requires visual experience during a circumscribed period in postnatal life (for reviews, see Movshon and Van Sluyters, 1981; Sherman and Spear, 1982). Cats deprived of normal visual experience during this critical period do not develop normal visual function and lack a normal complement of physiologically mature LGN Y-cells. While retinogeniculate axons arrive in the LGN and segregate in eye-specific layers well before birth (Shatz and Stryker, 1988), the final size and distribution of retinal arbors is determined by visually evoked activity during postnatal life (Garraghty et al., 1989; Sur et al., 1982). Manipulations of the visual system that prevent the normal maturation of Y-cell properties, including dark-rearing, neonatal monocular lid suture, and neonatal intraocular administration of tetrodotoxin, reduce Cat-301 immunoreactivity in the cat LGN (Hockfield et al., 1991; Sur et al., 1988).

The reduction in Cat-301 expression in the LGN is not tied simply to levels of neuronal activity, but expressly to neuronal activity during early postnatal life (Hockfield et al., 1989, 1990a). A reduction in neuronal activity in adult animals can produce a reduction in the level of a number of neural proteins

(Hendry and Kennedy, 1986; Hevner and Wong-Riley, 1990; Jones et al, 1990) without the profound and permanent effects on neuronal anatomy and physiology seen in neonates. However, deprivation of normal visual input in adult animals for extended periods of time has no effect on Cat-301 expression (Hockfield et al., 1990a; Sur et al., 1988).

Once the critical period for neuronal development has ended, abnormal features of a neuron produced by abnormal patterns of activity cannot be "rescued" by normal patterns of activity (Dubin et al., 1986; Sherman et al., 1972). Similarly, the reduction in Cat-301 expression following early visual deprivation cannot be reversed by normal visual activity. For example, in the LGN of animals that received intraocular injections of tetrodotoxin (which blocks Na^+ channels and, therefore, blocks neuronal conduction) for the first 7 weeks of life and then were allowed to survive (without tetrodotoxin or its effects) for another 17 weeks, there remains an almost complete depletion of Cat-301 from the LGN layers that receive input from the injected eye (Hockfield et al., 1990a, 1991).

The loss in Cat-301 immunoreactivity following deprivation could be due either to a reduction in the level of the antigen itself or to simply a masking or alteration of the epitope recognized by Cat-301. A second monoclonal antibody, Cat-304, recognizes the Cat-301 proteoglycan, but at a different site from that recognized by Cat-301 (Zaremba et al., 1989). Decreases in levels of immunoreactivity following visual deprivation is identical for both Cat-301 and Cat-304 (Guimaraes et al., 1990), strongly suggesting that the reduction in the Cat-301 proteoglycan following activity deprivation reflects a down-regulation of the proteoglycan itself and not simply a loss of the Cat-301 epitope.

4.2 Regulation of Cat-301 Proteoglycan Expression in the Neuromuscular System

Our studies on the regulation of expression of the Cat-301 proteoglycan in the visual system of cats have been confirmed and extended by studies in the rodent neuromuscular system (for review, see Kalb and Hockfield, 1992). In adult hamsters and rats all motor neurons with axons in the sciatic nerve express the surface-associated Cat-301 immunoreactivity by postnatal day 14 (Kalb and Hockfield, 1988). Manipulations of the neuromuscular unit that disrupt the normal pattern of motor neuron activity between postnatal days 5 and 21 prevent the normal development of the expression of the Cat-301 antigen. Sciatic nerve lesion, dorsal rhizotomy, decortication, and cordotomy performed during the early postnatal period all result in a marked reduction in the percent of sciatic motor neurons that are Cat-301–positive. When performed on adult animals, none of these lesions has any effect on Cat-301 expression (Kalb and Hockfield, 1988, 1990b). Cat-301 expression therefore defines a critical period for motor neuron development, during which alterations in activity of the neuromuscular unit influences the acquisition of mature molecular properties of motor neurons.

A third property of the Cat-301 proteoglycan that suggests a role in developmental plasticity is its regulation by the NMDA receptor. We have shown that large diameter, but not small diameter, primary afferents mediate activity-dependent Cat-301 expression on motor neurons (Kalb and Hockfield, 1990b). The neurotransmitter of some of the large diameter afferents is glutamate (Salt and Hill, 1983). Blockade of the NMDA subclass of glutamate receptor during the critical period inhibits Cat-301 expression on motor neurons (Kalb and Hockfield, 1990a).

5   ROLE OF NMDA RECEPTOR IN MATURATION OF THE VISUAL AND MOTOR SYSTEMS

These experiments provide evidence that NMDA-receptor mediated events are involved in activity-dependent maturation of motor neurons. The mechanisms of this process may be similar to other systems where the NMDA receptor has been implicated in mediating long-lasting, activity-dependent modifications of neuronal properties, including the segregation of retinotectal projections in the frog (Cline and Constantine-Paton, 1990; Cline et al., 1987) and the acquisition of response properties of visual cortical neurons in the developing cat (Bear et al., 1990). However, the role of NMDA receptors in development of the mammalian visual system is currently under some debate. In the cat visual cortex (Miller et al., 1989) a large component (perhaps the majority) of the excitatory drive to neurons is mediated by activation of the NMDA receptor, so that NMDA receptor blockade may be equivalent to a nonspecific inhibition of neuronal activity. In support of a role for the NMDA receptor in visual cortical plasticity are studies showing that a reduction in electrophysiologically identified NMDA receptors in layers 4–6 of cat visual cortex correlates with a decline in synaptic plasticity (Fox et al., 1989). Furthermore, dark-rearing, which has been reported to delay the close of the critical period (Cynader and Mitchell, 1980; Mower, 1991; Mower and Christen, 1985) also delays the down-regulation of NMDA receptor (Fox et al., 1991).

In contrast to the visual system, data in the spinal cord suggest that the major excitatory drive to motor neurons during development is mediated by activation of non-NMDA glutamate receptors. Our studies have shown that spinal cord motor neurons can be driven by segmental reflex pathways in the presence of NMDA receptor antagonists (Hockfield et al., 1990a). Others have shown that a substantial amount of excitation to motor neurons is carried by non-NMDA glutamate receptors in the prenatal and early postnatal period (Jahr and Yoshioka, 1986; Ziskind-Conhaim, 1990). NMDA antagonists do not, therefore, globally prevent synaptic activation of motor neurons.

Our recent experiments have shown that NMDA receptor expression in the spinal cord is developmentally regulated in a manner similar to that described in the developing visual cortex (Kalb et al., 1992). In the adult rodent spinal cord the highest levels of NMDA receptor exist in the dorsal horn in the substantia gelatinosa (Monaghan and Cotman, 1985). During the early postnatal period the distribution of NMDA receptors is markedly different with high levels of receptor present throughout the spinal gray matter (Kalb and Hockfield, 1991; Kalb et al., 1992). The loss of NMDA receptor from the ventral horn and the acquisition of the adult receptor distribution parallels the development of Cat-301 expression on motor neurons. These data suggest that the NMDA receptor participates in activity-dependent maturation of motor neurons. Activated NMDA receptors on target cells may regulate the expression of a class of neuronal proteins, of which Cat-301 is one example, that might subserve the anatomical and physiological consequences of activity-dependent development.

6 CONCLUSIONS

Together the results reviewed here suggest that the loss of synaptic plasticity during development is accompanied, and possibly subserved, by the elaboration of an ECM. This matrix could play a role in maintaining the mature, differentiated properties of neurons. The pattern of neuronal activity during a critical period in development may influence the acquisition of mature cellular phenotype by regulating the timing and selection of gene expression. Identification of molecules that differentiate mature, nonplastic neurons from immature, plastic neurons may lead to a more complete understanding of developmental synaptic plasticity and its reduction in adult animals.

It is important to remember that synaptic plasticity is not entirely limited to early periods in development. Reorganization of both motor and sensory maps in mature animals has been well documented (for review, see Kaas, 1991). The magnitude of stimulus-induced remapping is more limited in adult than in neonatal animals. As the cellular and molecular machinery underlying developmental plasticity is elucidated it will be interesting to learn if plasticity in adult animals makes use of the same cellular elements and molecular processes.

REFERENCES

Atoji, Y., Hori, Y., Sugimura, M., and Suzuki, Y. (1989) Extracellular matrix of the superior olivary nuclei in the dog. *J. Neurocytol.* 18:599–610.

Atoji, Y., Kitamura, Y., Suzuki, Y. (1990) Chondroitin sulfate proteoglycan in the extracellular matrix of the canine superior olivary nuclei. *Acta Anat. (Basel)* 139:151–153.

Bear, M.F., Kleinschmidt, A., Gu, Q. and Singer, W. (1990) Disruption of experience-dependent synaptic modifications in striate cortex by infusion of an NMDA receptor antagonist. *J. Neurosci.* 10:909–925.

Bode-Greuel, K. M., and Singer, W. 1989) The development of N-methyl-D-aspartate receptors in cat visual cortex. *Dev. Brain Res.* 46:197–204.

Bredt, D. S., and Snyder, S. H. (1992) Nitric oxide, a novel neuronal messenger. *Neuron* 8:3–11.

Brown, T. H., Kairiss, E. W., and Keenan, C. L. (1990) Hebbian synapses: Biophysical mechanisms and algorithms. *Annu. Rev. Neurosci.* 13:475–511.

Castejon, H. V. (1970) Histochemical demonstration of sulphated polysaccharides at the coat of nerve cells in the mouse central nervous system. *Acta Histochem.* 38:55–64.

Cline, H. T., and Constantine-Paton, M. (1990) NMDA receptor agonist and antagonists alter retinal ganglion cell arbor structure in the developing frog retinotectal projection. *J. Neurosci.* 10:1197–1216.

Cline, H. T., Debski, E. A., and Constantine-Paton, M. (1987) N-methyl-D-aspartate receptor antagonist desegregates eye-specific columns. *Proc. Natl. Acad. Sci. USA* 84:4342–4345.

Cynader, M, and Mitchell, D. E. (1980) Prolonged sensitivity to monocular deprivation in dark-reared cats. *J. Neurophysiol.* 43:1026–1040.

Daniels, J. D., Pettigrew, J. D., and Norman, J. L. (1978) Development of single-neuron responses in kitten's lateral geniculate nucleus. *J. Neurophysiol.* 41:1373–1393.

Dubin, M. W., Stark, L. A., and Archer, S. M. (1986) A role for action-potential activity in the development of neuronal connections in the kitten retinogeniculate pathway. *J. Neurosci.* 6:1021–1036.

Fox, K., Sato H., and Daw, N. (1989) The location and function of NMDA receptors in cat and kitten visual cortex. *J. Neurosci.* 9:2443–2454.

Fox, K., Daw, N., Sato, H., and Czepita, D. (1991) Dark-rearing delays the loss of NMDA-receptor function in kitten visual cortex. *Nature* 350:342–344.

Fryer, H. J., Kelly, G. M., Molinaro, L., and Hockfield, S. (1992) The high molecular weight Cat-301 chondroitin sulfate proteoglycan from brain is related to the large aggregating proteoglycan from cartilage, aggrecan. *J. Biol. Chem.*, 267:9874–9883.

Garraghty, P. E., Roe, A. W., Chino, Y. M., and Sur, M. (1989) Effects of convergent strabismus on the development of physiologically identified retinogeniculate axons in cats. *J. Comp. Neurol.* 289:202–212.

Guimaraes, A., Zaremba, S., and Hockfield, S. (1990) Molecular and morphological changes in cat lateral geniculate nucleus and visual cortex induced by visual deprivation are revealed by monoclonal antibodies Cat-301 and Cat-304. *J. Neurosci.* 10:3014–3024.

Hebb, D. O. (1949) *The Organization of Behavior.* John Wiley and Sons, New York.

Hendry, S. H. C., and Kennedy, M. B. (1986) Immunoreactivity for calmodulin-dependent protein kinase is selectively increased in macaque striate cortex after monocular deprivation. *Proc. Natl. Acad. Sci. USA* 83:1536–1541.

Hevner, R. F., and Wong-Riley, M. T. T. (1990) Regulation of cytochrome oxidase protein levels by functional activity in the macaque monkey visual system. *J. Neurosci.* 10:1331–1340.

Hockfield, S. (1990) Proteoglycans in neural development. *Semin. Dev. Biol.* 1:55–63.

Hockfield, S., and Kalb, R. G. (1993) Activity-dependent structural change during neuronal development. *Curr. Opinions Neurobiol.* 3:87–92.

Hockfield, S., and McKay, R. (1983) A surface antigen expressed by a subset of neurons in the vertebrate central nervous system. *Proc. Natl. Acad. Sci. USA* 80:5758–5761.

Hockfield, S., and Sur, M. (1990) Monoclonal antibody Cat-301 identifies Y-cells in the dorsal lateral geniculate nucleus of the cat. *J. Comp. Neurol.* 300:320–330.

Hockfield, S., McKay, R., Hendry, S. H. C., and Jones, E. G. (1983) A surface antigen that identifies ocular dominance columns in cortical area 17 and laminar features of the lateral geniculate nucleus. *Cold Spring Harbor Symp. Quant. Biol.* 48:877–889.

Hockfield, S., Kalb, R. G., and Guimaraes, A. (1989) Experience-dependent expression of neuronal cell surface molecules. In *Neuroimmune Networks: Physiology and Diseases*, E. J. Goetzl and N. H. Spector, eds., pp. 57–63. Alan R. Liss, New York.

Hockfield, S., Kalb, R. G., Zaremba, S., and Fryer, H. J. (1990a) Expression of neural pro-teoglycan correlates with the acquisition of mature neuronal properties in the mammalian brain. *Cold Spring Harbor Symp. Quant. Biol.* 55:505–514.

Hockfield, S., Tootell, R. B. H., and Zaremba, S. (1990b) Molecular differences among neurons reveal an organization of human visual cortex. *Proc. Natl. Acad. Sci. USA* 87:3027–3031.

Hockfield, S., Scheetz, A. J., and Dubin, M. W. (1991) Monocular action potential blockade reduces expression of the Cat-301 proteoglycan in the LGN of neonatal, but not adult, cats. *Invest. Ophthalmol. Vis. Sci.* 32:1035.

Jahr, C. E., and Yoshioka, K. (1986) Ia afferent excitation of motoneurons in the in vitro new-born rat spinal cord is selectively antagonized by kynurenate. *J. Physiol. (Lond).* 370:515–530.

Jones, E. G., Benson, D. L., Hendry, S. H. C., and Isackson, P. J. (1990) Activity-dependent regulation of gene expression in adult monkey visual cortex. *Cold Spring Harbor Symp. Quant. Biol.* 55:481–490.

Kaas, J. H. (1991) Plasticity of sensory and motor maps in adult mammals. *Annu. Rev. Neurosci.* 14:137–167.

Kalb, R. G., and Hockfield, S. (1988) Molecular evidence for early activity-dependent develop-ment of hamster motor neurons. *J. Neurosci.* 8:2350–2360.

Kalb, R. G., and Hockfield, S. (1990a) Induction of a neuronal proteoglycan by the NMDA receptor in the developing spinal cord. *Science* 250:294–296.

Kalb, R. G., and Hockfield, S. (1990b) Large diameter primary afferent input is required for expression of the Cat-301 proteoglycan on the surface of motor neurons. *Neuroscience* 34:391–401.

Kalb, R. G., and Hockfield, S. (1991) The distribution of spinal cord N-methyl-D-aspartate receptors is developmentally regulated. *Soc. Neurosci. Abstr.* 17:1534.

Kalb, R. G., and Hockfield, S. (1992) Activity-dependent development of spinal cord motor neurons. *Brain Res. Rev.* 17:283–289.

Kalb, R. G., Lidow, M. D., Halsted, M. J., and Hockfield, S. (1992) NMDA receptors are transiently expressed in the developing spinal cord ventral horn. *Proc. Natl. Acad. Sci. USA,* submitted.

Kennedy, M. B. (1989) Regulation of synaptic transmission in the central nervous system: long-term potentiation. *Cell* 59:777–787.

Luft, J. H. (1966) Fine structure of nerve and muscle cell membrane permeable to ruthenium red. *Anat. Rec.* 154:379.

Mangel, S. C., Wilson, J. R., and Sherman, S. M. (1983) Development of neuronal response properties in the cat dorsal lateral geniculate nucleus during monocular deprivation. *J. Neuro-physiol.* 50:240–262.

Miller, K. D., Chapman, B., and Stryker, M. P. (1989) Visual responses in adult cat visual cortex depend on N-methyl-D-aspartate receptors. *Proc. Natl. Acad. Sci. USA* 86:5183–5187.

Monaghan, D. T., and Cotman, C. W. (1985) Distribution of N-methyl-D-aspartate–sensitive L-[^{3}H]glutamate binding sites in rat brain. *J. Neurosci.* 5:2909–2919.

Movshon, J. A., and Van Sluyters, R. C. (1981) Visual neural development. *Annu. Rev. Psychol.* 32:477–522.

Mower, G. D. (1991) The effect of dark rearing on the time course of the critical period in cat visual cortex. *Dev. Brain Res.* 58:151–158.

Mower, G. D., and Christen W. G. (1985) Role of visual experience in activating critical period in cat visual cortex. *J. Neurophysiol.* 53:572–589.

Naegele, J. R., Arimatsu, Y., Schwartz, P., and Barnstable, C. J. (1988) Selective staining of a subset of GABAergic neurons in cat visual cortex by monoclonal antibody VC1.1. *J. Neurosci.* 8:79–89.

Nakanishi, S. (1983) Extracellular matrix during laminar pattern formation of neocortex in normal and reeler mutant mice. *Dev. Biol.* 95:305–316.

Peters, A., S. L. Palay, and H. deF. Webster (1976) The Fine Structure of the Nervous System: *The Neurons and Supporting Cells.* Saunders, Philadelphia.

Purves, D., and Lichtman, J. W. (1985) *Principles of Neural development.* Sinauer Associates, Sunderland, MA.

Reh, T. A., and Constantine-Paton, M. (1985) Eye specific segregation requires activity in 3 eyed *Rana pipiens. J. Neurosci.* 5:1132–1143.

Ruoslahti, E. (1989) Proteoglycans in cell regulation. *J. Biol. Chem.* 264:13369–13372.

Salt, T. E., and Hill, R. G. (1983) Neurotransmitter candidates of primary afferent somatosensory fibers. *Neuroscience* 10:1083–1103.

Shatz, C. J. (1990) Impulse activity and the patterning of connections during CNS development. *Neuron* 5:745–756.

Shatz, C. J., and Stryker, M. P. (1988) Prenatal tetrodotoxin infusion blocks segregation of retinogeniculate afferents. *Science* 242:87–89.

Sherman, S. M., and Spear, P. D. (1982) Organization of visual pathways in normal and visually deprived cats. *Physiol. Rev.* 62:738–855.

Sherman, S. M., Hofmann, K. P. and Stone, J. (1972) Loss of a specific cell type from dorsal lateral genicurate nucleus in visually deprived cats. *J. Neurophysiol.* 35:532–541.

Sur, M., Humphrey, A.L., and Sherman, S. M. (1982) Monocular deprivation affects X- and Y-cell retinogeniculate terminations in cats. *Nature* 300:183–185.

Sur, M., Humphrey, A. L., and Sherman, S. M. (1982) Monocular deprivation affects X- and Y-cell retinogeniculate terminations in cats. *Nature* 300:183–185.

Sur, M., Frost, D., and Hockfield, S. (1988) Expression of a cell surface antigen on Y-cells in the cat lateral geniculate nucleus is regulated by visual experience. *J. Neurosci.* 8:874–882.

Udin, S. B., and Keating, M. J. (1981) Plasticity in a central nervous system pathway in *Xenopus*: Anatomic changes in the isthmo-tectal projection after larval eye rotation. *J. Comp. Neurol.* 203:575–594.

Watanabe, E., Fujita, S. C., Murakami, F., Hayashi, M., and Matsumura, M. (1989) A monoclonal antibody identifies a novel epitope surrounding a subpopulation of the mammalian central neurons. *Neuroscience* 29:645–657.

Zaremba, S., Guimaraes, A., Kalb, R. G., and Hockfield, S. (1989) Characterization of an activity-dependent, neuronal surface proteoglycan identified with monoclonal antibody Cat-301. *Neuron* 2:1207–1219.

Zaremba, S., Kelly, G., Kalb, R. G., and Hockfield, S. (1990a) Keratan sulfate proteoglycans associated with neuronal surfaces in CNS. *Soc. Neurosci. Abstr.* 16:496.

Zaremba, S., Naegele, J. R., Barnstable, C. J., and Hockfield, S. (1990b) Multiple high molecular weight surface glycoconjugates defined by monoclonal antibodies Cat-301 and VC1.1. *J. Neurosci.* 10:2985–2995.

Zaremba, S., Fryer, H. J., Kalb, R. G., Kelly, G. M., and Hockfield, S. (1992) Development and distribution of keratan sulfate immunoreactivity on subsets of neurons in the mammalian CNS. submitted.

Ziskind-Conhaim, L. (1990) NMDA receptors mediate poly- and monosynaptic potentials in motoneurons of rat embryos. *J. Neurosci.* 10:125–135.

2 Molecular Sorting in Neurons: Cell Biological Processes that Play a Role in Synapse Growth and Plasticity

Oswald Steward

1 INTRODUCTION

Ever since the recognition of the basic circuit organization of the brain during the last century, hypotheses about the mechanisms of information storage have focused on the interconnections between neurons as the most likely site of plasticity. The earliest of these connectionistic hypotheses were those of Ramón y Cajal (Ramón y Cajal, 1911) and Tanzi (Tanzi, 1893), who proposed that use promoted the formation of new circuits or strengthened existing circuits. The more modern formulation which underlies much current thinking was that of Hebb (Hebb, 1949), who proposed more specific rules for synapse modification based on relationships between presynaptic and postsynaptic activity. These rules have proved to be remarkably prophetic for two of the best characterized forms of synaptic plasticity (long-term potentiation and the adjustments in visual circuitry during development as a result of experience). Both of these processes are now thought to follow "Hebbian" rules. These hypotheses were the intellectual ancestor of current hypotheses that posit that information storage occurs as a result of changes in the strength of synaptic connections between neurons (that is, long-term synaptic plasticity), and which define the rules for modification in terms of membrane events, ion fluxes, and electrical currents.

Despite the long-standing interest in the question of how information is stored, there are few cases in which the mechanism of storage is known. The exceptions are the well-studied forms of learning in *Aplysia*; here, there is evidence that both short- and long-term information storage involves changes in synapses, and that long-term storage involves actual synapse growth (Glanzman et al., 1990; Schacher et al., 1990). In the case of information storage in the mammalian CNS, neither the sites nor the mechanisms of change have been clearly defined. The synapse is certainly considered the most likely site of change, but there is less agreement about the types of change that might occur. There are several possibilities: Plasticity could involve (1) a *structural change in synapses* (increases or decreases in synapse size, formation of new synapses or elimination of existing ones, or changes in the configuration of spines); (2) *changes in the molecular composition of existing synapses* (incorporation of new molecular species or changes in the blend of the different molecules of the synapse); or (3) *changes in the state of the existing molecules* of the synapse (changes in phosphorylation state, or other post-translational modifications). Common features of most of these possibilities are that individual synapses are modified, and for (1) and (2), that the modifications require the delivery of new molecular constituents to the synaptic site.

The role that any of the above mechanisms plays in various forms of information storage must still be defined. However, the questions of how the molecular constituents of synapses are synthesized, delivered to synaptic sites, assembled, replaced as needed, modified on site (by posttranslational modifications), and degraded are likely to be key to our final understanding. These basic questions about the cell biology of neurons also obviously have broad implications for other important processes (for example, the formation of synaptic connections during development, the maintenance of connections throughout the life of the organism, and the loss of connections with aging or disease).

The present chapter reviews some of the cell biological issues related to the synthesis of the molecular constituents of synapses on CNS neurons, and the delivery of these molecular constituents to individual synaptic sites. I begin by defining what must be explained, based on what is known about the molecular composition of CNS synapses. I then outline several possible cellular mechanisms that could play a role in targeting molecules to synaptic sites, focusing especially on our recent work, which indicates that some molecular constituents of CNS synapses are synthesized on-site by a special protein synthetic apparatus that is selectively positioned beneath postsynaptic sites on CNS neurons. It will become clear that there are more questions than answers. Thus, an important goal of this chapter is to define what we do *not* know, and indicate some research strategies that might answer key questions.

2   MOLECULAR COMPOSITION OF SYNAPSES ON CNS NEURONS

Putting the task that neurons face in constructing and maintaining their synapses in perspective requires a consideration of neuronal synaptology. Most neurons give rise to a single axon which may form large numbers of synapses with other neurons or target cells. Most neurons of the CNS also receive a large number of inputs, often of different types. For example, neurons in the cerebral cortex may be contacted by tens of thousands of synapses, and neurons in the cerebellar cortex receive an even larger number of inputs.

Different problems are involved in making presynaptic terminals vs. postsynaptic sites. The principal difference is the degree of heterogeneity. Although the molecular composition of a presynaptic terminal is complex, all of the axon terminals from a single neuron are thought to have similar molecular properties (since all terminals from an individual neuron are thought to use the same transmitter or mix of neurotransmitters). In contrast, the different postsynaptic sites that form the receptive surface vary depending on the type of contact. For this reason, I will focus on what is the most difficult problem—how neurons construct and maintain their very complex postsynaptic receptive surface.

2.1 Molecular Heterogeneity of the Postsynaptic Cell's Receptive Surface

In considering the receptive surface of CNS neurons, the first point to make is that not only the type of neurotransmitter, but also the structure and site of the synaptic contact on the postsynaptic cell may be quite different for different classes of synapses. Structural differences between synapses have been known since the advent of electron microscopy. Thus, there are synapses with prominent postsynaptic membrane specializations (type I), and those where the postsynaptic membrane specialization is less prominent (type II); there are spine synapses, shaft synapses, and so forth. More recently, it has become clear that different types of synapse also have a different molecular composition. This means that the postsynaptic receptive surface is a mosaic of different membrane domains, each of which is associated with an individual synapse.

This molecular heterogeneity has several important features. First, the types of molecules that are present at the postsynaptic site differ depending on the type of transmitter that is used by the presynaptic element. At a minimum, each synapse must have the receptors and second messenger systems that are appropriate for the neurotransmitter used by the associated presynaptic element. In principle, neurons could position neurotransmitter receptors nonselectively, so that every synaptic site would have an entire complement of receptors for every possible type of neurotransmitter. In fact, however, at least some neurotransmitter receptors are differentially distributed, so that the receptors appropriate for the neurotransmitter used by a particular presynaptic element are present, and receptors for other neurotransmitters are not.

The most convincing evidence for a selective localization of receptors comes from electron microscopic immunocytochemical studies using antibodies to glycine receptors. These studies have shown that glycine receptors are highly concentrated at symmetric synapses that are apposed by terminals containing flattened vesicles, and absent from nearby asymmetric synapses on the same cells (Seitanidou et al., 1988; Triller et al., 1985). Until recently, antibodies for other receptors have not been available. However, the recent success in cloning receptors has made it possible to produce antibodies to synthetic fragments of the receptor proteins. Antibodies suitable for immunocytochemistry are now available for subunits of the glutamate receptor (Petralia and Wenthold, 1992; Rogers et al., 1991), and GABA receptor (Killisch et al., 1991). Electron microscopic studies have been carried out evaluating the subcellular localization of different glutamate receptors (Petralia and Wenthold, 1992). Immunostaining for these receptors was present throughout the dendritic cytoplasm of immunostained neurons, but was especially heavy over the postsynaptic membrane specializations of synapses that are thought to be glutamatergic. These authors did not comment on whether synapses that are thought to be nonglutamatergic were unstained. This may be because the immunocytochemical studies were carried out in the hippocampus and cerebral cortex, where the proportion of glutamatergic synapses is high.

Light microscopic studies of the distribution of pharmacologically defined binding sites also suggest a differential distribution of receptors along the postsynaptic membrane. This can be clearly seen in laminated structures such as the hippocampus. The distribution of some binding sites seems to correspond to the distribution of particular afferent systems (Monaghan et al., 1983). In other cases, however, a relationship between the binding sites and the particular afferent systems is less obvious. It may be significant that there appears to be less precise localization of pharmacologically defined binding sites, whereas precise localization at particular synapses has been demonstrated when receptors have been localized using immunocytochemistry.

At the simplest level, then, neurons could sort the molecular constituents of postsynaptic sites based simply on the neurotransmitter released by the presynaptic elements. In fact, however, the situation is more complex, because there may be different receptor systems for the same neurotransmitter. For example, several different classes of receptors for excitatory amino acids can be distinguished on the basis of agonist binding. The distribution of these pharmacologically distinct binding sites indicates a differential distribution of the sites on the postsynaptic membrane of individual neurons. Again, this is best seen in laminated structures such as the hippocampus; kainate-binding sites are concentrated in some afferent laminae and absent from others, NMDA-binding sites have a different distribution, and AMPA-binding sites have yet a third distribution (Monaghan et al., 1983, 1989).

Neurotransmitter receptors are only part of the story. In association with neurotransmitter receptors themselves are a host of other molecules that determine neurotransmitter action. This is especially true in the case of receptors that activate second messenger pathways, in which the final response to the neurotransmitter requires specific G-proteins, catalytic enzymes, compartmentalized second messengers, kinases, and kinase substrates. All of these systems must be in place for the synapse to operate properly. It is currently not known whether these molecules are selectively positioned according to classes of synapses or whether they are more broadly distributed.

3 SYNTHESIS AND DELIVERY OF THE MOLECULAR CONSTITUENTS OF SYNAPSES

Most of our current understanding of how the molecular constituents of synaptic junctions are synthesized, delivered, and assembled has come from studies of the neuromuscular junction. It is now clear, for example, that the cytoplasm underlying the postsynaptic membrane specialization is highly organized and quite different from the remainder of the muscle cytoplasm. In fact, this portion of the cytoplasm seems to be specialized for the synthesis, delivery, and assembly of molecular constituents of the synaptic site. For example, the mRNAs for some of the key protein constituents of the synaptic junction (including the acetylcholine receptor) are selectively localized beneath the postsynaptic membrane, in contrast to the mRNAs for nonsynaptic proteins, which are generally distributed throughout the muscle fiber (Changeux et al., 1990; Fontaine et al., 1988; Merlie and Sanes, 1985; Phillips et al., 1991). Also, other cellular machinery that is important for protein processing (the Golgi apparatus) is also present. The key elements of this complex cellular machinery are now being defined, and the molecules that play a role in assembly are being identified.

Despite these important discoveries, it is clear that many of the principles that are being defined from studies of neuromuscular synapses will not apply to neurons. There are two reasons for this conclusion: (1) muscle fibers receive only one input, and thus must construct a postsynaptic membrane appropriate for only a single type of synapse. In contrast, some CNS neurons receive tens of thousands of independent inputs, many of which use different neurotransmitters. (2) Muscle fibers are multinucleate. This is important because important aspects of molecular sorting in muscles are due to regulation of transcription by individual nuclei. For example, the local concentration of mRNA for the acetylcholine receptor in the subsynaptic cytoplasm is apparently due at least in part to the fact that the nuclei near the synaptic junction are specialized to produce the mRNA for the acetylcholine (ACh) receptor, whereas other nuclei are not (Changeux et al., 1990; Phillips et al., 1991; Sanes et al., 1991). In contrast, the thousands of individual synaptic sites on CNS neurons must be supplied by molecules that are encoded by genes in a single centrally located nucleus. This means that the synthesis, sorting and delivery of the molecular constituents of synapses in neurons must be much more complex than in muscles, and may require different mechanisms.

3.1 Constructing the Receptive Surface of Neurons

Given that each postsynaptic site on a neuron is a microdomain with a distinct molecular composition, and that there are a large number of these microdomains, what mechanisms could account for the construction of the many different sites? There are essentially three possibilities: (1) highly selective *targeted transport* systems to deliver molecules from the site of synthesis to postsynaptic sites; (2) a *selective docking and/or selective insertion* of molecules at particular synaptic sites; (3) a *selective retrieval* of molecules from the plasma membrane that are initially inserted ubiquitously, leaving only the molecules that are appropriate for the particular synaptic site; (4) a *local synthesis* of particular molecular constituents on-site. The latter mechanism requires the delivery of protein synthetic machinery and mRNA to synaptic sites. As will become clear, these are not mutually exclusive possibilities; different molecules may be targeted by different mechanisms, and the final assembly of synapses could involve a combination of mechanisms (see 5 Conclusions).

Targeted Transport Systems   Despite a wealth of information about axonal transport in neurons, very little is known about targeted transport systems that could deliver molecules to different intracellular destinations. There is, however, information about targeted transport in other types of cells which are "polarized" (that is, cells that have distinct plasma membrane domains with different molecular constituents). The prototype of this class of cell and the one that has been studied most extensively is the polarized epithelial cell (for a recent review, see Mostov et al., 1992).

Epithelial cells have two distinct membrane domains. An *apical domain* faces the environment or the lumen of an organ; other regions of the epithelial cell membrane that are apposed to neighboring cells comprise the *basolateral domain*. The two domains are separated by a region in which there are tight junctions. Tight junctions interconnect the external leaflets of the plasma membranes of adjacent cells, and prevent the diffusion of integral membrane proteins from one domain to another.

The protein compositions of the apical and basolateral domains are quite different. For example, depending on the type of epithelial cell, the apical domain may contain proteins that function as transporters for particular molecules (similar to the transporters responsible for selective uptake of neurotransmitters in neurons). The apical domain may also have structural specializations such as microvilli. The basolateral domain generally contains proteins that play a role in cell-cell interactions. The tight junctions between epithelial cells represent one such cell-cell interaction. The different protein composition of the two domains implies the existence of sorting mechanisms that permit the selective targeting of different molecules to the different domains.

How molecular sorting occurs in epithelial cells is currently a topic of considerable interest in cell biology. There appear to be at least two mechanisms. In one case, molecules are incorporated into vesicles, and the vesicles are transported differentially to one domain or the other after exiting the trans-Golgi network. In the second mechanism, proteins are transported initially to one domain. Proteins that are destined for the opposite domain are then retrieved by endocytosis into vesicles, and the endocytosed vesicles are delivered to the opposite surface by "transcytosis." In this mechanism, selectivity is conferred by the selective retrieval of particular membrane proteins from the domains in which they do not belong.

The initial studies of the mechanisms of protein sorting evaluated how epithelial cells sort viral proteins. When viruses infect cells, their RNA is released into the cytoplasm and is rapidly replicated. The viral RNA is then translated by the protein synthetic machinery of the host cell, producing proteins of two sorts: (1) envelope glycoproteins, and (2) capsid proteins which interact with and encapsulate the viral RNA. Envelope proteins are synthesized on the rough endoplasmic reticulum, whereas capsid proteins are synthesized on ribosomes that are not membrane-bound. The envelope proteins are then transported to the Golgi apparatus, where they are glycosylated. Vesicles containing the viral glycoproteins bud from the trans-Golgi network and are then transported to the plasma membrane. Capsid proteins remain in the cytoplasm where they bind with and encapsulate the viral RNA. Once the envelope proteins reach the plasma membrane, the newly formed capsids are wrapped in a portion of plasma membrane containing the envelope proteins, and the free virus "buds" from the cell. Budding requires the presence of the envelope proteins in the membrane. Thus, budding can only occur from portions of the plasma membrane that contain the envelope proteins.

The key to the studies of protein sorting is that the envelope proteins from different viruses are sorted to different plasma membrane domains. As a result, different viruses bud from different surfaces of epithelial cells. For example, influenza virus buds only from the apical surface; vesicular stomatitis virus buds only from the basolateral surface (figure 2.1). By tracing the localization of the proteins synthesized by these two virus using antibodies, it was found that the proteins destined for the two locations were co-localized at least through the trans-Golgi network. This implied that sorting took place when the vesicles containing the proteins separated from the trans-Golgi network.

Although the studies of viral protein sorting have been important, the most detailed information about the molecular signals for sorting in epithelial cells has come from studies of the sorting of intrinsic proteins. There have been two key strategies: (1) portions of proteins that are thought to contain the signal have been mutated, and the effects of the mutation on sorting have been evaluated; and (2) genetic engineering techniques have been used to construct DNA encoding fusion proteins that contain putative sorting signals along with some other reporter protein. These genes have then been introduced into epithelial cells by transfection to evaluate whether the putative signals lead to the predicted sorting of the fusion proteins.

The first sorting signal to be reasonably well characterized using these strategies is the so-called glycosyl-phosphatidylinositol (GPI) anchor. The GPI anchor is found on the carboxy-terminus of some proteins that are destined for delivery to the apical surface of epithelial cells. This is the portion of the membrane-spanning glycoprotein that faces the lumen when these proteins are present in vesicles. When a GPI anchor is transferred to a protein that is normally restricted to the basolateral domain, the protein is redirected to the apical surface (for a review, see Mostov et al., 1992). This is definitive evidence that the GPI anchor is sufficient to direct proteins to the apical surface. It is noteworthy, however, that the GPI anchor is on the luminal side. In this position, it cannot interact directly with the machinery in the cytoplasm that is presumably responsible for vectorial transport. Thus, the GPI anchor may interact with other specific transmembrane proteins with cytoplasmic domains that are responsible for the selective association with the vectorial transport machinery.

Signals for targeting to the basolateral surface of epithelial cells are less clear. Several studies have examined the sorting of basolateral proteins with mutations in their cytoplasmic domains. In several cases, mutations or deletions of the cytoplasmic domain result in these proteins being targeted to the apical surface (for a review, see Mostov et al., 1992). However, the molecular nature of the basolateral signals are less well defined.

Protein sorting in neurons Similar strategies have been applied to study protein sorting in neurons. These studies have provided hints that the mechanisms for the targeting of molecules to different cellular compartments (axons vs. dendrites) are very similar to those that operate in epithelial cells.

These studies evaluated the distribution of different viral glycoproteins in neurons in culture using antibodies and immunofluorescence. When neurons were infected with viruses whose envelope proteins are targeted to the apical surface of epithelial cells (the hemagglutinin protein of influenza virus), the viral glycoprotein was targeted primarily to axons. In contrast, a viral protein that is normally targeted to the basolateral surface of epithelial cells (vesicular stomatitis virus glycoprotein) was targeted to dendrites (Dotti and Simons, 1990; Dotti et al., 1991). A simple hypothesis that arises from these observations is that from the point of view of protein sorting, dendrites are analogous to the basolateral surface of polarized epithelial cells, whereas axons are analogous to the apical surface (figure 2.1). An easy mnemonic is that in epithelial cells, molecules that are important for cell-cell interactions (like receptors) are delivered to the basolateral surface, which is in contact with other cells; transporters (like those present in axon terminals) are delivered to the apical surface. It is possible that the relationships recalled by this mnemonic also imply something about the cellular mechanisms involved in protein sorting. However, even in epithelial cells, these statements may oversimplify the situation, especially because the composition of the membrane domains depends to some extent on the type of epithelial cell. In any case, these studies indicate that mechanisms for protein sorting are present in neurons, and that some of the same targeting signals may operate as in epithelial cells.

There have been some initial attempts to evaluate the signals for sorting of neuronal proteins by constructing DNAs encoding fusion proteins. One interesting protein that is differentially targeted in neurons is GAP-43 (also known as F1, B50, and neuromodulin), a protein that has been implicated in both axon regeneration (Skene, and Willard, 1981) and long-term potentiation (Routtenberg et al., 1985). GAP-43 protein is localized primarily in axons. It is present in especially high concentrations in axonal growth cones (Goslin et al., 1990). Studies that have attempted to define the location of the signal for targeting using fusion proteins have produced confusing results. For example, when PC12 cells were transfected with genes encoding fusion proteins containing the N-terminus of GAP-43 and a reporter protein that is normally not expressed in neurons (chloramphenicol acetyltransferase), the fusion proteins accumulated in the growth cone-like termini of the neuritic processes (Zuber et al., 1989). These results suggest that a signal for targeting exists in the N-terminus of the molecule. Similar experiments have been carried out by transfecting neurons in culture using fusion proteins composed of different parts of the GAP-43 protein together with the reporter protein beta-

NEURON

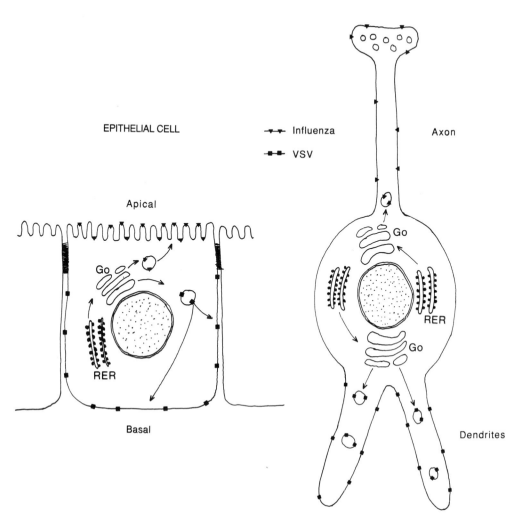

EPITHELIAL CELL

Influenza
VSV

Apical

Go

RER

Basal

Axon

Go

RER

Go

Dendrites

Figure 2.1 Targeted transport of proteins in epithelial cells and neurons. In epithelial cells, different types of proteins are delivered to different membrane domains by targeted (vectorial) transport systems. This has been well documented by studies of the targeting of viral proteins (for a review, see Mostov et al., 1992). For example, membrane glycoproteins of influenza virus are targeted to the apical membrane; glycoproteins of vesicular stomatitus virus (VSV) are targeted to the basolateral membrane. The same type of sorting occurs in neurons. Influenza virus glycoproteins are targeted to the axon, whereas VSV glycoproteins are targeted to the basolateral membrane (Dotti et al., 1990a, 1991). RER, rough endoplasmic reticulum; Go, Golgi apparatus; VSV, vesicular stomatitus virus.

A Selective Docking

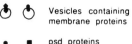

Vesicles containing
membrane proteins

psd proteins

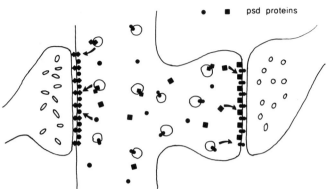

B Selective Retrieval

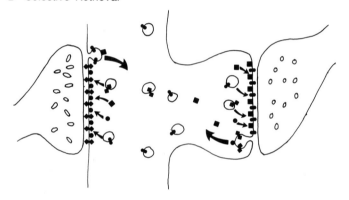

C. Delivery of Molecular Assemblies

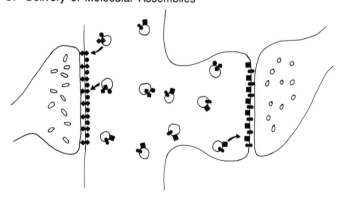

galactosidase. In the neurons, the fusion proteins became localized in neurites only when the protein included the full-length GAP-43 peptide (Liu et al., 1991). Although these results indicate that some targeting signal resides in the protein sequence, the location and nature of the targeting signal is not yet clear.

Sorting based on vectorial transport systems is appealing as a mechanism for delivering molecules to a few different domains such as the apical and basolateral membrane domains of epithelial cells or to axonal vs. dendritic compartments of neurons. It is difficult, however, to imagine how separate vectorial transport systems could exist for the selective delivery of molecules to the tens of thousands of different microdomains which comprise the post-synaptic receptive surface. The number of different transport systems that would be required is staggering. More appealing is the possibility that vectorial transport systems deliver molecules into the principal *compartments* of the neuron (cell bodies, axons, and dendrites for example), and that some other mechanism is then responsible for the subsequent targeting of molecules to individual synapses. It is in this regard that some selective docking or selective retrieval mechanisms come to mind.

Site-specific Construction Based on Selective Docking of Molecules
Targeting as a result of selective docking would require that the molecules in question arrive at a location near postsynaptic sites. The molecules that are appropriate for a given synapse would selectively associate with given postsynaptic sites via some sort of selective *docking* or *molecular trapping* mechanism, whereas those that are not appropriate would not (figure 2.2).

In principle, the molecules could exist in pools in either the underlying cytoplasm or in the plane of the plasma membrane. Trapping of molecules diffusing in the plane of the membrane is one of the mechanisms that has been proposed for the accumulation of ACh receptors at the neuromuscular junction (Andersen and Cohen, 1977). Indeed, this is the mechanism for which the term *molecular trapping* has previously been used. Although there is evidence for a trapping of mobile ACh receptors, most of the ACh receptors that accumulate at newly formed receptor clusters appear to be newly synthesized and inserted from a cytoplasmic pool (Dubinsky et al., 1989).

There are other reasons to think that molecules are inserted into postsynaptic sites on neurons from a cytoplasmic pool. A mechanism based

Figure 2.2 Some possible mechanisms of protein targeting to postsynaptic sites. (A) Molecular targeting based on selective binding of molecules in a mixed pool (a molecular trap mechanism). Molecules of the type that are appropriate to the synapse selectively bind; those that are not appropriate do not. (B) Constructing membrane domains of different composition by selectively retrieving inappropriate molecules. Molecules in a mixed pool associate randomly; inappropriate molecules are removed by selective retrieval (endocytosis). (C) Targeting of molecular assemblies. In this mechanism, molecules that are destined for different types of synapses are prepackaged. Targeting can then be based on an address marker present in only one of the molecules of the assembly.

on the trapping of molecules diffusing in the plane of the plasma membrane would require two things: (1) diffusion of the molecules in the lipid bilayer; and (2) a highly effective trapping mechanism (to account for the high concentration of molecules at the synaptic site). Free diffusion of proteins within the postsynaptic membrane seems unlikely given the highly structured nature of the postsynaptic receptive surface. An important feature of the dendritic membrane is the prominent association with the underlying cytoskeleton, which would be likely to restrict diffusion. Moreover, it seems very unlikely that it would be possible for a protein to diffuse from its site of synthesis in the neuronal cell body to a synaptic site on a distal dendrite without being trapped by one of the tens of thousands of synaptic sites in its diffusional path. In contrast, if the molecules were in the cytoplasm, they could be delivered into the appropriate domains (dendrites) by transport systems, and then released so as to be available for docking. In any case, the principles involved in the selective docking would be the same regardless of the location of the pool.

The docking or trapping of particular proteins would presumably depend upon some association of the proteins with elements that were uniquely present at the postsynaptic site. Presumably, such an association would require the presence of recognition signals on the parts of the molecules that could come into apposition. One interesting implication that is made evident by figure 2.2A is that sorting mechanisms based on molecular trapping of molecules in a pool become more difficult to imagine the further the trapping mechanism lies from the available pool. For example, if the molecular trap exists in the postsynaptic membrane itself, movement of molecules into spines would be required for trapping to occur. How this could occur in the case of very elongated spines is not clear unless the concentration of the molecules to be trapped was very high.

Another possible location of a molecular trap is within the subsynaptic cytoplasm or cytoskeleton. For example, both the spine apparatus (when present) and the actin-based microfilament network beneath the synapse span the distance between the dendritic cytoplasm and the postsynaptic membrane specialization. Either of these elements could possess recognition sites that extend into the dendrite where they could operate as molecular traps. Given the distribution of the microfilament network and the spine apparatus, either could also play a role in delivering the trapped molecules to the synaptic site.

One final point is worth noting. Figure 2.2A illustrates the selective docking of vesicles that contain only the proteins that are appropriate for one or the other of the synapses. This would require the production of transport vesicles specific to given types of synapses. It is also possible, however, that proteins for different types of synapses could be included in the vesicles, and that molecules that were inappropriate would not be incorporated, either diffusing away in the plane of the lipid bilayer, or being removed by endocytosis.

Site-specific Construction Based on Selective Retrieval of Inappropriate Molecules   Constructing postsynaptic sites of unique molecular composition on the basis of selective retrieval would operate analogously with the transcytosis system in epithelial cells described above. In this process, both appropriate and inappropriate molecules would be incorporated at the site; molecules that were inappropriate would then be removed by endocytosis (figure 2.2B). The requirements for this sort of mechanism are similar to those described above for selective docking, in that the molecular constituents of all types of synapses would be present in a mixed pool.

The signal for selective retrieval could be of several forms. One possibility is a negative signal—the absence of key interactions with other molecules at the synaptic site. That is, molecules that belonged at the site would interact with other molecules of the particular synaptic junction, form oligomers, and so on. Molecules that did not belong would not experience the appropriate intermolecular interactions, and would thus be targeted for removal. The same result could be achieved if the molecules that were not integrated simply diffused away from the synaptic site (moving within the plane of the lipid bilayer).

To what extent might the components of synapses be delivered as assemblies? Most of the preceding discussion has considered the delivery and assembly of the molecules of the synapse as if each molecular constituent were delivered separately. However, it is possible that assemblies of molecules appropriate for different types of synapses are packaged and delivered to the synaptic site (figure 2.2C).

There are important differences between the delivery of individual molecules and the delivery of molecular assemblies. A useful analogy is the difference between a "stick-built" house, which is assembled entirely on-site, and a "prefabricated" house in which entire portions of the structure are delivered in an assembled form. On-site assembly of components provides an opportunity for essentially unlimited fine-tuning of the molecular composition and fine structure of the synapse based on local conditions. In contrast, there would be less opportunity for such fine-tuning if synaptic components were delivered as molecular assemblies. Moreover, one could not mix and match components. On the other hand, preassembly would presumably guarantee a greater uniformity in the final product.

One important implication of a mechanism that allowed the delivery of assembled structures is that not all molecular constituents in that assembly would have to possess targeting signals. The preassembled package could be delivered as a result of an *address marker* on one key molecule. Nevertheless, some signals would still be necessary to allow the "follower" molecules to be appropriately sorted into the proper packages along with the key molecules with the address marker. Thus, a mechanism that allowed the delivery of molecular assemblies does not significantly reduce the complexity of the targeting problem.

Although selective docking and/or selective retrieval mechanisms are conceptually appealing as mechanisms for constructing membrane domains of different composition, evidence for the existence of such mechanisms in neurons is lacking. In the absence of such mechanisms, however, it is difficult to envision how domains of unique molecular composition could be established unless all of the unique molecules were synthesized on-site. On-site synthesis of all the molecular constituents of individual synapses seems unlikely because of the number of different molecules involved. Thus some form of molecular targeting based on selective docking or selective retrieval seems almost certain to exist.

Local Synthesis of Some Molecular Constituents of Synapses A third possible mechanism for constructing local domains with a different protein composition involves a local synthesis of proteins "on site." This hypothesis had its roots in the discovery that polyribosomes are preferentially localized beneath postsynaptic sites on the dendrites of CNS neurons (Steward, 1983b; Steward and Fass, 1983; Steward and Levy, 1982). At synapses on dendritic spines, polyribosomes are most often found at the base of the spine (figure 2.3). At other synapses (e.g., those on dendritic shafts and axonal initial segments) polyribosomes are localized beneath the postsynaptic membrane specialization (Steward and Ribak, 1986). The polyribosomes beneath synapses are often juxtaposed to membranous cisterns (figure 2.3) (Steward and Reeves, 1988). It is not known if this represents a functional association equivalent to that between polyribosomes and the rough endoplasmic reticulum. The cisterns in turn are often connected with a spine apparatus if one is present (Steward et al., 1988). Synapse-associated polyribosomes are particularly prominent during periods of synapse growth, suggesting that the polyribosomes

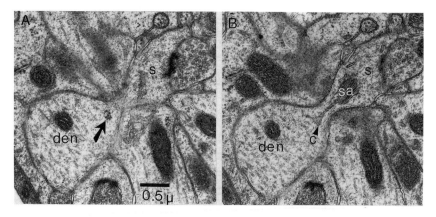

Figure 2.3 Polyribosomes associated with spine synapses on the dendrites of CNS neurons. These photomicrographs illustrate two serial sections through the dendrite of a granule cell of the dentate gyrus that illustrate the typical configuration of the protein synthetic machinery at spine synapses. The polyribosomes are most often present at the base of the spine (slanted arrow in A); these can be seen to lie very near a membranous cistern (c, visible in B), which is true of about 50% of the polyribosomes at spine synapses. The cistern in turn appears to be connected with a spine apparatus (small arrow in B). den, dendrite; s, spine; sa, spine apparatus; (From Steward and Banker, 1992.)

might synthesize components of the postsynaptic junction (Palacios-Pru et al., 1981; Steward, 1983a; Steward and Falk, 1986).

The discovery of polyribosomes in dendrites led to the question of how these elements were delivered. Some information on this question has been provided by studies of the translocation of recently synthesized RNA from the nucleus after pulse-labeling with RNA precursors (Davis et al., 1987, 1990). Recently synthesized RNA can be labeled by pulse-labeling neurons in culture with ^{3}H-uridine, which is incorporated into RNA in the nucleus. Autoradiographic analyses can then be used to trace the subsequent migration of the recently synthesized RNA through the cytoplasm. When neurons were fixed immediately after a 1-hr pulse-labeling period, labeled RNA was restricted almost exclusively to the nucleus. If the cells were returned to media with excess cold uridine for various periods of time, the label was found progressively further into the dendrites, so that by about 12 hr, the entire dendritic tree was labeled (figure 2.4).

In young neurons (before the time that dendrites acquire their characteristic features), recently synthesized RNA is transported into both axons and dendrites (R. Kleiman, G. Banker, and O. Steward, in preparation). However, in well-differentiated neurons, axons are only occasionally labeled. These results

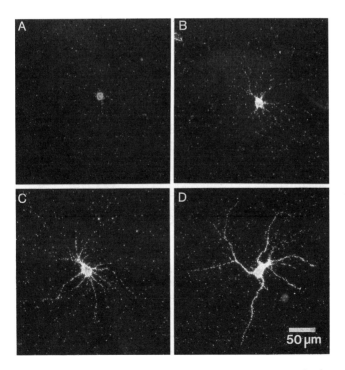

Figure 2.4 Selective dendritic transport of recently synthesized RNA. Hippocampal neurons in culture were pulse-labeled with ^{3}H-uridine for 1 hr, and then fixed immediately or returned to a chase medium containing an excess of unlabeled uridine. The intracellular distribution of the recently synthesized RNA was determined autoradiographically. (A) A neuron fixed at the end of the 1-hr pulse. (B–D) Neurons fixed at 3, 6, and 24 hr respectively. (From Steward et al., 1988.)

Molecular Sorting in Neurons

suggest that after the neurons have developed their characteristic polarity, RNA transport is selective to dendrites.

By measuring the average distance of labeling at different time intervals, it was determined that the rate of dendritic transport was about 0.25−0.5 mm/day (roughly comparable to slow axonal transport). Interestingly, the rate of transport seems to vary between individual dendrites depending on the length of the dendrite and its branching characteristics (Davis et al., 1990).

There is also some information about the nature of the transport process. For example, dendritic transport of RNA has been found to be sensitive to metabolic poisons like sodium azide (Davis et al., 1987), and microtubule poisons such as nocodozole (R. Kleiman, G. Banker, and O. Steward, in preparation). These observations suggest that RNA transport involves microtubules. Also, much of the recently synthesized RNA that is present in dendrites is resistant to detergent extraction, suggesting that it is bound to the cytoskeleton (Davis et al., 1987). Other properties of this selective RNA transport system remain to be defined.

4 WHAT TYPES OF PROTEINS ARE LOCALLY SYNTHESIZED?

Two lines of research have provided some indications about what proteins are synthesized by the dendritic polyribosomes. The first line of evidence comes from in situ hybridization analyses of the distribution of mRNA within neurons. The second comes from biochemical studies of proteins that are synthesized in subcellular fractions containing pinched-off dendrites and synaptic terminals.

4.1 Localization of Particular mRNAs in Dendrites

A casual glance at most published in situ hybridization studies in which the cellular distribution of mRNA can be assessed reveals that the majority of neuronal mRNAs are localized primarily or exclusively in neuronal cell bodies. This can be easily seen when evaluating the distribution of mRNA in laminated structures such as the cerebellum or hippocampus; in these areas, the labeling for most mRNAs is found predominantly over the cell body laminae.

In dramatic contrast, in situ hybridization studies of the distribution of two neuronal mRNAs have revealed substantial amounts of mRNA in laminae that contain dendrites but few neuronal cell bodies (for example, the neuropil layers of the hippocampus and cerebral cortex). The initial report of such neuropil labeling was of the mRNA encoding the high-molecular-weight form of the high-molecular-weight microtubule-associated protein MAP2 (Garner et al., 1988). This was of considerable interest because MAP2 is considered to be a marker for the dendritic cytoskeleton (Goedert et al., 1991; Matus et al., 1981). Subsequent studies revealed that the mRNA encoding the alpha-subunit of Ca^{2+}/calmodulin−dependent protein kinase (CaM II kinase) was also present in dendritic laminae, especially in the hippocampus (Burgin et al., 1990). In addition, a nontranslated RNA, termed BC1, has approximately the same distribution as the mRNAs for MAP2 and the alpha subunit of CaM II kinase (Tiedge et al., 1991b). This RNA is a polymerase III transcript of unknown function (see below).

Although in situ hybridization studies using tissue sections are suggestive, caution is needed in attempting to infer the subcellular distribution of mRNAs in such material. Falsely positive conclusions are possible in the case of mRNAs that are present in the glia in neuropil layers. In addition, some mRNAs that appear to be confined to cell bodies in tissue sections may actually be present at low levels in dendrites. For example, probes that hybridize with ribosomal RNA (rRNA) primarily label cell bodies, with little indication of labeling in dendritic laminae (Phillip et al., 1987); however, electron microscopic studies clearly reveal that ribosomes are present in dendrites. Thus, labeling due to RNAs present in dendrites at relatively low levels may not be readily distinguishable from background in tissue sections.

To circumvent these difficulties, in situ hybridization has recently been applied to neurons in culture, where the subcellular distribution of mRNA can be visualized directly. These studies confirmed the differential distribution of mRNA suggested by studies of tissue sections. Most mRNAs, including those encoding actin, tubulin, a neurofilament subunit, and GAP-43 are largely restricted to neuronal cell bodies. In contrast, the mRNA encoding MAP2 is present at high levels in dendrites (Bruckenstein et al., 1990; Kleiman et al., 1990; see figure 2.5). Studies are in progress to evaluate the intracellular distribution of mRNA for CaM II kinase. Ribosomal RNA can also be readily detected in the dendrites of cultured neurons (R. Kleiman, G. Banker, and O. Steward, unpublished), as can poly-A$^+$ RNA (Bruckenstein et al., 1990)

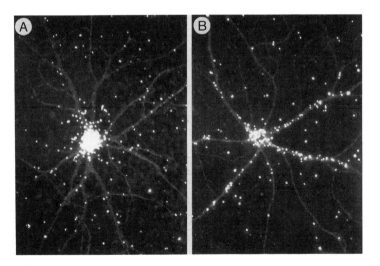

Figure 2.5 Differential distribution of mRNAs in neurons. (A) Distribution of the mRNA for the 68 kD neurofilament protein as revealed by in situ hybridization. (B) Distribution of the mRNA for MAP2. Most neuronal mRNAs have a distribution like that of the mRNA for neurofilament protein. A few mRNAs, including the mRNA for MAP2, are present throughout the dendritic arbor. (From Kleiman et al., 1990.)

and the polymerase III transcript BC1 (Tiedge et al., 1991a). These results indicate that an mRNA sorting mechanism exists in neurons which permits the targeting of different types of mRNA to different intracellular locations. How fine this targeting system is remains to be determined.

There is also evidence that the mRNA for amyloid precursor protein is present in part of the dendritic arbor of neurons in culture (Strong et al., 1990). This is surprising because the localization of this mRNA in tissue sections does not suggest a dendritic localization (Higgins et al., 1988; Lewis et al., 1988). This may be another example (like ribosomal RNA) of an RNA that is present in dendrites at low levels, but is difficult to detect in studies using tissue sections.

4.2   Evidence that Some Protein Constituents of the Postsynaptic Junction Are Locally Synthesized

Another approach to the question of what proteins are synthesized in dendrites evaluates proteins that are synthesized within subcellular fractions enriched in pinched off presynaptic terminals and dendrites (synaptodendrosomes) (Rao and Steward, 1991a). It has been known since the mid-1960s that synaptodendrosome fractions exhibit protein synthesis (Autilio et al., 1968; Morgan and Austin, 1968). Initially, the protein synthesis was thought to occur within presynaptic terminals. However, autoradiographic studies revealed that the synthesis was actually occurring primarily in fragments of dendrites and contaminating cell bodies (Gambetti et al., 1972).

The major difficulty in using synaptodendrosomes to study dendritic protein synthesis is that the fractions are contaminated with fragments of neuronal and presumably glial cell bodies as well as mitochondria. There are, however, strategies that can be used to deal with these confounding variables. The contribution of mitochondria to protein synthesis can be evaluated using protein synthesis inhibitors which block either mitochondrial or eucaryotic ribosomal protein synthesis (chloramphenicol and cycloheximide respectively). The problem of protein synthesis within fragments of neuronal and glial cell bodies can be circumvented by focusing on the proteins that are assembled into synaptic structures. Thus, the experimental strategy was to allow synaptodendrosomes to synthesize proteins in the presence of labeled precursors (^{35}S-methionine), and then use subcellular fractionation techniques to isolate components of the synapse (synaptic plasma membranes and synaptic junctional complexes, which are the insoluble components that remain after detergent extraction of synaptic plasma membranes [Rao et al., 1991a]. The proteins that were synthesized within the synaptodendrosomes and that had become associated with synaptic plasma membranes (SPM) and synaptic junctional complexes (SJC) were then characterized by polyacrylamide gel electrophoresis and fluorography.

The results from these experiments suggested that a relatively small number of protein components of the synaptic junction were locally synthesized within dendrites. Fluorographs of polyacrylamide gels of proteins from SPM

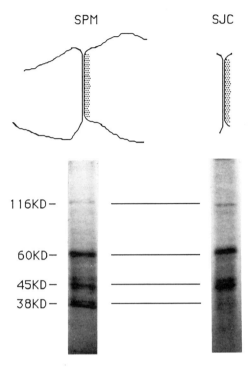

The Major labeled bands in the synaptic plasma
membrane and synaptic junctional complex fractions

Figure 2.6 Evidence that some proteins of the postsynaptic junction are locally synthesized. Synaptodendrosomes were pulse-labeled with ^{35}S-methionine to label proteins that were synthesized within elements in the synaptodendrosome fraction. Subcellular fractions enriched in synaptic plasma membranes and synaptic junctional complexes were prepared. Proteins from these fractions were electrophoresed on polyacrylamide gels, and the gels were dried onto filter paper and exposed to photographic film in order to obtain fluorographs, so as to identify proteins that were synthesized during the pulse-labeling period. Several labeled bands are evident in the fluorograph prepared from synaptic plasma membranes (SPM). The doublet at an apparent molecular weight of 38 kD was removed when the synaptic plasma membranes were treated with Triton X-100 in order to solubilize the plasma membranes leaving synaptic junctional complexes (SJC). The identity of the labeled proteins is not yet known. (From Rao et al., 1991a.)

and SJC fractions revealed a few prominently labeled bands (figure 2.6), in contrast to the large number of labeled bands that were evident in fluorographs prepared from unfractionated synaptodendrosomes. This labeling was inhibited by cycloheximide but not by chloramphenicol, indicating that the labeling was the result of eucaryotic ribosomal protein synthesis. These results suggested that at least some of the protein constituents of synaptic junctions were locally synthesized within the dendritic fragments, presumably by subsynaptic polyribosomes. Interestingly, the most prominent bands did not seem to correspond either to MAP2 or to the alpha-subunit of CaM II kinase, suggesting that other proteins synthesized at synaptic sites are quantitatively more important than the two proteins whose mRNAs have thus far been found in dendrites.

An obvious goal for the future is to isolate and clone dendritic mRNAs. One obvious potential source of dendritic mRNA is the synaptodendrosome preparation (Chicurel et al., 1990). However, it will be essential to develop a way to sort dendritic mRNAs from the mRNA present in contaminants of the fraction, including glial cells (Rao and Steward, 1991b; submitted). Another promising approach follows from the development of a cell culture technique for harvesting axons and dendrites free of contamination by neuronal and glial cell bodies (Torre and Steward, 1992). This technique has allowed an unequivocal demonstration that isolated dendrites exhibit local protein synthesis (and thus have translationally competent mRNA) (Torre and Steward 1992). This finding is important in its own right, because it is the first definitive evidence that the polyribosomes that are present in dendrites are active in protein synthesis. More importantly, this preparation should provide a source of uncontaminated dendritic RNAs that can be amplified using the polymerase chain reaction and cloned.

4.3   Sorting, Intradendritic Transport, and Docking of mRNA at Synapses

Taken together with the earlier morphological work, the recent discoveries on the differential distribution of RNA within neurons suggest the existence of three previously unknown processes: (1) a sorting mechanism that determines whether particular RNAs will be transported into dendrites or will remain in the cell body; (2) a mechanism for transporting RNA selectively into dendrites (and presumably initial segments of axon); and (3) a mechanism that docks mRNA and associated translational machinery (ribosomes) beneath post-synaptic sites (figure 2.7). Experimental strategies are available to begin to investigate these mechanisms.

Sorting of mRNA   Sorting of mRNA to dendrites and neuronal cell bodies could occur in one of three ways: (1) there could be signals that target mRNA for transport into dendrites, and mRNAs without the signal would remain in the cell body; (2) there could be signals that target mRNAs to sites in the cell body, and mRNAs without the signal would be transported; (3) there could be separate targeting signals for both sites. There are also at least two different possibilities about the nature of the molecular signals. (1) the signal could lie in the protein encoded by the particular mRNA; (2) the signal could lie in the mRNA itself.

The hypothesis that sorting depends upon a signal in the protein is based on analogy with the signal sequence mechanism that leads to the association of mRNA with the rough endoplasmic reticulum. In the case of mRNAs targeted to the endoplasmic reticulum, protein synthesis is initiated on free ribosomes, but becomes arrested when the initial portion of the nascent polypeptide (signal sequence) is recognized by and binds to a signal recognition

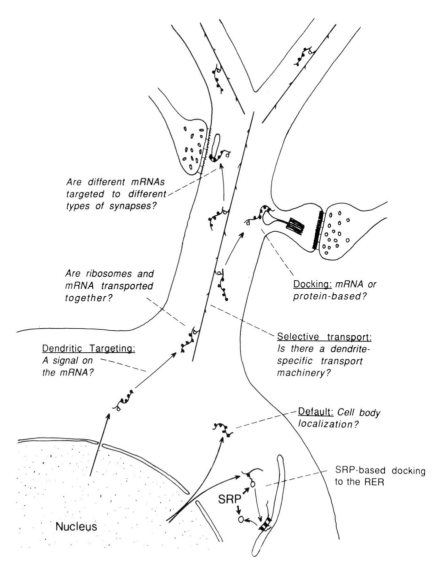

Are different mRNAs
targeted to different
types of synapses?

Are ribosomes and
mRNA transported
together?

Docking: mRNA or
protein-based?

Dendritic Targeting:
A signal on
the mRNA?

Selective transport:
Is there a dendrite-
specific transport
machinery?

Default: Cell body
localization?

SRP-based docking
to the RER

SRP

Nucleus

Figure 2.7 Possible mechanisms of mRNA sorting, intracellular transport, and docking in neurons. Messenger RNA synthesized in the nucleus can be targeted to the rough endoplasmic reticulum by a signal sequence mechanism, or targeted for dendritic transport. In the absence of a targeting signal (default) the RNA presumably remains in the cell body. RNA is transported selectively into dendrites, implying that the dendritic transport machinery has different properties than the transport machinery of the axon. Polyribosomes are selectively docked beneath synaptic sites. Unresolved questions regarding these mechanisms are indicated. SRP, signal recognition particle. (From Steward and Banker, 1992.)

particle (see figure 2.7). Interaction between the signal recognition particle and its receptor in the rough endoplasmic reticulum mediates the binding of the ribosome and mRNA to the rough endoplasmic reticulum, which in turn leads to release of the signal recognition particle and resumption of protein synthesis. A similar mechanism might operate to target mRNA to the dendritic transport machinery.

The hypothesis that sorting depends on a signal in the mRNA comes from studies of the mechanisms of mRNA sorting in other cell types. For example, in cells ranging from oocytes to migrating fibroblasts, the 3' noncoding regions of mRNAs that are differentially distributed contain signals that are sufficient for differential sorting. In this regard, it is of interest that both of the mRNAs that are delivered into dendrites (MAP2 and CaM II kinase) have long noncoding sequences.

The experiments needed to identify mRNA sorting signals are in principle straightforward. Chimeric cDNAs can be constructed using a portion of a dendritic mRNA fused with a portion of a somatic mRNA. These artificial genes can be introduced into neurons, and the sorting of the chimeric mRNAs encoded by the cDNAs can be evaluated using in situ hybridization. Then, depending on the results, the putative signal region can be narrowed down further. If the signals are found to lie within coding regions, this approach could also be used to determine if translation is necessary for sorting; for example, start sites could be mutated or stop codons could be inserted.

This approach has already been used successfully to define the mechanisms of mRNA sorting in *Xenopus* oocytes. A number of maternal mRNA species are differentially distributed along the animal-vegetal axis of the oocyte. The best characterized of these is Vg1, which encodes a peptide growth factor that appears to be a member of the transforming growth factor β (TGFβ) family that may play a role in mesoderm induction (Melton, 1991). Vg1 is initially distributed uniformly in the oocyte. As the oocyte matures, it is actively translocated to the vegetal pole—a process that is blocked by drugs that disrupt microtubules (Melton, 1987). The signal responsible for Vg1 localization appears to be part of the 3' untranslated portion of the mRNA. Chimeric mRNAs that include the 3' untranslated sequence of the Vg1 mRNA are localized like native Vg1, whereas chimeras lacking this region are not (Yisraeli and Melton, 1988). Subsequent studies have narrowed the signal to a segment of the 3' untranslated region that is 340 nucleotides long (Mowry and Melton, 1991).

Another well-characterized example of mRNA sorting occurs in Drosophila embryos. One message that has been studied extensively is the product of the bicoid gene, termed bcd, which is concentrated at the anterior pole of the oocyte (Frigerio et al., 1986). During embryogenesis, bcd protein comes to be localized in a concentration gradient along the anterior-posterior axis of the embryo. The bcd protein acts as a transcription factor that activates subordinate gene(s) in a concentration-dependent fashion (Driever and Nusslein-Volhard, 1989), thus specifying position along the anterior-posterior axis (MacDonald and Struhl, 1986).

The differential localization of bcd also depends on a signal in the mRNA. Chimeric mRNAs containing a 630-nucleotide-long portion of the 3' untranslated region are properly localized; however, localization is disrupted when 100–150 nucleotides are removed from either end of this segment (MacDonald and Struhl, 1988). Identifying the signals that determine mRNA targeting in neurons should also provide a means to alter mRNA localization experimentally, and hence test the role of mRNA sorting in neuronal function.

While conceptually straightforward, these experiments may be technically difficult. There are two problems: (1) having the chimeric mRNAs survive in the cells long enough to be transported; and (2) having well-differentiated neurons in which sorting can be evaluated.

In principle, one could either inject chimeric mRNAs or transfect cells with chimeric DNAs that encode the mRNAs. The injection approach may be problematic for three reasons: (1) it may be technically difficult to inject sufficient quantities of the artificial mRNAs; (2) injected mRNAs may be rapidly degraded; and (3) targeting may require that the mRNAs be synthesized by the cell. For example, it may be that RNA targeting requires that the mRNAs begin their journey at the nuclear pore. For this reason, transfection approaches are more appealing.

There are, however, a different set of problems associated with transfection approaches. Valid sorting assays will require the use of differentiated cells with well-developed dendrites. This implies the use of primary cultures, which may be difficult to transfect. Also, mRNA half-life will have to be considered. Some mRNAs may be restricted to cell bodies simply because they are too short-lived to be transported into dendrites. This possibility must be kept in mind when comparing mRNAs that are transported with those that are not, and when introducing genetically modified mRNAs into cells during the search for putative targeting signals, especially since sequences within the 3' untranslated regions are thought to govern mRNA degradation.

One added complication is that mRNA targeting may depend not on a limited nucleotide or amino acid sequence but on secondary structure determined by sequences that are broadly distributed throughout the molecule. The proposal that sorting signals are based on secondary structure comes from studies of the differential localization of mRNAs in *Drosophila* embryos. For example, the mRNA for bcd is appropriately localized in different drosophila species despite the fact that there is less than 50% sequence homology in the portion of the mRNA that is thought to contain the localization signal (MacDonald, 1990). However, the predicted secondary structure of the mRNA is similar across species. If the signal for mRNA sorting is the secondary structure of the mRNA rather than the specific nucleotide sequence, characterization of the signal may be more difficult.

mRNA Transport and Docking at Synaptic Sites   Possible approaches to the mechanisms of RNA transport and docking are less obvious. RNA transport is selective to dendrites, and detergent extraction experiments have revealed that the RNA that is present in dendrites is bound to the cytoskeleton

(Davis et al., 1987). Thus, mRNA targeting may depend on interactions between the mRNA and dendrite-specific cytoskeletal elements. If this is the case, then the elucidation of the signals for sorting will also reveal the nature of the interaction between RNA and the dendritic transport machinery.

The other issue is docking. Docking is strongly implied by the highly selective localization of polyribosomes beneath synapses (Steward, 1983b; Steward and Levy, 1982). A key issue is whether different mRNAs are positioned beneath different types of synapses. Intuitively, it seems unlikely that transport and docking both rely on the same signals—seemingly, the two processes call for mutually opposing effects. The most likely possibility for docking would seem to be some interaction with the cytoskeletal network that is present beneath synapses. Electron microscopic studies suggest that the subsynaptic cytoskeleton is different from the cytoskeleton in other parts of the neuron, which may provide the basis for such docking. Experiments involving the construction of chimeric mRNAs may provide important hints about mRNA-cytoskeletal interactions. However, it will be necessary to develop assays for docking before these experiments can be carried out.

Untranslated RNAs in Dendrites

Another interesting RNA present in dendrites does not encode a protein. This RNA, called BC1, is a small RNA (152 nucleotides) that lacks a protein-coding sequence. It was first identified in rats as a result of its high abundance in brain and its absence in most other tissues (hence the name brain cytoplasmic RNA) (DeChiara and Brosius, 1987; Sutcliff et al., 1984). In situ hybridization studies of the distribution of BC1 in brain (Tiedge et al., 1991b) and in neurons in culture (Tiedge et al., 1991a) reveal that it has about the same distribution in dendrites as MAP2 and CaM II kinase mRNAs. The human counterpart of BC1, termed BC200, was recently cloned (H. Tiedge, H., Chen, W., and. Brosius, J., personal communication). This RNA shares only limited sequence homology with rodent BC1, but its pattern of expression is very similar, including its distribution in dendrites.

BC1 and BC200 are transcribed by RNA polymerase III, which also synthesizes several other small stable untranslated RNAs including tRNAs and 7SL RNA (an RNA component of the signal recognition particle) (DeChiara and Brosius, 1987). Like 7SL RNA, BC1 associates with proteins to form a ribonucleoprotein particle (Kobayashi et al., 1991; Tiedge et al., 1991b). In addition, both BC1 and BC200 contain a consensus sequence that is similar to the consensus sequence in 7SL RNA responsible for the binding of a protein component of the signal recognition particle that arrests translation. These findings are consistent with the hypothesis BC1 and BC200 play some role in mRNA targeting or translation in dendrites (Tiedge et al., 1991b). On the other hand, if these RNAs have such a role, the limited sequence similarity between rodent and human varieties of the molecule is surprising; other small RNAs that function in protein synthesis, including tRNAs and 7SL RNA, are highly conserved in evolution (Gundelfinger et al., 1984).

It is not clear how BC1 and BC200 themselves are targeted and transported into dendrites. Because they do not encode proteins, they cannot be targeted by a signal sequence mechanism. The most likely possibility is that targeting sequences lie within the BC1 and BC200 RNA or the proteins with which BC1 and BC200 associate.

Why Are Some Synaptic Proteins Synthesized Locally?

This is perhaps the most important question of all, although answers so far are only speculative. Obviously local synthesis provides the opportunity for constructing local domains with a unique protein composition. However, the evidence suggests that some of the most important molecular components that are unique to particular classes of synapse are *not* synthesized locally. Specifically, in situ hybridization analyzes have revealed that the mRNAs for neurotransmitter receptors are largely restricted to neuronal cell bodies (Boulter et al., 1990; Ito and Sugiyama, 1991; Keinanen et al., 1990; Sakimura et al., 1990; Sommer et al., 1990). There is as yet no evidence that any of these mRNAs are localized in dendrites. It is important to note, however, that the distribution of receptor mRNAs has not yet been evaluated in neurons in culture, where it is possible to define the subcellular distribution of mRNAs more precisely. Nevertheless, it is clear that the mRNAs for receptors are not present in high concentrations in dendrites. These results suggest that receptors are delivered via targeted transport or selective docking/retrieval.

What other functions might local synthesis serve? One attractive possibility is that the localization of particular mRNAs and associated protein synthetic machinery at postsynaptic sites provides the opportunity for regulating the amount of key proteins synthesized at different times in response to local conditions. Given that the most obvious way to influence the local postsynaptic microenvironment is through signals generated by synaptic activity, this mechanism seems ideally suited to play a role in activity-dependent synaptic plasticity. In this regard, it is certainly of interest that both MAP2 and CaM II kinase have been implicated in neuronal growth and plasticity. In this regard, it is noteworthy that protein synthetic activity within synapto-dendrosome fractions is modified by depolarization (Weiler and Greenough, 1991; Weiler et al., 1991).

Obviously, all of these possibilities are purely speculative. An understanding of the significance of dendritic protein synthesis will almost certainly require the identification of the proteins that are synthesized within dendrites and an elucidation of the functional role that these proteins play in synaptic function.

5 CONCLUSIONS

The three possible mechanisms for molecular sorting described above are speculative, but are based on current cell biological knowledge. It is again important to emphasize that the different mechanisms are not mutually exclusive; in fact they probably operate in concert. For example, in the comparatively simple case of targeting of proteins to axons, there is evidence to suggest that vectorial transport is responsible for bringing the proteins into the axon, while molecular trapping leads to the accumulation of particular proteins at different sites such as the growth cone (Sheetz et al., 1990).

The construction of the postsynaptic receptive surface must be more complex, and probably involves all three mechanisms. Synapses are undoubtedly composed of many molecules that are present ubiquitously, and a few molecules that are unique to the particular class of synapse. It would seem efficient to deliver the common molecules as molecular assemblies. The delivery of molecules that are unique to the class of synapse would have to be more closely regulated. These may be targeted individually after synthesis in a central location (as may be the case with neurotransmitter receptors based on available evidence about the distribution of mRNAs for receptors) or synthesized locally at the synaptic site. The analogy with prefabricated buildings is again useful. If a prefabricated building is delivered to a site, it is still necessary to prepare the building site, attach utilities, build a foundation, attach the different components together, and complete the interior decoration according to the tastes of the future occupant. These sorts of fine adjustments may be the ones that involve the targeted delivery or local synthesis of individual molecules on site. Obviously, all of this is currently speculation. Until the molecular constituents of synaptic junctions are more completely characterized, and their site of assembly identified, these questions will remain open.

The goal of this chapter was to define what neurons presumably must do to construct, maintain, and modify their synapses. As indicated, there are many more questions than answers. It is clear that we do not know enough about the basic cell biology of neurons to even pose some of the key questions at this time. Some of the important gaps in our knowledge are:

• We do not yet know enough about the molecular composition of synapses on CNS neurons. An important issue is how much of the junctional material is generic and how much is unique to a particular class of synapse. The answer to this question will define the extent of the molecular sorting which must occur.

• We do not yet know enough about the way that synaptic sites are assembled, especially the important issue of how much of the junction is constructed on site from individual molecules, and how much (if any) is delivered in preassembled form. The answer to this question will help to define the nature of the sorting process.

• We do not yet know enough about the turnover of the important functional molecules of the synapse or of the synapses themselves. If molecular constituents are replaced individually, this implies a complex molecular targeting. If the constituents are replaced as assemblies, then the sorting problem is somewhat easier. If entire synaptic sites turn over, a different type of process is implied.

• We do not yet know the link between activity at the synapse and changes in synapse structure or function. If activity leads to changes in the molecular composition of synapses, then there must be some intracellular signaling pathways to accomplish such changes.

• We do not yet know whether the molecular composition of individual synapses can be changed in response to local conditions at that synapse (for example, in response to activity) or whether any changes that are induced are more widespread. The answer to this question has important implications for the mechanisms for molecular assembly that must operate, and the degree of specificity that can be expected for the changes that occur.

Taken together, answers to these questions are likely to be pivotal to an understanding of the cellular and molecular mechanisms of synaptic plasticity. Perhaps by defining some of the key issues, the present chapter will help to focus future research efforts.

ACKNOWLEDGMENTS

Thanks to Paula M. Falk and Leanna Whitmore for technical help in our studies of the cell biology of synapse plasticity, to my colleague Gary Banker, who has collaborated on the studies of dendritic transport of RNA and RNA sorting in neurons and who has been an important source of ideas and discussions, and to L. Davis, R. Kleiman, A. Rao, and E. R. Torre, whose work is described herein. The author gratefully acknowledges the continuous generous support provided by National Institute of Health Research grants NS 12333 to the author, and NS 23094 to Gary Banker. Some of the material discussed in this chapter has been included in a previous review (Steward and Banker, 1992).

REFERENCES

Andersen, M. J., and Cohen, M. W. (1977) Nerve-induced and spontaneous redistribution of acetylcholine receptors on cultured muscle cells. *J. Physiol.* 268:757–773.

Autilio, L. A., Appel, S. H., Pettis, P., and Gambetti, P. (1968) Biochemical studies of synapses in vitro. 1. Protein synthesis. *Biochemistry* 7:2615–2622.

Boulter, J., Hollmann, M., O'Shea-Greenfield, A., Hartley, M., Deneris, E., Maron, C., and Heinemann, S. (1990) Molecular cloning and functional expression of glutamate receptor subunit genes. *Science,* 249:1033–1037.

Bruckenstein, D. A., Lein, P. J., Higgins, D. and Fremeau, R. T. (1990) Distinct spatial localization of specific mRNAs in cultured sympathetic neurons. *Neuron* 5:809–819.

Burgin, K. E., Washam, M. N., Rickling, S., Westgate, S. A., Mobley, W. C., and Kelly, P. T. (1990) In situ hybridization histochemistry of CA^{++}/calmodulin-dependent protein kinase in developing rat brain. *J. Neurosci,* 10:1788–1798.

Changeux, J. P., et al. (1990) Compartmentalization of acetylcholine receptor gene expression during development of the neuromuscular junction. *Cold Spring Harbor Symp. Quant. Biol.* 55:381–396.

Chicurel, M. E., Terrian, D. M., and Potter, H. (1990) Subcellular localization of mRNA: Isolation and characterization of mRNA from an enriched preparation of hippocampal dendritic spines. *Soc. Neurosci. Abstr.* 16:353.

Davis, L., Banker, G. A., and Steward, O. (1987) Selective dendritic transport of RNA in hippocampal neurons in culture. *Nature* 447–479.

Davis, L., Burger, B., Banker, G. and Steward, O. (1990) Dendritic transport: Quantitative analysis of the time course of somatodendritic transport of recently synthesized RNA. *J. Neurosci.* 10:3056–3058.

DeChiara, T. M., and Brosius, J. (1987) Neural BC1 RNA: cDNA clones reveal nonrepetitive sequence content. *Proc. Natl. Acad. Sci. USA* 84:2624–2628.

Dotti, C. G. and Simons, K. (1990) Polarized sorting of viral glycoproteins to the axons and dendrites of hippocampal neurons in culture. *Cell* 62:63–72.

Doni, C. G., Parton, R. G. and Simons, K. (1991) Polarized sorting of glypiated proteins in hippocampal neurons. *Nature* 349:158–161.

Driever, W., and Nusslein-Volhard, C. (1989) Determination of spatial domains of zygotic gene expression in the *Drosophila* embryo by the affinity of binding sites for the bicoid morphogen. *Nature* 340:363–367.

Dubinsky, J. M., Loftus, D. J., Fischbach, G. D., and Elson, E. L. (1989) Formation of acetylcholine receptor clusters in chick myotubes: Migration or new insertion? *J. Cell Biol.* 109:1733–1743.

Fontaine, B., Sassoon, D., Buckingham, M., and Changeux, J. P. (1988) Detection of the nicotinic acetylcholine receptor alpha-subunit mRNA by in situ hybridization at neuromuscular junctions of 15-day-old chick striated muscles. *EMBO J.* 7:603–609.

Frigerio, G., Burri, M., Bopp, D., Baumgartner, S., and Noll, M. (1986) Structure and segmentation gene paired and the *drosophila* PRD gene set as part of a gene network. *Cell* 47:735–746.

Gambetti, P., Autilio-Gambetti, L. A., Gonatas, N. K., and Shafer, B. (1972) Protein synthesis in synaptosomal fractions: Ultrastructural radioautographic study. *J. Cell Biol* 52:526–535.

Garner, C. C., Tucker, R. P., and Matus, A. (1988) Selective localization of messenger RNA for cytoskeletal protein MAP2 in dendrites. *Nature* 336:674–677.

Glanzman, D. L., Kandel, E. R., and Schacher, S. (1990) Target-dependent structural changes accompanying long-term synaptic facilitation in *Aplysia* neurons. *Science* 249:799–801.

Goedert, M., Crowther, R. A., and Garner, C. C. (1991) Molecular characterization of microtubule-associated proteins tau and MAP2. *Trends Neurosci.* 14:193–199.

Goslin, K., Schreyer, D. J., Skene, J. H. P., and Banker, G. (1990) Changes in the distribution of GAP-43 during the development of neuronal polarity. *J. Neurosci.* 10:588–602.

Gundelfinger, E. D., Di Carlo, M., Zopf, D., and Melli, M. (1984) Structure and evolution of the 7SL component of the signal recognition particle. *EMBO J.* 10:2325–2332.

Hebb, D. O. (1949) *The Organization of Behavior.* New York: John Wiley and Sons.

Higgins, G. A., Lewis, D. A., Bahmanyar, S., Goldgaber, D., Gajdusek, D. C., Young, W. G., Morrison, J. H., and Wilson, M. C. (1988) Differential regulation of amyloid β-protein mRNA expression within hippocampal neuronal subpopulations in Alzheimer disease. *Proc. Natl. Acad. Sci USA* 85:1297–1301.

Ito, I., and Sugiyama, H. (1991) Roles of glutamate receptors in long-term potentiation at hippocampal mossy fiber synapses. 2:333–336.

Keinanen, K., Wisden, W., Sommer, B., Werner, P., Herb, A., Verdoorn, T. A., Sakmann, B., and Seeburg, P. H. (1990) A family of AMPA-sensitive glutamate receptors. *Science* 249:556–249.

Killisch, I., Dotti, C. G., Laurie, D. J., Luddens, H., and Seeburg, P. H. (1991) Expression patterns of GABA$_A$ receptor subtypes in developing hippocampal neurons. *Neuron* 7:927–936.

Kleiman, R., Banker, G., and Steward, O. (1990) Differential subcellular localization of particular mRNAs in hippocampal neurons in culture. *Neuron* 5:821–830.

Kobayashi, S., Goto, S., and Anzai, K. (1991) Brain-specific small RNA transcript of the identifier sequences is present as a 10 S ribonucleoprotein particle. *J. Biol. Chem.* 266:4726–4730.

Lewis, D. A., Higgins, G. A., Young, W. G., Goldgaber, D., Gajdusek, D. C., Wilson, M. C., and Morrison, J. H. (1988) Distribution of precursor amyloid β-protein messenger RNA in human cerebral cortex: Relationship to neurofibrillary tangles and neuritic plaques. *Proc. Natl. Acad. Sci. USA* 85:1691–1695.

Liu, Y., Chapman, E. R., and Storm, D. R. (1991) Targeting of neuromodulin (GAP43) fusion proteins to growth cones in cultured rat embryonic neurons. *Neuron* 6:411–420.

MacDonald, P. M. (1990) Bicoid mRNA localization signal: Phylogenetic conservation of function and RNA secondary structure *Development* 110:161–171.

MacDonald, P. M., and Struhl, G. (1986) A molecular gradient in early *Drosophila* embryos and its role in specifying the body pattern. *Nature* 324:537–545.

MacDonald, P. M., and Struhl, G. (1988) Cis-acting sequences responsible for anterior localization of bicoid mRNA in *Drosophila* embryos. *Nature* 336:595–598.

Matus, A., Bernhardt, R., and Hugh-Jones, T. (1981) HMW proteins are preferentially associated with dendritic microtubules in brain. *Proc. Natl. Acad. Sci. USA* 78:3010–3014.

Melton, D. A. (1987) Translocation of a localized maternal mRNA to the begetal pole of *Xenopus* oocytes. *Nature* 328:80–82.

Melton, D. A. (1991) Pattern formation during animal development. *Science* 252:224–241.

Merlie, J. P., and Sanes, J. A. (1985) Concentration of acetylcholine receptor mRNA in synaptic regions of adult muscle fibers. *Nature* 317:66–68.

Monaghan, D. T., Holets, V. R., Toy, D. W., and Cotman, C. W. (1983) Anatomical distributions of four pharmacologically distinct ^{3}H-L-glutamate binding sites. *Nature* 306:176–179.

Monaghan, D. T., Bridges, R. J. and Cotman, C. W. (1989) The excitatory amino acid receptors: their classes, pharmacology, and distinct properties in the function of the central nervous system. *Annu. Rev. Pharmacol. Toxicol.* 29:365–402.

Morgan, I. G., and Austin, L. (1968) Synaptosomal protein synthesis in a cell-free system. *J. Neurochem.* 15:41–51.

Mostov, K., Apodaca, G., Aroeti, B. and Okamato, C. (1992) Plasma membrane protein sorting in polarized epithelial cells. *J. Cell Biol.* 116:577–583.

Mowry, K., and Melton, D. A. (1991) Localization of mRNA in frog oocytes and eggs. *J. Cell Biol.* 115:123A.

Palacios-Pru, E. L., Palacios, L., and Mendoza, R. V. (1981) Synaptogenetic mechanisms during chick cerebellar cortex development. *J. Submicros. Cytol.* 13:145–167.

Petralia, R. S., and Wenthold, R. J. (1992) Light and electron immunocytochemical localization of AMPA-selective glutamate receptors in the rat brain. *J. Comp. Neurol.* 318:329–354.

Phillips, L. L., Nostrandt, S. J., Chikaraishi, D. M., and Steward, O. (1987) Increases in ribosomal RNA within the denervated neuropil of the dentate gyrus during reinnervation: Evalation by in situ hybridization usihng DNA probes complementary to ribosomal RNA. *Mol. Brain Res.* 2:251–261.

Phillips, W. D., Kopta, C., Blount, P., Gardner, P. D., Steinbach, J. H., and Merlie, J. P. (1991) ACh Receptor-rich membrane domains organized in fibroblasts by recombinant 43-kilodalton protein. *Science* 251:568–570.

Ramón y Cajal, S. (1911) *Histologie du système nerveux de l'homme et des vertébrés*. Paris: A. Maloine.

Rao, A., and Steward, O. (1991a) Evidence that protein constituents of postsynaptic membrane specializations are locally synthesized: Analysis of proteins synthesized within synaptosomes. *J. Neurosci.* 11:2881–2895.

Rao, A., and Steward, O. (1991b) Synaptosomal RNA: Assessment of contamination by glia and comparison with total RNA. *Soc. Neurosci. Abstr.* 17:379.

Rao, A., and Steward, O. (in press) Evaluation of RNAs present in synaptodendrosomes: Dendritic, glial and neuronal cell body contribution. *J. Neurochem.*

Rogers, S. W., Hughes, T. E., Holimann, M., Gasic, G. P., Deneris, E. S., and Heinemann, S. (1991) The characterization of the glutamate receptor subunit GluR1 in the rat brain. *J. Neurosci.* 11:2713–2724.

Routtenberg, A., Lovinger, D. M., and Steward, O. (1985) Selective increase in phosphorylation state of a 47 KD protein (F1) directly related to long-term potentiation. *Behav. Neural Biol.* 43:3–11.

Sakimura, K., Bujo, H., Kushiya, E., Araki, K., Yamazaki, M., Yamazaki, M., Meguro, H., Warashina, A., Numa, S, and Misha, M. (1990) Functional expression from cloned cDNAs of glutamate receptor species responsive to kainate and quisqualate. *FEBS* 272:73–80.

Sanes, J. R., Johnson, Y. R., Kotzbauer, P. T., Mudd, J., Hanley, T., Martinou, J.-C., and Merlie, J. P. (1991) Selective expression of an acetylcholine receptor-lacZ transgene in synaptic nuclei of adult muscle fibers. *Development* 113:1181–1191.

Schacher, S., Glanzman, D., Barzilai, A., Dash, P., Grant, S. G. N., Keller, F., Mayford, M., and Kandel, E. R. (1990) Long-term facilitation in *Aplysia*: Persistent phosphorylation and structural changes. *Cold Spring Harbor Symp. Quant. Biol.* 55:187–202.

Seitanidou, T., Triller, A., and Korn, H. (1988) Distribution of glycine receptors on the membrane of a central neuron: An immunoelectron microscopy study. *J. Neurosci.* 8:4319–4333.

Sheetz, M. P., Baumrind, N. L., Wayne, D. B., and Perlman, A. L. (1990) Concentration of membrane antigens by forward transport and trapping in neuronal growth cones. *Cell* 61:231–241.

Skene, J. H. P., and Willard, M. (1981) Axonally transported proteins associated with axon growth in rabbit central and peripheral nervous systems. *J. Cell Biol.* 89:96–103.

Sommer, B., Keinanen, K., Verdoorn, T.A., Wisden, W., Burnashev, N., Herb, A., Kohler, M., Takagi, T., and Sakmann, B. (1990) Flip and flop: A cell-specific functional switch in glutamate-operated channels of the CNS. *Science* 249:1580–1585.

Steward, O. (1983a) Alterations in polyribosomes associated with dendritic spines during the reinnervation of the dentate gyrus of the adult rat. *J. Neurosci.* 3:177–188.

Steward, O. (1983b) Polyribosomes at the base of dendritic spines of CNS neurons: Their possible role in synapse construction and modification. *Cold Spring Harbor Symp. Quant. Biol.* 48:745–759.

Steward, O., and Banker, G. A. (1992) Getting the message from the gene to the synapse: Sorting and intracellular transport of RNA in neurons. *Trends Neurosci.* 15:180–186.

Steward, O. and Falk, P. M. (1986) Protein synthetic machinery at postsynaptic sites during synaptogenesis: A quantitative study of the association between polyribosomes and developing synapses. *J. Neurosci.* 6:412–423.

Steward, O., and Fass, B. (1983) Polyribosomes associated with dendritic spines in the denervated dentate gyrus: Evidence for local regulation of protein synthesis during reinnervation. *Prog. Brain Res.* 58:131–136.

Steward, O., and Levy, W. B.(1982) Preferential localization of polyribosomes under the base of dendritic spines in granule cells of the dentate gyrus. *J. Neurosci.* 2:284–291.

Steward, O., and Reeves, T. M. (1988) Protein synthetic machinery beneath postsynaptic sites on CNS neurons: association between polyribosomes and other organelles at the synaptic site. *J. Neurosci.* 8:176–184.

Steward, O. and Ribak, C. E. (1986) Polyribosomes associated with synaptic sites on axon initial segments: Localization of protein synthetic machinery at inhibitory synapses. *J. Neurosci.* 6:3079–3085.

Steward, O., Davis, L., Dotti, C., Phillips, L. L., Rao, A., and Banker, G. (1988) Protein synthesis and processing in cytoplasmic microdomains beneath postsynaptic sites on CNS neurons. *Mol. Neurobiol.* 2:227–261.

Strong, M. J., Svedmyr, A., Gajdusek, D. C., and Garruto, R. M. (1990) The temporal expression of amyloid precursor protein mRNA in vitro in dissociated hippocampal neuron cultures. *Exp. Neurol.* 109:171–179.

Sutcliffe, J. G., Milner, R. J., Gottesfeld, J. M., and Reynolds, W. (1984) Control of neuronal gene expression. *Science* 225:1308–1315.

Tanzi, E. (1893) I fatti e le induzioni nell'odierna istologia del sistema nervoso. *Riv. sperim. freniatria medic. leg.* 19:419–472.

Tiedge, H., Banker, G. A., and Brosius, J. (1991a) (Expression of BC1 RNA in developing hippocampal neurons in culture. *Soc. Neurosci. Abstr.* 17:539.

Tiedge, H., Fremeau, R. T., Jr., Weinstock, P. H., Arancio, O., and Brosius, J. (1991b) Dendritic location of neural BC1 RNA. *Proc. Natl. Acad. Sci. USA,* 88:2093-2097.

Torre, E. R., and Steward, O. (1992) Demonstration of local protein synthesis within dendrites using a new cell culture system that permits the isolation of living axons and dendrites from their cell bodies. *J. Neurosci.* 12:762–772.

Triller, A., Cluzeaud, F., Pfeiffer, F., Betz, H., and Korn, H. (1985) Distribution of glycine receptors at central synapses: An immunoelectron microscopy study. *J. Cell Biol.* 101:683–688.

Ullu, E., and Tschudi, C. (1984) Alu sequences are processed 7SL genes. *Nature* 312:171–172.

Weiler, I. J., and Greenough, W. T. (1991) Potassium ion stimulation triggers protein translation in synaptoneuronsomal polyribosomes. *Mol. Cell. Neurosci.* 2:305–314.

Weiler, I. J., Davenport, W. J., and Greenough, W. T. (1991) Depolarization-dependent stimulation of polyribosome loading in synaptoneurosomes. *Soc. Neurosci. Abstr.* 17(605.9):1516.

Yisraeli, J. K., and Melton, D. A. (1988) The maternal mRNA *Vg1* is correctly localized following injection into *Xenopus* oocytes. *Nature* 336:592–595.

Zuber, M. X., Strittmatter, S. M., and Fishman, M. C. (1989) A membrane-targeting signal in the amino terminus of the neuronal protein GAP-43. *Nature* 347:345–348.

3

Neuroplasticity of the Hippocampus and Striatum: Models for Aging and Neurodegenerative Disease

Caleb E. Finch and Thomas H. McNeill

1 INTRODUCTION

Neuroplasticity may be viewed as the ability of neurons to adapt or modify their structure in response to changes in intrinsic and/or extrinsic environmental cues. These phenotypic alternatives are fundamental in the formation of neuroanatomical networks during development in mammals (reviewed in Black, 1978; Black et al., 1984; Purves and Litchman, 1985) because the vertebrate brain is characterized by a stochastic pattern of cell survival during development (Davidson, 1991), which implies a high degree of plasticity in the formation of nervous system connections. By contrast, nematodes and some other species show little evidence of neural plasticity during development, since the developmental fates of individual cells are much more rigidly determined during early differentiation.

In the adult vertebrate brain, synaptic plasticity is considered to be critical for the day-to-day maintenance of normal brain function (Greenough, 1984; Lichtman et al., 1987; Purves and Lichtman, 1985; Purves et al., 1986). This view recognizes the ability of target neurons to remodel their neuronal circuitry in response to naturally occurring phenomena such as cell loss and/or partial neuronal deafferentation and focuses on the importance of neuronal plasticity in maintaining the functional integrity of the CNS in normal aging (Coleman and Flood, 1986, 1987; Coleman et al., 1990; Cotman and Anderson, 1988). By contrast, impaired or aberrant neuronal plasticity in these same pathways has been demonstrated anatomically, and is hypothesized to be a factor in the cognitive, motor, and behavioral deficits associated with neurodegenerative diseases of the central nervous system such as Alzheimer's disease (AD) (reviewed in Coleman and Flood, 1986, 1987; De Ruiter and Uylings, 1987; Flood and Coleman, 1991; Geddes et al., 1985; Gertz et al., Represa et al., 1988; Stroemberg et al., 1990). However, while many deficits observed in AD are intensified variations of what occurs during normal aging, it is important to emphasize that AD is not simply an intensification of the normal aging process since we do not fully understand the cellular and molecular changes that could be a general basis for changes in brain functions during aging.

2.1 Normal Neurocircuitry

Hippocampus The entorhinal cortex (EC, Brodmann's synonym for his eponymous area 28 in the human), septum/diagonal band, and locus ceruleus are interconnected with the hippocampus proper (i.e., Ammmons' horn) and dentate gyrus through sets of neurochemically defined projection pathways arranged in parallel, well-defined laminae. For details of anatomy and species differences, see Amaral and Insausti (1990); Cotman and Nadler (1978); Cotman et al. (1981); Cowen et al. (1980); Rosene and Van Hoesen (1987). Specifically, the EC receives afferents from several neocortical regions and sends major projections to the hippocampus through the perforant path (figure 3.1; table 3.1).

While the EC is a multilaminar structure, like other parts of the neocortex, it differs from most other neocortical regions in its patterns of layers and cell composition (Amaral and Insausti, 1990). Unlike other regions of the neocortex, the EC lacks an internal granule neuron layer, which in the EC is occupied by the lamina dissecans, an acellular neuropil region that reacts intensely with silver stains. There are also many species differences in the EC between rodents, primates, and humans, in particular, the extent of association with the amygdala and characteristics of layers and cytoarchitectonic fields.

The major projection of the EC to the hippocampus is the perforant pathway, which arises mainly from pyramidal and stellate neurons in layers II and III. The perforant pathway terminates on dendrites of granule cells in the outer two thirds of the molecular layer of the dentate gyrus and in the stratum lacunosum molecular layer of the CA1 and CA3 pyramidal neurons in Ammon's horn (figure 3.1). Terminal degeneration studies found that about 85% of the terminal boutons in the outer two thirds of the molecular layer of the dentate gyrus arise from perforant path fibers from the ipsilateral EC. In addition, cells from the lateral regions of the EC project to the most superficial portions of the outer molecular layer of the dentate, while more medially placed cells project to the deeper regions of the perforant path projection field.

The remaining afferents to the hippocampus are also organized into well-defined lamina and originate from projection neurons with distinct neurotransmitter characteristics (table 3.1): the septum/diagonal band (cholinergic); locus ceruleus (noradrenergic); dorsal raphe nucleus (serotonin); contralateral EC (glutamatergic), and hippocampal interneurons (GABA). In addition, granule cells of the dentate gyrus also receive afferents from glutamatergic ipsilateral (associational) and contralateral (commissural) CA3 pyramidal cells that terminate in the inner one third of the molecular layer and do not overlap with projections from the EC.

In turn, granule neurons in the dentate gyrus send their axons (mossy fibers) to the hilus of the dentate and to the stratum lucidum and pyramidale of CA3 pyramidal neurons in Ammon's horn. Afferent fibers from CA3 pyra-

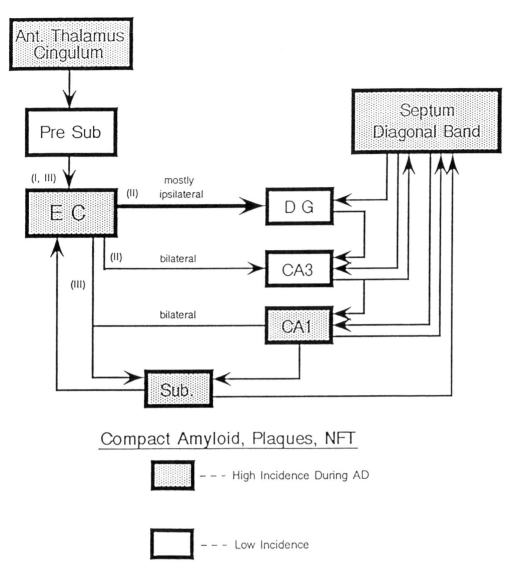

Figure 3.1 Schematic diagram of the principal afferent connections to the hippocampus. Layer II and III neurons from entorhinal cortex (EC) projects via the perforant pathway to granule cells of the dentate gyrus (DG) and CA1 and CA3 pyramidal neurons of Ammon's horn. DG, CA1 and CA3 neurons also receive cholinergic input from the septum and diagonal band, as well as noradrenergic input from the locus ceruleus. Mossy fiber axons from dentate granule neurons project to CA3, while CA3 pyramidal cells project via Schaffer collaterals to CA1. In turn CA1 projects to the subiculum and EC. The shaded boxes indicate the tendencies of neurons in these circuits for degeneration, as judged by the presence of neurofibrillary tangles (NFT) and neuritic plaques with compact β-amyloid (aggregated Aβ peptide fragments; Akiyama et al., 1990; Ball et al., 1985; Braak and Braak, 1991). A working hypothesis is that Alzheimer's disease causes disconnection of the hippocampus, through degeneration of the perforant path, which is a major afferent from the EC to the dentate gyrus (Hyman et al., 1984). This is supported, for example by correlations between the densities of plaques in the outer molecular layer of the dentate and the density of NFTs in the EC (Senut et al., 1991).

Table 3.1 Comparison of Basal Ganglia and Hippocampus Circuitry and Their Response to Cortical Deafferentation and Aging

Striatum	Hippocampus
Neurotransmitter Composition of Afferent Input	
Frontal cortex: glutamate	Entorhinal cortex: glutamate
Thalamus: glutamate	Commissural/associational: glutamate
Substantia nigra: dopamine	Septum/diagonal band: acetylcholine
Dorsal raphe: serotonin	Dorsal raphe: serotonin
Locus ceruleus: norepinephrine	Locus ceruleus: norepinephrine
Anatomical Organization of Afferent Input on Postsynaptic Dendrite	
Interdigitated mosaic	Parallel lamina
Reactive Response to Deafferentation of Primary Afferent System	
Homotypic innervation by the contralateral cortex via paraterminal sprouting	Heterotypic innervation via commissural/associational, septum; Homotypic innervation via contralateral EC via collateral sprouting
Influence of Age and Hormonal Manipulation	
Reactive response fails to slow with age	Reactive response slows with age
Glial hypertrophy not associated with aging	Glial hypertrophy characteristic of aging
Striatum moderately sensitive to hormonal manipulation	Hippocampus and reactive synaptogenesis extremely hormone sensitive (glucocorticoid and gonadal)

midal neurons project via the Schaffer collateral system to the stratum radia-tum, pyramidale, and oriens of CA1 pyramidal neurons. Subsequently, the efferent axons of CA1 pyramidal cells project back to the lower cell layers of the EC and subiculum, completing the hippocampal circuit.

While the distribution of hippocampal afferents is anatomically arranged into distinct sets of adjacent lamellae, we note that the three-dimensional connectivity and processing of information within the hippocampus is made possible because of prominent interconnections of these adjacent lamellar circuits through the longitudinal projections of the basket cells and other neurons (Amaral and Insausti, 1990).

Striatum In contrast with the hippocampus, where dentate granule and pyramidal neurons are arranged in well-defined rows and form the basis of the laminar organization of the afferent input, target neurons in the striatum are not arranged in any well-defined anatomical pattern. The principal cell type found in the striatum is the medium spiny I (MSI) neuron. MSI neurons represent approximately 95% of all neurons found in the striatum (DiFiglia et al., 1976; Kemp and Powell, 1970) and form synaptic specializations with afferent axons from distinct sets of topographically and neurochemically de-

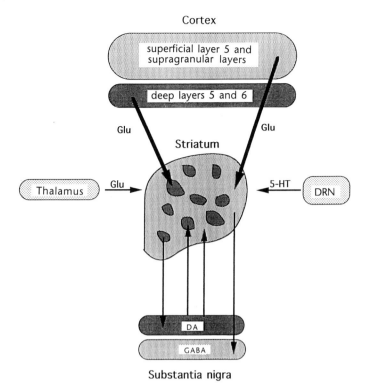

Figure 3.2 Schematic diagram of the principal afferent projection systems to the striatum. These include: glutamatergic (Glu) fibers from the cortex and thalamus; dopaminergic (DA) fibers from the substantia nigra, pars compacta; and serotonergic (5-HT) axons from the dorsal raphe nucleus (DRN) of the midbrain. See text for detail of functional compartmentalization related to patch-matrix and organization of the corticostriatal and striatonigral pathways. GABA, gamma aminobutyric acid.

fined projection neurons from the cortex, thalamus, and midbrain as well as numerous interneurons (figure 3.2). MSI neurons are distributed throughout the neuropil and all use GABA as their primary neurotransmitter. However, certain GABA MSI neurons also contain either enkephalin or substance P as a possible cotransmitter (Graybiel and Ragsdale, 1983). In addition, MSI neurons form aggregates of cells within the striatum that may contain up to 60 contiguous cells (Paskevich et al., 1991). These appear to correspond to reports of cell clusters (Mensah, 1977) and cellular islands (Goldman-Rakic, 1982) in the striatum; however, the functional significance of these anatomically linked neurons is unclear.

Morphological differences also exist in the anatomical orientation of the primary dendrites of target neurons in the hippocampus and striatum. In contrast to the hippocampus, where the apical dendrites of dentate granule neurons are oriented away from the cell body in only one direction, dendrites of MSI neurons radiate from the cell soma in all directions. Nonetheless, synaptic inputs to a single dendrite show a distinct proximal-to-distal distribution of afferent inputs reminiscent of the laminar organization of hippocampus. In general, afferents from projection neurons from outside the striatum, such as the cortex, thalamus, and midbrain, contact the more distal parts of the dendritic tree of MSI neurons. while inputs from local interneurons are distributed on the intermediate and most proximal parts of MSI dendrites (Smith and Bolam, 1990).

Furthermore, unlike the hippocampus where cortical input from different layers of the EC cells are not localized to topographically arranged compartments in the hippocampus, glutamatergic neurons from different layers of the neocortex give rise to afferents that terminate in different subcompartments of the striatum, termed the patch and matrix (figure 3.2) (Gerfen, 1989, 1992; Graybiel and Ragsdale, 1983). Specifically, neocortical afferents from the deep layer V and layer VI neurons project to the patch compartment, whereas neurons from the superficial layer V and the supragranular cortex project to the matrix (Gerfen, 1989, 1992; Graybiel and Ragsdale, 1983).

The patch-matrix organization is important functionally in the striatum, because matrix neurons project directly to GABAergic neurons in the substantia nigra, pars reticulata (SNR), whereas the neurons of the patch project directly to the DAergic neurons of the substantia nigra compacta (SNC). Thus, the patch-matrix compartments of the striatum provide an important level of functional organization in the striatum by segregating cortical outputs from different subcortical lamina into two parallel pathways, through which projections from distinct layers of the cortical neurons can target information to select populations of DAergic and/or GABAergic neurons in the substantia nigra (Gerfen, 1992).

A second functional level of compartmentalization also exists in the striatum which is related to the tonic, GABA-mediated inhibitory effect of basal ganglia output nuclei on the firing rate of thalamic neurons (Gerfen, 1992). Specifically, striatal projection neurons modulate the firing rate of thalamic neurons by sending topographically organized GABAergic efferent fibers via direct and indirect pathways to the major output nuclei of the basal ganglia, i.e. the substantia nigra, pars reticulata (SNR), and internal segment of the globus pallidus (GPi) (Parent, 1990). In particular, MSI neurons that co-contain the neurotransmitters GABA and substance P (Gale et al., 1977; Hong et al., 1977; Parent et al., 1987) form the "direct" pathway (Alexander and Crutcher, 1990) that terminates in SNR; while MSI GABA neurons with enkephalin as a neuropeptide cotransmitter (DiFiglia et al., 1982; Haber, 1986) project to the external segment of the globus pallidus to form the initial link in the "indirect" pathway. Together, the "direct" and "indirect" pathways form two opposing but parallel circuits that regulate the firing rate of target nuclei in the thalamus through the differential modulation of inhibitory GABAergic neurons in the SNR and GPi.

Other projections to the ST include axons from: DAergic perikarya from the SNC (Freund et al., 1984; Hokfelt and Ungerstedt, 1973; Veening et al., 1980) putative glutamatergic cells from the intralaminar nuclei of the thalamus (Kemp and Powell, 1971; Powell and Cowen, 1956); and serotonergic neurons of the dorsal raphe which synapse on both spiny and aspiny striatal cells

(Steinbusch et al., 1980, 1981). In addition, numerous other synaptically active molecules such as somatostatin, NPY, neurotensin, and ACh mediate actions of the complex network of interneurons within the ST, and serve to integrate the regulation of motor function in the ST (Graybiel and Ragsdale, 1983; Lehmann and Langer, 1983).

2.2   Hippocampal Reorganization in Response to Perforant Path Lesions

Lesions of rats that damage the perforant path, the major glutamatergic input to the hippocampus, are a major model for studying reactive synaptogenesis in the hippocampus and the effects of aging (reviewed in Cotman and Anderson, 1988; Cotman et al., 1981; see chapter 2). Two lesions are used: unilateral electrolytic ablation of the EC, which does extensive damage to EC layers, or the more discrete knife-cut lesions of the angular bundle of the perforant path (Gibbs et al., 1985). The electrolytic EC lesions are the most widely used and remove 86% of the synaptic input to the outer two thirds of the molecular layer of the dentate gyrus (Matthews et al., 1976). However, electrolytic EC lesions product more damage to surrounding tissues at the lesion site than do discrete knife cuts of the angular bundle, and the early responses to the larger damage from electrolytic EC lesions show greater glial and inflammatory responses in surrounding tissues (N. Laping and Finch, unpublished).

In response to neuronal deafferentation, surviving afferents show two general modes of axonal sprouting, collateral and paraterminal spouting, which are distinguished by the origin of the branch point between the newly formed axon and the parent fiber (reviewed in Cotman and Nadler, 1978) (figure 3.3). In *collateral sprouting*, new axon collaterals originate along the shaft of the existing axon and grow out into a region of the deafferented target that was previously unoccupied by the parent fiber. Collateral axons typically establish new synaptic contacts at some distance from the original axon. Examples of

INTACT   LESION

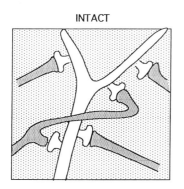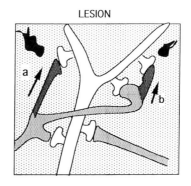

Figure 3.3   Schematic representation of two possible mechanisms of axonal sprouting in reactive synaptogenesis. Arrows indicate direction of new growth. a, collateral sprouting; b, paraterminal sprouting.

collateral sprouting are found throughout the peripheral nervous system and in some lamina of the hippocampus after unilateral EC lesions, as described below. In contrast, during *parerminal sprouting*, there is either (1) an enlargement of preexisting axon terminals to form multiple presynaptic contacts with adjacent dendritic spines or (2) the formation of small terminal buds that grow out of parent axon terminals to form new synapses with an adjacent dendritic spine or a part of a nearby dendrite that is within a few microns of the original terminal. Paraterminal sprouting is most likely to occur in brain regions where surviving afferent axons already exist in the deafferented target zone and are in contact with the partially denervated target cell.

In the hippocampus, the loss of perforant path projections induces reactive synaptogenesis in the surviving afferent fibers of the commissural/associational, septohippocampal, locus ceruleus, and crossed-perforant pathways. The reorganization of the synaptic input into the hippocampus within several months after a EC lesion establishes a new pattern of synaptic innervation. While this new pattern of contact is similar to that in the unlesioned animal, it is not identical.

Specifically, collaterals from the commissural/associational pathway axons expand outward to make new synaptic contacts (Lynch et al., 1977; Scheff et al., 1977) and replace lost synapses derived from the most medial component of the perforant pathway (Lynch et al., 1976). Additionally, new synaptic contacts are formed by both collateral and paraterminal sprouting of existing axons from the septohippocampal, locus ceruleus, and crossed perforant path that are concentrated in the outer half of the dentate molecular layer (Lynch et al., 1972; Steward et al., 1974, 1976).

Moreover, synaptic reorganization after an EC lesion alters the distribution of the specific subtypes of glutamatergic receptors, including NMDA, quisqualate, and kainate (Ulas et al., 1990a, b). Specially, the lesion-induced expansion of the commissural/associational pathway into the outer molecular layer is paralleled by a similar expansion of kainate receptors into the same region (Ulas et al., 1990a). Changes also occur in the distribution of hippocampal NMDA and quisqualate receptors after an EC lesion. However, the pattern of changes in hippocampal NMDA and quisqualate receptors differs from the time course for kainate, which suggests that the different subtypes of glutamate receptors are differentially regulated in the hippocampus in response to an EC lesion and the subsequent synaptic reorganization.

2.3 Hippocampus and Alzheimer's Disease

Alzheimer's disease (AD) involves a selective degeneration of neurons in parts of the neocortical-hippocampal circuits (figure 3.1). The selectivity is remarkable, since adjacent cell groups may be spared. The EC, for example, shows extensive degeneration of neurons in layers II and V, but not of neurons in layers III and VI (Hyman et al., 1984). Layer II is a major source of afferents to the hippocampus via the perforant path. Other examples of selective degeneration include the hippocampus, in particular, the sparing of dentate gyrus granule layer neurons and the CA3 neurons in Ammon's horn. In contrast, CA1 neurons, the major output neurons of the hippocampus are extensively lost during AD.

In general, neurons in the EC, subiculum, and CA1 neurons commonly show more extensive degeneration at early stages of Alzheimer's disease than those in the presubiculum and granule layer (dentate gyrus). However, some specimens show neurofibrillary tangles (NFTs) in granule neurons at end stages of Alzheimer's disease (Braak and Braak, 1991). Although individual specimens vary widely in the locations of neurodegeneration, the hippocampal pyramidal neurons are widely regarded as a preferential target in Alzheimer's disease. However, postmortem analysis of some individuals with severe clinical dementia at advanced ages and extensive NFTs in the neocortex nonetheless showed relatively few NFTs in the hippocampus (Dickson and Clark, 1992). These and other cases challenge concepts that Alzheimer's disease is exclusively a hippocampal neurodegenerative condition.

The loss of EC afferents is a good explanation for the reactive synaptogenesis and aberrant sprouting observed in the hippocampus during AD (Geddes et al., 1985; Gertz et al., 1987). The presentation of reactive synaptogenesis in the dendritic zones (molecular layer) of the dentate gyrus during AD qualitatively resembles that in adult rodents following EC lesioning by three criteria: (1) AChE staining from septal afferent, (2) kainate (glutamatergic) receptors from the commissural/associational fibers, and (3) the increase of mRNA for tubulin-α_1 (table 3.2).

However, changes in the hippocampus during AD may involve other afferents as well as the predominant degeneration of the perforant path, for example, concomitant degeneration of afferents from the noradrenergic locus ceruleus and septohippocampal cholinergic pathways that are typical of AD. Kainate receptor histochemistry indicates that expansion of commissural/associational fibers by 73% into the outer molecular layer of the dentate gyrus in AD brain may exceed the 57% expansion in unilaterally EC-lesioned rats (Geddes et al., 1985). These data suggest that effects of the loss of glutamatergic inputs from the EC on neurite outgrowth may be enhanced by the loss of afferents from the locus ceruleus or septohippocampal pathways (McNeill et al., 1991b) However, little is known about responses of afferent axons and dendrites to combined lesions of the EC, septum/diagonal band, and locus ceruleus.

It is unclear whether the new pattern of synaptic innervation formed after combined deafferentation lesions found in AD is functionally equivalent to those that are lost or whether the new synapses form an aberrant neural circuit that may increase the vulnerability of surviving dentate granule and pyramidal neurons to excitotoxic injury and impair neuronal plasticity. Evidence to support the later hypothesis was found in postmortem AD brain using Golgi staining methods (Coleman and Flood, 1986, 1987; Flood and Coleman, 1991). The typical patterns of compensatory dendritic growth in response to cell loss and partial deafferentation are either impaired with age or lost in specific neuron populations of both the HC and parahippocampal cortex in

Table 3.2 Descriptions of mRNA Species that Show Changes in Response to Deafferenting Lesions

	Source	Functions/Associations	References
1. ApoE[a]	Astrocytes	Recycling of membranes after neural injury	Poirier et al., 1991a,b
2. Ferritin[a]	?	Iron storage protein	Day et al., 1992
3. GFAP[a]	Astrocytes	Intermediate filament increased with reactive astrocytosis	Bignami & Rueger, 1980; Steward et al., 1990; Laping et al., 1991a
4. SGP-2[b]			May & Finch, 1992 (for review)
	Prostate	Cell death	Buttyan et al., 1989
	Testis	Spermatogenesis	Collard & Griswold, 1987
	Astrocytes	Ibotenic lesions	Pasinetti & Finch, 1991
	Astrocytes	Deafferentation	May et al., 1990; Day et al., 1990
	Astrocytes	Adrenalectomy-induced neuron death in postpubertal hippocampus	McNeill et al., 1991a
Clusterin	Testis	Sertoli cell aggregation	Fritz et al., 1983
TRPM-2	Prostate	Cell death	Buttyan et al., 1989
CLI	Blood	Complement-lysis inhibition	Jenne et al., 1991
SP-40,40	Blood	Complement-lysis inhibition	Kirszbaum et al., 1989
pADHC-9	Neuron (?)	Alzheimer's disease	May et al., 1990; Duguid et al., 1989
GP-III	Adrenal medulla	Secretion	Fischer-Colbrie et al., 1984; Palmer & Christie, 1990
ApoJ	Blood	Lipid transport	da Silva et al., 1990
5. TGF-β1[c]	Microglia	Modifies extracellular matrix; chemoattractant	Nichols et al., 1991; Pasinetti et al., 1993b; Morgan et al., 1993
6. Tubulin-α1[a]	Neurons	Embryonic isoform	Geddes et al., 1990; Poirier et al., 1991a

Sources: [a] Cloned from young rat hippocampus after EC lesions. [b] Cloned from hippocampus of humans with AD. cCloned from young rat hippocampus after adrenalectomy.

Abbreviations: ApoE, apolipoprotein E; GFAP, glial fibrillary acidic protein; SGP-2, sulfated glycoprotein-2; TRPM-2, testosterone-repressed prostatic messenger; CLI, complement lysis inhibitor; SP-40,40, serum protein-40,40; pADHC-9, AD hippocampus clone #9; GP-III, glycoprotein III; ApoJ, apolipoprotein J; TGF-β1, transforming growth factor β1.

AD. For example, significant reductions in dendritic length in AD were found in granule neurons of the dentate gyrus (Flood et al., 1985, 1987), layer II pyramidal neurons in the parahippocampal gyrus (Buell and Coleman, 1979, 1981), layer III pyramidal neurons of the subiculum (Flood, 1991), and CA1 pyramidal neurons of the HC (Hanks and Flood, 1991).

2.4 Aging and Hippocampal Responses to Perforant Path Lesions

While the use of young rats with perforant path lesions appears to be a useful model for specific aspects of AD, we emphasize that there are species differences as well as similarities in the pathobiology of aging between rodents and humans. First, humans, but not mice or rats, develop the intraneuronal neurofibrillary tangles at advanced ages that are a characteristic of AD; these have not been found in any other animal. Second, lab rodents do not develop cerebral vascular or parenchymal deposits of the β/A4 amyloid fragment found to increase during aging in humans and more so in AD. Vascular deposits of β/A4 amyloid, however, accumulate during aging in dogs, monkeys, and other mammals of intermediate life span (Selkoe et al., 1987).

Despite these major differences in brain pathology, many other features of the patterns of aging are quite similar and occur in corresponding fractions of the life span. Among general aging changes that are shown by rodents (> 20 mo) and humans (> 70 yr) are astrocytic hyperactivity with increased glial fibrillary acidic protein (GFAP) (Goss et al., 1991; Hansen et al., 1987; Landfield et al., 1987; Nichols et al., in press) and the loss of the striatal D2 receptor (Morgan et al., 1987).

Effects of aging on responses to an EC lesion are most characterized in rats. In senescent rats, the reactive response is slower than in young adults, although eventually the same density of synapses is recovered by 3 months post lesion (Hoff et al., 1982a, b; Scheff et al., 1980; Vijayan and Cotman, 1983). There is also a delay in removing the degenerative debris from the lesion site, which involves reactions by astrocytes and microglia.

Hormonal changes during aging may interact with reactive synaptogenesis. Elevations of plasma corticosterone that occur in many rat strains during aging (DeKosky et al., 1984; Sapolsky, 1992) may be a cause of slowed reactive synaptogenesis. In young rats with EC lesions, elevated corticosterone slowed synaptogenesis, removal of debris (Scheff et al., 1986) and altered elevations of astrocyte mRNAs (Laping et al., 1991a). Thus, the delayed response of senescent rats to deafferenting lesions may be an epiphenomenon of adrenal hyperactivity. Gonadal steroids in both genders also alter the schedule of reactive synaptogenesis and interact with adrenal steroids (Morse et al., 1992; Scheff et al., 1988). There are no studies of how gonadal age changes alter synaptogenesis.

Normal humans show evidence for sprouting of mossy fiber collaterals (projections from granule to CA3) at later ages. Comparison of three brains (72–79 yr) with younger (48–61 yr) by the Timm's stain for mossy fibers showed a new zone of staining in the supragranular zone of the older brains, which suggests the sprouting of mossy fiber collaterals (Cassell and Brown, 1984). Such Timm's staining is seen in rats after lesions of the perforant path or the CA3 neurons (Laurberg and Zimmer, 1981; Nadler et al., 1980), which are both damaged during AD.

In summary, the evidence for sprouting during AD and the ability to complete sprouting responses in old rats indicate that these compensatory responses are basically maintained during aging and AD.

2.5   Striatal Reorganization after Decorticating Lesions

While many studies examined responses of surviving target neurons and afferent axons to glutamatergic afferent fibers to the hippocampus, few studies have addressed similar questions in the striatum. Kemp and Powell (1977) reported a persistent loss of dendritic spines on MSI neurons in the striata of adult cats and kittens following unilateral lesions of the cortex and/or thalamus up to 52 weeks post pesion. In contrast to the cat, mice showed considerable synaptic recovery. Unilateral corticostriate lesions caused a transient loss of dendritic spine density on MSI neurons in the ipsilateral striatum at 3 and 10 days post lesion, which was followed by synaptogenesis with a return to 80% of control levels by 20 days post lesion. Spine loss occurred along both the proximal and distal portions of the dendrite and ranged from 31%–47% at 3 days post lesion to 39–53% at 10 days post-lesion.

No age changes were found in the schedule of spine loss and regrowth in senescent mice (25 mo) (Cheng, 1989; Cheng et al., 1988, in prep.), in contrast to the slowed responses observed in the rat hippocampus. Specifically, spine loss occurred along all segments of spiny dendrites at 3 and 10 days post lesion, ranging from an average of 28% at 3 days post lesion to a maximum of 47% at 10 days post lesion. Thus, there was full recovery by 20 days post lesion. Moreover, aging did not alter the length of striatal dendrites after decorticating lesions.

To determine whether remaining homotypic fibers from the contralateral cortex or heterotypic fibers from the thalamus played a role in inducing spine growth after unilateral decortication, a second lesion was placed in either the contralateral cortex or ipsilateral thalamus 10 days after the first lesion. Mice were examined 15 days later, or a total of 25 days after the first lesion (Cheng, 1989). These cases showed losses in all segments of the spiny dendrites, which ranged from 34% to 45% of their normal spine density values in age-matched controls. The data resemble those obtained from mice allowed to survive for 10 days after a unilateral cortical lesion, which suggests that the second lesion of the contralateral cortex had prevented regrowth of dendritic spines after the unilateral cortical lesion. In contrast, the combined cortex and thalamus lesions caused an average spine loss of 21% of normal control values (range 12–28%). These values are like those at 20 days postlesion in unilaterally decorticated mice.

2.6 Striatal Changes During AD and AD-Parkinson's Disease

Because AD involves extensive damage to the neocortex, it is of interest to consider effects of AD on the striatum. In one study of AD brains, there were correlations of glutamate binding in striatum with the density of senile plaques in the neocortex; this correlation was interpreted as a supersensitization response to the loss of corticostriatal afferents (Pearce et al., 1984). Moreover, in brains of subjects with Parkinson's disease (PD) with dementia and with AD associated with parkinsonism, the striatum showed astrocytic hyperactivity in small foci and bulk atrophy; however, these changes did not occur in AD without parkinsonism (de la Monte et al., 1989).

Little is known about the corticostriatal pathways in AD. There is no distinctive loss of D2 receptors in the striatum during AD relative to age-matched nondemented and non-PD controls (Morgan et al., 1987). A subpopulation of D2 receptors is located on the corticostriatal terminals; the normal age-related loss of D2 receptors in the striata of humans and rodents could include this D2 subpopulation. While we did not find differences in D2 receptors between AD and age-matched control groups, others found further deficits of D2 receptors in AD (reviewed in Morgan et al., 1987).

2.7 General Discussion of Anatomical Findings

Comparisons of Striatum and Hippocampus   Unilateral glutamatergic deafferentation of hippocampus or striatum causes a transient loss of dendritic spines and ultrastructurally defined synapses from the granule neurons in hippocampus or the MSI neurons in striatum. The regrowth of dendritic spines after deafferentation is attributed to the sprouting of axons that preexisted in the deafferented zone in both striatum and hippocampus. In the hippocampus, the replacing synapses are formed from several sources through both collateral and parateminal sprouting. However, in the striatum, synaptogenesis after unilateral cortical lesions is due almost entirely to homotypic parateminal sprouting of axons from the contralateral cerebral cortex. Thus, striatal responses to cortical deafferentation differ importantly from those of the hippocampus, since the striatum forms new synapses without the ingrowth of new axons. This difference may have a counterpart in astrocytic molecular responses, which follow a different time course in the striatum than hippocampus.

Effects of Aging   While the capacity for eventual recovery of lost synapses through compensatory sprouting in the brains of old rodents is preserved in both the hippocampus and striatum, the recovery of dendritic spine density is slower in the aging rat hippocampus than in the aging mouse striatum. We consider several mechanisms which are not mutually exclusive.

First, adaptive responses of old animals to deafferenting lesions or other injuries may be affected differentially by brain region. Alternatively, there may be species differences. We note that aging C57BL/6 mice used in these studies do not show elevated corticosterone during aging (Latham and Finch, 1976), in contrast to most studies of rats, which show progressive increases of plasma corticosterone during aging (De Kosky et al., 1984; Landfield et al., 1978; Sapolsky, 1992).

Age changes in the cellular properties could influence synaptogenesis. Astrocytes are implicated in early responses to deafferentation, as scavengers of debris and as possible sources of trophic factors. Both the striatum and hippocampus show astrocytic hyperactivity during aging in the absence of experimental injury, as characterized by an increase in cell size and content of GFAP (Goss et al., 1990; Hoff et al., 1982a, b; Landfield et al., 1977; O'Callaghan and Miller, 1991; Scheff et al. 1980). Although few studies have directly compared aging changes in hippocampus and striatum, both regions show similar increase during aging in GFAP mRNA (Goss et al., 1990; Nichols et al., 1993).

We note that both hippocampus and striatum of rats show a similar age change in sensitivity of muscarinic regulation, which could be pertinent to the sprouting of septal cholinergic fibers. Studies from different laboratories indicate similar loss of sensitivity to muscarinic regulation in aging rats, of DA release in striatum (Joseph et al., 1990) and ACh release in hippocampus (Araujo et al., 1990). In hippocampus, old mice show an increased postsynaptic excitability with commensurate increases in electrotonic coupling of neurons (Barnes et al., 1987). These authors suggest that these changes could be compensations for loss of perforant path input during aging, for which there is some anatomical evidence from rats (Geinisman and Bondareff, 1976; Geinisman et al., 1986). To date, there is no evidence for a similar change in electrical activities of neurons in the striatum.

Moreover, the differential effect of aging on the rate of recovery of spine density and new synapse formation in hippocampus and striatum, following deafferentation might reflect differences in the form of presynaptic sprouting involved in the formation of new synaptic contacts at the lesion site. Recall that axonal sprouting can be of two types: collateral sprouting and paraterminal sprouting. Data from Hoff et al. (1982a, b) and McNeill et al. (1991) suggest an inverse relationship between the type of axonal sprouting required to form new synaptic contacts following neuronal deafferentation and the influence of age on the reinnervation process. For example, old rats following EC lesion showed a 13-day delay in the reinnervation index, RI_{50}, the time required after the lesion to recover 50% of the synapses found in controls (Hoff et al., 1982a). This delayed RI_{50} occurred in the *middle* molecular layer of the dentate gyrus, which is dependent on the *collateral* sprouting of axons from the commissural/associational pathway in the inner molecular layer of the dentate. In contrast, old rats showed only a 5-day delay in the RI_{50} in the *outer* molecular layer of the dentate gyrus, a location of both *collateral and paraterminal sprouting* of existing axons in the terminal field. Conversely, our data suggest that reinnervation of the striatum via paraterminal sprouting of homotypic fibers from the contralateral cortex showed no delay in the recovery of dendritic spine density to preoperative levels. While circumstantial, these data suggest that the type of axonal sprouting used to form new synaptic contacts after neuronal deafferentation influences the effects of aging on the schedule synaptogenesis.

3   MOLECULAR RESPONSES TO DEAFFERENTATION IN HIPPOCAMPUS AND STRIATUM

To understand the molecular basis for responses to deafferenting lesions in the HC and ST, we must learn the mechanisms whereby the brain performs the following types of recognition:

1. Identification of debris from degenerating axons for selective removal. This process involves astrocytes, microglia, and probably other cell types, some of which, particularly microglia, may be hematogenous (i.e., immigrated from the blood). Inflammatory mediators such as the cytokines and complement may be involved. One model may be peripheral macrophages, which are closely related in functions and cell-type markers to microglia, which preferentially phagocytose apoptotic cells (Savill et al., 1989). It is unknown to what extent the brain protects healthy neurons from damage or how this is accomplished. We are also investigating a molecule that has activities as a complement lysis inhibitor (SGP-2, table 3.2), which may serve to protect innocent bystander cells during complement-mediated responses in the brain.

2. Recruiting of new afferents to replace the degenerating axons. This process requires outgrowth of new axons in homotypic and collateral sprouting and of new terminals in paraterminal sprouting. These processes must involve regulation of the cytoskeleton and growth cone. We find increases in mRNA for an embryonic isoform of tubulin (α1-T). BDNF and other trophic factors are implicated in responses to EC (Beck et al., 1993).

3. Where new axons outgrow into the denervated zone, there must be chemotactic signals to direct the migration. These are unknown. In either (2) or (3), it is unknown what changes in nuclear gene activity may occur in presynaptic neurons. It seems likely that there will be changes in the macromolecules on the surface of outgrowing and target neurons, and in the extracellular matrix.

4. Specification of synapses. The postsynaptic cells must form new postsynaptic complexes with appropriate specificity to the ingrowing presynaptic apparatus. This clearly requires macromolecular reorganization.

Some information on these complex processes is already available from the work of Steward and colleagues on the polysomes in the dendritic spines of granule neurons (chapter 2). Dendritic polysomes are found in many types of hippocampal synapses and are of high interest for their potential role in the molecular specification of synaptogenesis (Steward and Ribak, 1986). The EC lesions induce a major redistribution of polysomes within dendritic zones before the arrival of new afferent terminals and sprouting (Steward, 1983). EC lesions also increase the amount of ribosomal RNA and [^{3}H]leucine incorporation in the dendritic zone (Phillips et al., 1987). The proteins made locally by these dendritic polysomes are unknown. The dendrites of unlesioned hippo-

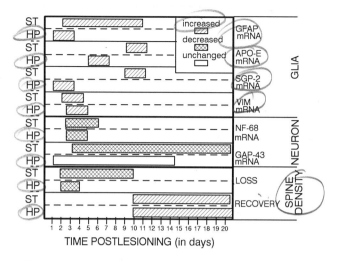

Figure 3.4 Comparisons of responses in the hippocampus (HC) and striatum (ST) to deafferenting lesions. HC deafferentation was by electrolytic lesions of the entorhinal cortex (Poirier et al., 1991a,b); ST deafferentation was by removal of the parietal and cingulate cortex (medial and lateral agranular cortex) (Pasinetti et al. 1993a). (Data are presented in these references and in Cheng, 1990. This diagram was kindly provided by G. M. Pasinetti. Adapted from Pasinetti et al., 1993a.)

campal granule neurons make proteins of diverse sizes, as studies in synaptosomes from the dendritic zone (Rao and Steward, 1991).

Next we describe the regulation of mRNAs in the hippocampus and striatum in response to the decorticating lesions which were anatomically characterized above. To identify mRNAs that change during deafferenting lesions, we screened 2-d gel translation products (Poirier et al., 1990) and hippocampal cDNA libraries from humans (May et al., 1990) and rats (Day et al., 1992; Poirier et al., 1991a, b). These efforts gave new mRNA markers for responses to deafferenting lesions. The mRNAs discussed below have been identified for cell type (table 3.2). Other hippocampal mRNAs that responded to EC lesioning but have not been identified for cell type distribution include sequences related to ferritin, SNAP-25, and the neuroendocrine peptide 7B-2 (Day et al., 1992). The present data are restricted to young male rats. Figure 3.4 summarizes the schedules for anatomical and mRNA changes in hippocampi from rats and striata from mice. The mRNA data are derived from separate studies of the hippocampus and striatum in rats.

3.1 Neurons

A least two cytoskeletal mRNAs show marked changes. The mRNA for α_1-tubulin, a developmental isoform (table 3.2), increased threefold by 6 days post ECL in hippocampus (Geddes et al., 1990; Poirier et al., 1991a). In contrast, NF-68 mRNA (neuronal intermediate neurofilament 68 kDa) decreased on about the same schedule in striatum (Pasinetti et al., 1992) and hippocampus (Laping, Day and Finch, in preparation) after cortical deafferentation (figure 3.4). The northern blot data do not resolve if these cytoskeletal mRNAs changed simultaneously in the same neurons.

The neuronal marker GAP-43 is prominent in growth cones during development and is implicated in axonal growth and synaptic plasticity (table 3.2). In striatum after cortical deafferentation, GAP-43 mRNA decreased by more than 50% and did not recover by 27 days post lesioning (Pasinetti et al., 1991, 1992). However, in the hippocampus, GAP-43 mRNA did not change after unilateral EC lesioning (Nichols et al. 1991) (figure 3.4). This difference between striatum and hippocampus in the changes in GAP-43 mRNA could arise from differences, because the striatum has more paraterminal sprouting than the hippocampus.

3.2 Astrocytes

Deafferentation by cortex lesions transiently causes major changes in astrocytic activities as judged morphologically (see above) and by the prevalence of astrocytic mRNAs. The best known responses are in GFAP-mRNA, which encodes an intermediary filament that is associated with morphological transitions of astrocytes. We also discovered two other astrocyte-specific mRNAs that change during responses to lesions: ApoE (apolipoprotein E), a putative lipoprotein carrier; and SGP-2 (sulfated glycoprotein-2), a multifunctional protein with activities that may include lipoprotein transport and inhibition of complement (table 3.2).

GFAP-mRNA showed peak elevations in hippocampus by 2–4 days post lesion in parallel with astrocytic responses and corticohippocampal terminal degeneration (Hoff et al., 1982). The increased SGP-2 mRNA in the hippocampus was localized to reactive astrocytes (Day et al., 1990). However, SGP-2 was also distributed as punctate deposits at the site of degenerating perforant path afferents (Lampert-Etchells et al., 1991). Similar immunoreactive deposits were found in the deafferented striatum after frontal cortex ablation (Pasinetti et al., 1992) or excitoxin lesions (Pasinetti and Finch, 1991). Synaptic density in the outer molecular layer of the dentate recovered to 65% of control values by 14 days post lesion and dendritic spine density on the denervated HC targets reached 80% of control values by 30 days post lesioning. A similar schedule for the recovery for dendritic spine density was also found in the striatal frontal cortex ablation (Cheng et al., 1992). This coordination of astrocyte activities supports the view that astrocytes have a key role in synaptogenesis.

The overlapping schedules of GFAP and SGP-2 mRNA elevation and afferent fiber degeneration both in striatum and hippocampus immediately before the initiation of synaptic sprouting suggests an important role for astrocytes in removal of debris, but also in synaptic reorganization. In response to deafferentation in striatum, GFAP and SGP-2 mRNA returned toward controls by 30 days post lesioning as also shown in hippocampus after EC lesion (Pasinetti et al., 1992, 1993a; Poirier et al., 1991a, b).

SGP-2 appears to be the rat homolog of the human protein complement lysis inhibitor (CLI) (table 3.2), so called because the serum protein blocks complement (C)-mediated cytolysis of the membrane attack complex (Jenne and Tschopp, 1989; Kirszbaum et al., 1989; Murphy et al., 1988). Complement-mediated neurotoxicity is little investigated in the brain. Frontal cortex ablation elevated C1qB mRNA (first component of complement protein) in activated microglia by 10 days post lesion in striatum (Pasinetti et al., 1992). ECL also induced C1qB mRNA by 2–4 days in hippocampus (Johnson et al., 1992).

SGP-2 is also similar to the human apolipoprotein J (ApoJ; numerous acronyms include CLI, Sp 40, 40, and pADHC-9), which is a component of specific subclasses of high-density lipoprotein (HDL) (May and Finch, 1992) (table 3.2). Apolipoprotein E (ApoE) mRNA, which encodes another HDL-associated apolipoprotein, also increases in hippocampal astrocytes by 6 days postlesioning (Poirier et al., 1991a). The hippocampus in AD also shows major increases of SGP-2 (CLI) mRNA (Duguid et al., 1989; May et al., 1990). A greater than fivefold elevation of ApoE mRNA was also found in striatum 10 days after frontal cortex ablation (G. M. Pasinetti, unpublished) (figure 3.4). A function of SGP-2 during responses to deafferentation could also be related to membrane lipid redistribution during synaptic remodeling.

In summary. three astrocyte mRNAs (GFAP, SGP-2, ApoE) respond more slowly to deafferenting lesions in the striatum than in the hippocampus, which suggests coordinate expression of these three genes. The coordination could program cytoskeletal changes in the astrocyte through GFAP that increase contact with degenerating terminals, whereas membrane recycling might be mediated by ApoE and ApoJ (SGP-2). We hypothesize that the paraterminal sprouting in the striatum requires a different schedule of coordinated astrocytic functions than the heterosynaptic replacement in the hippocampus.

3.3 Microglia: TGF-β1

The activation of the complement cascade in reactive microglia may trigger immune-inflammatory responses which could also stimulate astrocytic proliferation (Giulian, 1990). As noted above, striatal microglia make C1q mRNA in responses to decortication (Pasinetti et al., 1992).

Recent work shows intriguing involvement of TGF-β1 mRNA in responses to lesions. Transforming growth factor β1 (TGF-β1) is a multifaceted cytokine involved in cell differentiation and proliferation. TGF-β1 mRNA is increased in hippocampus (Nichols et al., 1991) and striatum after deafferentation (Pasinetti et al., 1993b). Combined in situ and immunocytochemistry show that striatal microglia contain TGF-β1 mRNA (Pasinetti et al., 1992). Like interleukin-1 (IL-1) (Giulian, 1990), TGF-β1 may also modulate inflammatory responses (Wahl et al., 1991) and stimulate astrocytosis and GFAP mRNA (Laping et al., 1991b, Lindholm et al. 1990, 1992). TGF-β1 may also regulate synthesis of nerve growth factor (NGF) as well as of TGF-β1 itself (Lindholm et al., 1990; Pasinetti et al., 1993b).

The role of NGF in the adult brain is best established for its ability to rescue septohippocampal cholinergic neurons after axotomy (Hefti and Lapchak, 1992). However, local injury to ST from a cannula penetration promoted an increase of NGF receptors, which was increased by infusion of NGF and partly blocked by infusion of antibodies to NGF (Gage et al., 1989). These findings, which suggest that NGF can be produced locally by tissue injury, are consistent with our results that deafferenting lesions increase NGF mRNA in striatum, in association with degenerating terminals.

There may be relationships between TGFβ-1, NGF, and IL-1. There is evidence that IL-1 can release TGF-β1 from several brain cells, in the order: oligodendroglia > microglia > astrocytes (da Cunha et al., 1991). Initially released IL-1 could thereby stimulate the release of TGF-β1 by local brain cells. In primary astrocyte cultures, TGF-β1 is a positive regulator of its own transcription as well as NGF (Lindholm et al., 1990). The potential for self-amplifying cascades of TGF-β1 noted in other cells (e.g., Kim et al., 1990) might yield a self-amplifying surge of TGF-β1, around regions of tissue damage or deafferentation. Finally, intraventricular infusion of IL-1 caused a major increase of NGF-mRNA in hippocampus (Spranger et al., 1990). Together, these findings suggest an interactive regulatory network of lymphokines and neurotropins that govern the synthesis of macromolecules during reactive synaptogenesis.

4   CONCLUSIONS

In summary, we discussed anatomical and molecular responses to cortical deafferentation lesions in the rat hippocampus and striatum in relation to general questions of neural plasticity and the effects of aging. The loss of dendritic spines and ultrastructurally defined synapses from dentate granule and striatal MSI neurons following unilateral glutamatergic deafferentation lesions is a transient phenomenon. The regrowth of dendritic spines after deafferentation may be attributed to the sprouting of surviving axons that already exist in the lesioned target. The reorganization of new synaptic circuits in hippocampus involves collateral and paraterminal sprouting of surviving presynaptic axons from several afferent pathways including those from the contralateral entorhinal cortex, septum, and commissural/association pathways. However, the synaptic reformation in the striatum after cortical ablation is accomplished almost entirely by paraterminal sprouting of axons from the contralateral cerebral cortex. Likewise, the schedules of astrocytic responses to axonal degeneration are different in the striatum and hippocampus. These differences are not easily explained by the schedules of dendritic spine loss and replacement, which occur at about the same times in both regions.

Moreover, there are regional or possibly species difference in the effects of aging on recovery of synapses after deafferenting lesions. The male rat hippocampus shows age-related delay in the reformation of new synaptic contacts following lesions of the entorhinal cortex. However, the recovery of dendritic spine density to preoperative levels in the striatum of mice in response to unilateral lesion of the corticostriatal pathway is not affected by aging. Although the cellular mechanisms that contribute to the preservation of the capacity of the aged striatum to restore synaptic connections following a corticostriatal lesion are unknown, it is clear that deafferentation lesions in both the hippocampus and striatum involve the reactivation of developmental gene programs of astrocytes and neurons that can affect the ability of reactive glia to remove degenerative debris from the lesion site as well as facilitate the neurite outgrowth. While it is difficult to estimate the relative contribution of any single factor in reactive synaptogenesis, we suggest that the form of axonal sprouting used in the formation of new synaptic contacts following neuronal deafferentation (paraterminal vs. collateral sprouting) may play some role in the influence of aging on the reinnervation process.

REFERENCES

Akiyama, H., Tago, H., Itagaki, S., and McGeer, P. L. (1990) Occurrence of diffuse amyloid deposits in the presubicular parvopyramidal layer in Alzheimer's disease. *Acta Neuropathol.* 79:539–544.

Alexander, G. E., and Crutcher, M. D. (1990) Functional architecture of basal ganglia circuits: Neural substrates of parallel processing. *Trends Neurosci.* 13:266–271.

Amaral, D. G., and Insausti, R. (1990) In *The Human Nervous System*, G. Paxinos (ed.), pp. 711–756, Academic Press, San Diego.

Araujo, D. M., Lapchak, P. A., Meany, M. J., Collier, B., and Quirion, R. (1990) Effects of aging on nicotinic and muscarinic autoreceptor function in the rat brain: Relationship to presynaptic cholinergic markers and binding sites. *J. Neurosci.* 10:3069–3078.

Ball, M. J., Hachinsky, V., and Fox, A. (1985) A new definition of Alzheimer's disease: A hippocampal dementia. *Lancet* 1:14–16.

Barnes, C. A., Rao, G., and McNaughton, B. L. (1987) Increased electronic coupling in aged rat hippocampus: A possible mechanism for cellular excitability changes. *J. Comp. Neurol.* 259:549–558.

Beck, K. D., McNeill, T. H., Finch, C. E., Hefti, F., and Day, J. R. (1993) Induction of truncated trk B neurotrophin receptors in hippocampal glial cells during injury-induced axonal sprouting. (in preparation)

Bignami, A., and Rueger, D. G. (1980) Glial fibrillary acidic GFA protein in normal neural cells and in pathological conditions. *Adv. Cell. Neurobiol.* 1:285–310.

Black, I. B. (1978) Regulation of autonomic development. *Annu. Rev. Neurosci.* 1:183–214.

Black, I. B., Adler, J. E., Dreyfus, C. F., Jonakait, G. M., Katz, D. M., LaGamma, E. F., and Markey, K. M. (1984) Neurotransmitter plasticity at the molecular level. *Science* 225:1266–1270.

Braak, H., and Braak, E. (1991) Neuropathological stageing of Alzheimer-related changes. *Acta Neuropathol.* 82:239–259.

Buell, S. J., and Coleman, P. D. (1979) Dendritic growth in the aged human brain and failure of growth in senile dementia. *Science* 206:854–856.

Buell, S. J., and Coleman, P. D. (1981) Quantitative evidence for selective dendritic growth in normal human aging but not in senile dementia. *Brain Res.* 214:23–41.

Buttyan, R., Olsson, C. A., Pintar, J., Chang, C., Bandyk, M., Ng, P. O., and Sawczuk, I. S. (1989) Induction of the TRPM-2 gene in cells undergoing programmed cell death. *Mol. Cell Biol.* 9:3473−3481.

Cassell, M. D., and Brown, M. W. (1984) The distribution of Timm's stain in the nonsulphide-perfused human hippocampal formation. *J. Comp. Neurol.* 222:461−471.

Cheng, H. W. (1989) Dendritic plasticity in aging striatal neurons: Changes induced by de afferentation. Wayne State University, Detroit, Ph.D. thesis.

Cheng, H. W., Anavi, Y., Coshgarian, H., McNeill, T. H., and Rafols, J. A. (1988) Loss and recovery of striatal dendritic spines following lesions in the cerebral cortex of adult and aged mice. *Soc. Neurosci. Abstr.* 14:1292.

Cheng, H. W., Mori, N., and McNeill, T. H. (1991) Differential induction of SCG-10 and GAP-43 mRNA in the contralateral cortex following unilateral striatal deafferenation. *Soc. Neurosci. Abstr.* 17:735.

Cheng, H. W., Anavi, Y., Coshgarian, H., McNeill, T. H., and Rafols, J. A. (in prep.) Loss and regrowth of striatal spines in adult and aged mice following ipsilateral cortial lesion: A Golgi study.

Coleman, P. D., and Flood, D. G. (1986) Dendritic proliferation in the aging brain as a compensatory repair mechanism. *Prog. Brain Res.* 70:227−237.

Coleman, P. D., and Flood, D. G. (1987) Neuron numbers and dendritic extent in normal aging and Alzheimer's disease. *Neurobiol. Aging* 8:521−545.

Coleman, D. P., Rogers, E. K., and Flood, D. G. (1990) Neuronal plasticity in normal aging and deficient plasticity in Alzheimer's disease: A proposed intercellular signal cascade. *Prog. Brain Res.* 86:75−87.

Collard, M. W., and Griswold, M. D. (1987) Biosynthesis and molecular cloning of sulfated glycoprotein 2 secreted by rat Sertoli cell. *Biochemistry* 26:3297−3303.

Cotman, C. W., and Anderson, K. J. (1988) Synaptic plasticity and functional stabilization in the hippocampal formation: Possible role in Alzheimer's disease. In *Physiological Basis for Functional Recovery in Neurological Disease*, S. Waxman (ed.), pp. 313−336. Raven Press, New York.

Cotman, C. W., and Nadler, J. V. (1978) In *Neuronal Plasticity*, C. W. Cotman (ed.), pp. 227−271. Raven Press, New York.

Cotman, C. W., Nieto-Sampedro, M., and Harris, E. W. (1981) Synapse replacement in the nervous system of adult vertebrates. *Physiol. Rev.* 61:684−784.

Cowan, W. M., Stanfield, B. B., and Kishi, K. (1980) The development of the dentate gyrus. In *Current Topics in Developmental Biology*, A. A. Moscona and A. Monro (eds.), pp. 103−157. Academic Press, New York.

da Chunha, A., Jefferson, J., Jannotta, F. S., and Vitkovic, L. (1991) Specificity of interleukin-1-mediated induction of transforming growth factor-beta in glia. *Soc. Neurosci. Abstr.* 17:914.

da Silva, H. V., Harmony, J. A. K., and Stuart, W. D. (1990) Apolipoprotein J: Structure and tissue distribution. *Biochemistry* 29:5380−5389.

Davidson, E. H. (1991) Spatial mechanisms of gene regulation in metazoan embryos. *Development* 113:1−26.

Day, J. R., Laping, N. J., McNeill, T. H., Schreiber, S. S., Pasinetti, G. M., and Finch, C. E. (1990) Castration enhances expression of glial fibrillary acidic protein sulfated glycoprotein-2 in the intact and lesion-altered hippocampus of the adult male rat. *Mol. Endocrinol.* 4:1995−2002.

Day, J. R., Min, B. H., Laping, N. J., Martin, G., Osterburg, H. H., and Finch, C. E. (1992) New mRNA probes for hippocampal responses to entorhinal cortex lesions in the adult male rats: A preliminary report. *Exp. Neurol.* 117:97–99.

DeKosky S. T., Scheff, S. W., and Cotman, C. W. (1984) Elevated corticosterone levels: A possible cause of reduced axon sprouting in aged animals. *Neuroendocrinology* 38:33–38.

de la Monte, S., Wells, S. E., Hedley-Whyte, T. E., and Growdon, J. H. (1989) Neuropathological distinction between Parkinson's dementia and Parkinson's plus Alzheimer's disease (1989). *Ann. Neurol.* 26:309–320.

De Ruiter, J. P., and Uylings, H. B. M. (1987) Morphometric and dendritic analysis of fascia dentata granule cells in human aging and senile dementia. *Brain Res* 402:217–229.

Dickson, D. W., and Clark, A. W. (1992) Alzheimer's disease with relative hippocampal sparing. *Noteworthy Brains (CERAD Newsletter)* 2:1–2.

DiFiglia, M., Pasik, P., and Pasik, T. (1976) A Golgi study of neuronal types in the neostriatum of monkeys. *Brain Res.* 114:245–256.

Difiglia, M., Aronin, N., and Martin, J. B. (1982) Light and electron microscopic localization of immunoreactive leu-enkephalin in the monkey basal ganglia. *J. Neurosci.* 2:303–320.

Duguid, J. R., Boumont, C. W., Liu, N., and Tourtellote, W. (1989) Changes in brain gene expression shared by scrapie and Alzheimer disease. *Proc. Natl. Acad. Sci. USA* 86:7260–7264.

Fisher-Colbrie, R., Zangerle, R., Fritshen-schlager, I., and Weber, A. (1984) Isolation and immunological characterization of a glycoprotein from adrenal chromaffin granules. *J. Neurochem.* 42:1008–1016.

Flood, D. G. (1991) Region specific stability of dendritic extent in normal aging and regression in Alzheimer's disease. II. Subiculum. *Brain Res.* 540:83–95.

Flood, D. G., and Coleman, P. D. (1991) Hippocampal plasticity in normal aging and decreased plasticity in Alzheimer's disease. *Prog. Brain Res.* 83:435–443.

Flood, D. G., Buell, S. J., DeFiore, C. H., Horwitz, G. J., and Coleman, P. D. (1985) Age-related dendritic growth in dentate gyrus of human brain is followed by regression in the "oldest old." *Brain Res.* 345:366–368.

Flood, D. G., Buell, C. H., Horwitz, G. J., and Coleman, P. D. (1987) Dendritic extent in human dentate gyrus granule cells in normal aging and senile dementia. *Brain Res.* 402:205–216.

Freund, T. F., Powell, J. F., and Smith, A. D. (1984) Tyrosine hydroxylase-immunoreactive boutons in synaptic contact with identified striatonigral neurons, with particular reference to dendritic spines. *Neuroscience* 13:1189–1215.

Fritz, I. B., Burdzy, K., Setchell, B., and Blaschuk, A. (1983) Ram rete testis fluid contains a protein (clusterin) which influences cell-cell interactions in vitro. *Biol. Reprod.* 28:1173–1188.

Gage, F. H., Batchelor, P., Chen, K. S., Chin, D., Higgins, G. A., Koh, S., Deputy, S., Rosenberg, M. B., Fischer, W., and Bjorklund, A. (1989) NGF receptor reexpression and NGF-mediated cholinergic neuronal hypertrophy in the damaged adult neostriatum. *Neuron* 2:1177–1184.

Gale, K., Hong, J.-S., and Guidotti, A. (1977) Presence of substance P and GABA in separate striatonigral neurons. *Brain Res.* 136:371–375.

Garden, G. A., Bothwell, M., and Rubel, E. W. (1991) Lack of correspondence between mRNA expression for a putative cell death molecule (SGP-2) and neuronal cell death in the central nervous system. *J. Neurobiol.* 22:590–604.

Geddes, J. W., Monaghan, D. T., Cotman, C. W., Lott, I. T., Kim, R. C., and Chui, H. C. (1985) Plasticity of hippocampal circuitry during Alzheimer's disease. *Science* 230:1179–1181.

Geddes, J. W., Wong, J., Choi, B. H., Kim, R. C., Cotman, C. W., and Miller, F. D. (1990) Increased expression of the embryonic form of a developmentally regulated mRNA in AD. *Neurosci. Lett.* 109:54−61.

Geinisman, Y. and Bondareff, W. (1976) Decrease in number of synapses in the senescent brain: A quantitative electron microscopic analysis of the dentate gyrus molecular layer in the rat. *Mech. Aging Dev.* 5:11−23.

Geinisman, Y., de Toledo-Morrell, L., and Morrell, F. (1986) Loss of perforated synapses in the dentate gyrus: morphological substrate of memory deficit in aged rats. *Proc. Natl. Acad. Sci. USA* 83:3027−3031.

Gerfen, C. R. (1989) The neostriatal mosaic: Striatal patch-matrix organization is related to cortical lamination. *Science* 246:385−388.

Gerfen, C. R. (1992) The neostriatal mosaic: Multiple levels of compartmental organization. *Trends Neurosci.* 15:133−138.

Gertz, H. J., Cervos-Navarro, J., and Ewald, V. (1987) The septo-hippocampal pathway in patients suffering from senile dementia of Alzheimer's type. Evidence for neuronal plasticity? *Neurosci. Lett.* 76:228−232.

Gibbs, R. B., Harris, E. W., and Cotman, C. W. (1985) Replacement of damaged cortical projections by homotypic transplants of entorhinal cortex. *J. Comp. Neurol.* 237:47−64.

Giulian, D. (1990) Microglia, cytokines, and cytotoxins: Modulators of cellular responses after injury to the central nervous system. *J. Immunol. Immunopharmacol.* 10:15−21.

Goldman-Rakic, P. (1982) Cytoarchitectonic heterogeneity of the primate neostriatum: Subdivision into island and matrix cellular compartments. *J. Comp. Neurol.* 205:398−413.

Goss, J. R., Finch, C. E., and Morgan, D. G. (1990) GFAP RNA prevalence is increased in aging and in wasting mice. *Exp. Neurol.* 108:266−268.

Goss J., Finch, C. E., and Morgan, D. G. (1991) Age-related changes in glial fibrillary acidic protein mRNA in the mouse brain. *Neurobiol. Aging* 12:165−170.

Graybiel, A. M., and Ragsdale, C. W. (1983) Biochemical anatomy of the striatum. In *Chemical Neuroanatomy*, P. C. Emson (ed.), pp. 427−504, Raven Press, New York.

Greenough, W. T. (1984) Structural correlates of information storage in the mammalian brain: A review and hypothesis. *Trends Neurosci.* 7:229−33.

Haber, S. N. (1986) Neurotransmitters in the human and nonhuman primate basal ganglia. Human Neurobiol. 5:159−168.

Hanks, S. D., and Flood, D. G. (1991) Region specific stability of dendritic extent in normal aging and regression in Alzheimer's disease. I. CA1 of hippocampus. *Brain Res.* 540:63−82.

Hansen, L. A., Armstrong, D. M., and Terry, R. D. (1987) An immunohistochemical quantification of fibrous astrocytes in the aging human cerebral cortex. *Neurobiol. Aging* 8:1−6.

Hefti F., and Lapchak, P. A. (1993) Pharmacology of nerve growth factor in the brain. *Adv. Pharmacol.* 24:239−273.

Hoff, S. F., Scheff, S. W., and Cotman, C. W. (1982a) Lesion-induced synaptogenesis in the dentate gyrus of aged rats: I. Loss and reacquisition of normal synaptic density. *J. Comp. Neurol.* 205:246−252.

Hoff, S. F., Scheff, S. W., and Cotman, C. W. (1982b) Lesion-induced synaptogenesis in the dentate gyrus of aged rats: II. Demonstration of an impaired clearing response. *J. Comp. Neurol.* 205:253−259.

Hokfelt, T., and Ungerstedt, U. (1973) Specificity of 6-hydroxydopamine induced degeneration of central monoamine neurons: An electron and fluorescence microscopic study special reference to intracerebral injection of the nigrostriatal dopamine system. *Brain Res.* 60:269–297.

Hong, J.-S., Yang H. Y., Racagni, G., and Costa, E. (1977) Projections of substance-P containing neurons from neostriatum to substantia nigra. *Brain Res.* 122:541–544.

Hyman, B. T., Van Hoesen, G. W., Damasio, A. R., and Barnes, C. L. (1984) Alzheimer's disease: Cell-specific pathology isolates the hippocampal formation. *Science* 225:1168–1170.

Jenne, D. E., Lowin, B., Peitsch, M. C., Bottcher, A., Schmitz, G., and Tschopp, J. (1991) Clusterin (Complement Lysis Inhibitor) forms a high density lipoprotein complex with apolipoprotein A-I in human plasma. *J. Biol. Chem.* 266:11030–11036.

Johnson, S., Lampert-Etchells, M., Painetti, G., Rozovsk, I., and Finch, C. E. (1992) Complement mRNA in the mammalian brain: Responses to Alzheimer's disease and experimental brain lesioning. *Neurobiol. Aging* 13:641–648.

Joseph, J. A., Roth G. S., and Strong, R. (1990) The striatum, a microcosm for the examination of age-related alterations in the CNS: A selected review. *Rev. Biol. Res. Aging* 4:181–199.

Kemp, J. M., and Powell, T. P. S. (1970) The cortico-striate projection in the monkey. *Brain* 93:525–546.

Kemp, J. M. and Powell, T. P. S. (1971) The termination of fibers from the cerebral cortex and thalamus upon dendritic spines in the caudate nucleus: A study with the Golgi method. *Philos. Trans. R. Soc. Lond. B.* 262:429–439.

Kesslak, J. P., Nito-Sampedro, M., Globus, J., and Cotman, C. W. (1986) Transplantation of purified astrocytes promotes behavioral recovery after frontal cortex ablation. *Exp. Neurol.* 92:377–390.

Kim, S.-J., Angel, P., Lafyatis, R., Hattori, K., Kim, K. Y., Sporn, M. B., Karin, M. B., and Roberts, A. B. (1990) Autoinduction of transforming growth factor $\beta 1$ in mediated by the AP-1 complex. *Mol. Cell. Biol.* 10:1492–1497.

Kirszbaum, L., Sharpe, J. A., Murphy, B., d'Apice A. J. F., Classon, B., Hudson, P., and D. Walker (1989) Molecular cloning and characterization of the novel, human complement-associated protein, SP-40, 40: A link between the complement and the reproductive system. EMBO J. 8:711–718.

Kunzle H. (1975) Bilateral projections from precentral motor cortex to the putamen and other parts of the basal ganglia. An autoradiographic study in *Macaca fascicularis. Brain Res.* 88:195–209.

Lampert-Etchells, M., McNeill, T. H., Laping, N. J., Zarow, C., Finch, C. E., and May, P. C. (1991) Sulfated glycoprotein-2 is increased in rat hippocampus following entorhinal cortex lesioning. *Brain Res.* 563:101–106.

Landfield, P. W., Rose, G., Sandles, L., Wohlstadter, T. C., and Lynch, G. (1977) Patterns of astroglial hypertrophy and neuronal degeneration in the hippocampus of aged memory-deficient rats. *J. Gerontol.* 32:3–12.

Landfield, P. W., Waymire, J. C., and Lynch, G. (1978) Hippocampal aging and adrenalcorticoids: Quantitative correlations. *Science* 202:1098–1102.

Laping, N. J., Nichols, N. R., Day, J. R., and Finch, C. E. (1991a) Corticosterone differentially regulates the bilateral response of astrocyte mRNAs in the hippocampus to entorhinal cortex lesions in male rats. *Mol. Brain Res.* 10:291–297.

Laping, N. J., Morgan, T. E., Nichols, N. R., and Finch, C. E. (1991b) Transforming growth factor-$\beta 1$ increases glial fibrillary acidic protein mRNA in the hippocampus of young adult male rats 24 hours after an intraventricular infusion. *Soc. Neurosci. Abstr.* 17:754.

Latham, K. R., and Finch, C. E. (1976) Hepatic glucocorticoid binders in mature and senescent C57BL/6J male mice. *Endocrinology* 98:1480−1489.

Laurberg, S., and Zimmer, J. (1981) Lesion-induced sprouting of hippocampal mossy fiber collaterals to the fascia dentata in developing and adult rats. *J. Comp. Neurol.* 200:433−459.

Lehmann, J., and Langer, S. Z. (1983) The striatal cholinergic interneuron: Synaptic target of dopaminergic terminalis. *Neuroscience* 10:1105−1120.

Lichtman, J. W., Magrassi, L., and Purves, D. (1987) Visualization of neuromuscular junctions over periods of several months in living mice. *J. Neurosci.* 7:1215−22.

Lindholm, D., Hengerer, B., Zafra, F., and Thoenen, H. (1990). Transforming growth factor-beta 1 stimulates expression of nerve growth factor in the rat CNS. *NeuroRep.* 1:9−12.

Lindholm, D., Castren, E., Kiefer, R., Zafra, F., and Thoenen, H. (1992) Transforming growth factor-beta 1 in the rat brain: Increase after injury and inhibition of astrocyte proliferation. *J. Cell Biol.* 117:395−400.

Lynch, G., Gall, C., Rose, G., and Cotman, C. W. (1976) Changes in the distribution of the dentate gyrus associational system following unilateral or bilateral entorhinal lesions in the adult rat. *Brain Res.* 110:57−71.

Lynch, G., Gall, C., and Cotman, C. W. (1977) Temporal parameters of axons "sprouting" in the brain of the adult rat. *Exp. Neurol.* 54:179−183.

Lynch, G. S., Matthews, D. A., Mosko, S., Parks, T., and Cotman, C. W. (1972) Induced acetylcholinesterase-rich layer in rat dentate gyrus following entorhinal lesions. *Brain Res.* 42:311−318.

Matthews, D. A., Cotman, C. W., and Lynch, G. (1976) An electron microscopic study of lesion-induced synaptogenesis in the dentate gyrus of the adult rat. I. Magnitude and time course of degeneration. *Brain Res.* 115:1−21.

May, P. C. and Finch, C. E. (1992) Sulfated glycoprotein-2: New relationships of this multifunctional protein in neurodegeneration. *Trends Neurosci.* 15:391−396.

May, P. C., Lampert-Etchells, M., Johnson S. A., Poirier, J., Masters, J. N., and Finch, C. E. (1990) Dynamics of gene expression for hippocampal glycoprotein elevated in Alzheimer's disease and in response to experimental lesions in rat. *Neuron* 8:831−839.

McNeill, T. H., Masters, J. N., and Finch, C. E. (1991a) Effect of chronic adrenalectomy on neuron loss and distribution of sulfated glycoprotein-2 in the dentate gyrus of prepubertal rats. *Exp. Neurol.* 111:140−144.

McNeill, T. H., Cheng, H.-W., Day, J. R., and Finch, C. E. (199b) Unilateral entorhinal cortex/ fimbria fornix lesion (EC/FF) encodes GAP-43 mRNA in the contralateral hippocampus. *Soc. Neurosci. Abstr.* 17:735.

Mensah, P. L. (1977) The internal organization of the mouse caudate nucleus: Evidence for cell clustering and regional variation. *Brain Res.* 137:53−66.

Morgan, D. G., May, P. C., and Finch, C. E. (1987) Dopamine and serotonin systems in human and rodent brain: Effects of age and neurodegenerative disease. *J. Am. Geriatr. Soc.* 35:334−345.

Morgan, T. E., Nichols, N. R., Pasinetti, G. M., and Finch, C. E. (1993) TGF-β1 mRNA increases in macrophage/microglia cells of the hippocampus in response to deafferentation and kainic acid-induced neurodegeneration. *Exp. Neurol.* 120:291−301.

Morse, J. K., DeKosky S. T., and Scheff, S. W. (1992) Neurotrophic effects of steroids on lesion-induced growth in the hippocampus. II. Hormone replacement. *Exp. Neurol.* 118:47−52.

Murphy, B. F., Kirszbaum, L., Walker, I. D., and d'Apice, A. J. F. (1988) SP-40, 40 a newly identified human serum protein found in the SC5b-9 complex of complement and and immune deposits in glomerular nephritis. *J. Clin. Invest.* 81:1858–1864.

Nadler, J. V., Perry, B. W., and Cotman, C. W. (1980) Selective reinnervation of hippocampal area CA1 and the fascia dentata after destruction of CA3-CA4 afferents with kainic acid. *Brain Res.* 182:1–9.

Nichols, N. R., Laping, N. J., Day, J. R., and Finch, C. E. (1991) Increases in transforming growth factor-beta mRNA in hippocampus during response to entorhinal cortex lesions in intact and adrenalectomized rats. *J. Neurosci. Res.* 28:134–139.

Nichols, N. R., Day, J. R., Laping, N. J., Johnson, S. A., and Finch, C. E. (1993) GFAP mRNA increases with age in rat and human brain. *Neurobiol. Aging*, in press.

O'Callaghan J. P., and Miller, D. (1991) The concentration of glial fibrillary acidic protein increases with age in the mouse and rat brain. *Neurobiol. Aging* 12:171–174.

O'Callaghan, J. P., Brinton, R. E., and McEwen, B. S. (1989) Glucocorticoids regulate the concentration of glial fibrillary acidic protein throughout the brain. *Brain Res.* 494:159–161.

Palmer, D. J., and Christie, D. L. (1990) The primary structure of glycoprotein III from bovine adrenal medullary chromaffin granules. *J. Biol. Chem.* 265:6617–6623.

Parent, A. (1990) Extrinsic connections of the basal ganglia. *Trends Neurosci.* 13:254–271.

Parent, A., Smith, Y., and M.-Y. Arsenault (1987) Chemical anatomy of basal gangalia neurons in primates In *The Basal Ganglia II. Structure and Function*, M. B. Carpenter, and A. Jyaraman, (eds.), *Adv. in Behavioral Biol.* Vol. 32, pp. 3–41. Plenum, New York.

Pasinetti, G. M., and Finch, C. E. (1991) Sulfated glycoprotein-2 (SGP-2) mRNA is expressed in rat striatal astrocytes following ibotenic acid lesions. *Neurosci. Lett.* 130:1–4.

Pasinetti, G. M., Kohama, S., Reinhard, J. F. Jr., Cheng, H. W., McNeill, T.H., and Finch, C. E. (1991) Striatal responses to decortication. I. Dopaminergic and astrocytic activities. *Brain Res.* 567:253–259.

Pasinetti, G. M., Johnson, S. A., Lampert-Etchells, M., Finch, C. E. (1992) Complement mRNAs and response to brain lesions. *Exp. Neurol.* 118:117–125.

Pasinetti, G. M., Cheng, H. W., Morgan, D. G., Lampert-Etchells, M., McNeill T. H., and Finch, C. E. (1993a) Astrocytic mRNA responses to striatal deafferentation in male rat. *Neuroscience* 53:199–211.

Pasinetti, G. M., Nichols, N. R., Tocco, G., Morgan, T., Laping, N., and Finch, C. E. (1993b) Transforming growth factor beta-1 (TGF-β1) and fibronectin mRNA in rat brain: Responses to injury and cell type localization. *Neuroscience* 54:893–907.

Paskevich P. A., Evans, H. K., and Domesick, V. B. (1991) Morphological assessment of neuronal aggregates in the striatum of the rat. *J. Comp. Neurol.* 305:361–369.

Pearce, B. R., Palmer, A. M., Bowen, D. M., Wilcock, G. K., Esiri, M. M., and Davison; A. L. (1984) Neurotransmitter dysfunction and atrophy of the caudate nucleus in Alzheimer's disease. *Neurochem. Pathol.* 2:221–232.

Phillips, L. L., Nostrand, S. J., Chikiraishi D. M., and Steward, O. (1987) Increases in ribosomal RNA within the denervated neuropil of the dentate gyrus during reinnervation: Evaluation by in situ hybridization using DNA probes complementary to ribosomal RNA. *Mol. Brain Res.* 2:251–261.

Poirier, J., May, P. C., Osterburg, H. H., Geddes, J., Cotman, C., and Finch, C. E. (1990) Selective alterations of RNA in rat hippocampus after entorhinal cortex lesioning. *Proc. Natl. Acad. Sci. USA* 87:303–307.

Poirier, J., Hess, M., May, P.C., and Finch, C. E. (1991a) Cloning of hippocampal poly(A) RNA sequences that increase after enthorhinal cortex lesion in adult rat. *Mol. Brain Res.* 9:191–195.

Poirier, J., Hess, M., May, P. C., and Finch, C. E. (1991b) Astrocytic apolipoprotein E mRNA and GFAP mRNA in hippocampus after enthorhinal cortex lesioning. *Mol. Brain Res.* 11:97–106.

Powell, T. P. S. and Cowen, W. M. (1956) A study of thalamostriate relations in the monkey. *Brain* 79:364–390.

Purves, D., and Lichtman, J. W. (1985) Maintenance and modifiability of synapses, In *Principles of Neural Development*, D. Purves, and J. W. Lichtman (eds.), pp. 301–328. Sinauer Associates, Sunderland, MA.

Purves, D., Hadley, R. D., and Voyvodic, J. T. (1986) Dynamic changes in the dendritic geometry of individual neurons visualized over periods of up to three months in the superior cervical ganglion of living mice. *Neuroscience* 6:1051–1060.

Rao A., and Steward, O. (1991) Evidence that protein constituents of postsynaptic membrane specializations are locally synthesized: Analysis of proteins synthesized within synaptosomes. *J. Neurosci.* 11:2881–2895.

Represa, A., Duyckaerts, C., Tremblay, E., Hauw, J.J., and Ben, A. Y. (1988) Is senile dementia of the Alzheimer's type associated with hippcampal plasticity? *Brain Res.* 457:355–359.

Rosene, D. L., and Van Hoesen, G. W. (1987) The hippocampal formation of the primate brain: A review of some comparative aspects of cytoarchitecture and connections. In *Cerebral Cortex*, E. G. Jones and A. Peters (eds.), pp. 345–456. Plenum Press, New York.

Sapolsky, R. M. (1992) *Stress, the Aging Brain, and the Mechanisms of Neuron Death.* The MIT Press, Cambridge, MA.

Savill, J. S., Wyellie, A. H., Henson, J. E., Walport, M. J., Henson, P. M., and Haslett, C. (1989) Macrophage phagocytosis of aging neutrophils in inflammation. Programmed cell death in the neutrophil leads to recognition by macrophages. *J. Clin. Invest.* 83:865–875.

Scheff, S., Benardo, L., and Cotman, C. W. (1977) Progressive brain damage accelerates axon sprouting in adult rat. *Science* 197:795–797.

Scheff, S. W., Bernardo, L. S., and Cotman, C. W. (1980) Decline in reactive fiber growth in the dentate gyrus of aged rats compared to young adult rats following entorhinal cortex removal. *Brain Res.* 199:21–38.

Scheff, S. W., Hoff, S. F., and Anderson, K. J. (1986) Altered regulation of lesion induced synaptogenesis by adrenalectomy and corticosterone in young adult rats. *Exp. Neurol.* 93:456–470.

Scheff, S. W., Morse, J. K, and DeKosky, S. T. (1988) Neurotrophic effects of steroids on lesion-induced growth in the hippocampus. I. The asteroidal condition. *Brain Res.* 457:246–250.

Schiffer, D., Giordana, M. T., Migheli, A., Giaccone, G., Pezzotta, S., and Mauro, A. (1986) Glial fibrillary acidic protein and vimentin in the experimental glial reaction of the rat brain. *Brain Res.* 374:110–118.

Selkoe, D. J., Bell, D. S., Podlisny, M. B., Price, D. L., and Cork, L. C. (1987) Conservation of brain amyloid proteins in aged mammals and humans with AD. *Science* 235:873–877.

Senut, M. C., Roudier, M., Fallet-Bianco, C., and Lamour, Y. (1991) Senile dementia of the Alzheimer type: Is there a correlation between entorhinal cortex and dentate gyrus lesions? *Acta Neuropathol.* 82:306–315.

Smith, D. A., and Bolam, J. P. (1990) The neural network of the basal ganglia as revealed by the study of synaptic connections of identified neurons. *Trends Neurosci.* 13:259–265.

Spranger, M., Lindholm, D., Bandtlow, C., Heumann, R., Gnahn, H., Naher-Noe, M., and Thoenen, H. (1990) Regulation of nerve growth factor (NGF) synthesis in rat central nervous system: Comparison between the effects of Interleukin-1 and various growth factors in astrocyte culture and in vivo. *Eur. J. Neurosci.* 2:69–76.

Steinbusch H. W. M., van der Kooy, D., Verhofstad, A. A. J., and Pellegrino, A. (1980). Serotonergic and non-serotonergic projections from the nucleus raphe dorsalis to the caudate-putamen complex in the rat, studied by a combined immunofluorescence and fluorescent retrograde axonal labeling technique. *Neurosci. Lett.* 19:137–142.

Steinbusch, H. W. M., Neiuwenhuys, R., Verhofstad, A. A. J., and van der Kooy, D. (1981) The nucleus raphe dorsalis of the rat and its projection upon the caudatoputamen: A combined cytoarchitectonic, immunohistochemical and retrograde transport study. *J. Physiol.* 77:157–174.

Steward, O. (1983) Alterations in polyribosomes associated with dendritic spines during the reinnervation of the dentate gyrus of the adult rat. *J. Neurosci.* 3:177–188.

Steward, O., and Ribak, C. E. (1986) Polyribosomes associates with synaptic sites on axon initial segments: Localization of protein synthetic machinery at inhibitory synapses. *J. Neurosci.* 6:3079–3085.

Steward, O., Cotman, C. W., and Lynch, G. S. (1976) A quantitative autoradiographic and electrophysiological study of the reinnervation of the dentate gyrus by the contralateral entorhinal cortex following ipsilateral entorhinal lesions. *Brain Res.* 114:181–200.

Steward, O., Torre, E. R., Phillips L. L., and Trimmer, P. A. (1990) The process of reinnervation in the dentate gyrus of adult rats: Time course of increases in mRNA for glial fibrillary acidic protein *J. Neurosci.* 10:2373–2384.

Stroemberg, I., Wetmore, C. J., Ebendal, T. Ernfors, P., Persson, H., and Olson, L. (1990) Rapid communication rescue of basal forebrain cholinergic neurons after implantation of genetically modified cells producing recombinant NGF. *J. Neurosci. Res.* 25:405–411.

Ulas, J., Monaghan, D. T., and Cotman, C. W. (1990a) Kainate receptors in the rat hippocampus: A distribution and time course of changes in response to unilateral lesions of the entorhinal cortex. *J. Neurosci.* 10:2352–2362.

Ulas, J., Monaghan, D. T. and Cotman, C. W. (1990b) Plastic response of hippocampal excitatory amino acid receptors to deafferentation and reinnervation. *Neuroscience* 34:9–17.

Veening, J. G., Cornelissen, F. M., and Lieven, P. A. J. (1980) The topical organization of the afferents to the caudato putamen of the rat. A horseradish peroxidase study. *Neuroscience* 5:1253–1268.

Vijayan, V. K., and Cotman, C. W. (1983) Lysosomal enzyme changes in young and aged control and entorhinal-lesioned rats. *Neurobiol. Aging* 4:13–23.

Wahl, S. M., Allen, J. B., and McCartney, F. N. (1991) Macrophage- and astrocyte-derived transforming growth factor beta as a mediator of central nervous system dysfunction in acquired immune deficiency syndrome. *J. Exp. Med.* 173:981–991.

4 Forms of Long-term Potentiation Induced by NMDA and non-NMDA Receptor Activation

Timothy Teyler and Leslie Grover

1 INTRODUCTION

Long-term potentiation (LTP) is an enduring increase in synaptic strength seen at monosynaptic junctions in the mammalian forebrain. It has been extensively studied in hippocampal tissues where insights regarding the mechanisms underlying its induction, expression, and maintenance have been uncovered. LTP has been proposed as a candidate neuronal mechanism underlying memory formation in the mammalian brain (Teyler and DiScenna, 1987). This is due, in part, to the properties that LTP displays (discussed below) and, in part, to the observation that a LTP-like phenomenon can be seen in the brains of animals successively learning a behavioral task (Berger, 1984; Sharp et al., 1985; Skelton et al., 1985). Similarly, pharmacologically blocking LTP induction interferes with the acquisition of behavioral learning (Morris et al., 1986).

LTP has been seen in a wide variety of structures in the mammalian brain. Although most extensively studied in the hippocampal formation synapses, it has also been documented at neocortical synapses, sensory relay nuclei, and brainstem structures (see review by Teyler and DiScenna, 1987). Thus, LTP is a relatively widespread phenomenon throughout the mammalian brain. It is generally associated with dendritic spines, particularly those employing the neurotransmitter glutamate. LTP is *induced* by repeatedly stimulating the afferents leading to the synapse under study. Entry of calcium into the postsynaptic neuron appears to be critical for the induction of LTP and LTD (long-term depression: a decrease in synaptic efficacy). LTP can be induced by tetanic stimulation of these afferents, by altering the chemical environment of the synapse (usually done in brain slice preparations), or by behavioral training techniques (in intact preparations). LTP is *expressed* as an increase in the postsynaptic response to constant test stimuli. Over a period of time the response magnitude increases, stabilizes, then generally begins to decay slowly, reaching baseline (in intact preparations) in about a week.

LTP assumes different forms in different areas of the brain and following different induction protocols. For example, LTP induced at the glutamatergic synapses in dentate gyrus or CA1 regions displays a relatively rapid onset peaking in about 5 min after tetanus, followed by a slow decay back to baseline. Neocortical long-term potentiation, in contrast, displays a prolonged onset, requiring 30–90 min for full expression, followed by little decay across the 8–9 hr after induction (in neocortical slice preparations) (Teyler et al., 1990). Whether these two extremes of LTP expression represent qualitatively different forms of synaptic plasticity mediated by different cellular machinery, or quantitative differences in the engagement of the same cellular machinery remains an unanswered question.

2 PROPERTIES OF LTP

Why believe that LTP may be the neuronal substrate of memory? There are a number of characteristics of LTP that make it a plausible candidate for a neuronal mechanism underlying information storage in the brain. The *magnitude* of LTP is a significant change above baseline. That is, the signal-to-noise ratio of a potentiated versus unpotentiated synapse is roughly 2:1. This means that the potentiated synapse displays a significantly enhanced activity with respect to baseline and should thus have a marked influence on the network in which it resides. The *duration* of LTP is long with respect to neurophysiological phenomena, but trivial with respect to the duration of behavioral memory. While neurophysiologists tend to find remarkable a physiological change that lasts for days, the behavioral scientist finds unremarkable a change that will not last for a significant fraction of the organism's life. Why then is LTP considered as a candidate underlying memory when the time course of the two do not match very well? There are several answers to this question. One answer is that it is currently the best candidate for the job. A better answer is that our knowledge of the properties of LTP comes in large part from artificial situations wherein LTP is initiated by synchronous electrical stimulation of a large population of afferents synapsing on the cells under study. This probably never occurs in nature and may give an unrealistic cast to the phenomenon of LTP. Experiments using intact preparations have varied the parameters of electrical stimulation used to induce LTP and find that "massed" vs. "distributed" stimulation results in a different time course in the decay of the LTP induced. The quickest decay was seen in the massed stimulation paradigm, whereas the slowest decay was observed in the distributed stimulation situation (Teyler and DiScenna, 1984). Thus the longevity of LTP is, in part, a function of the parameters used to elicit it. Behavioral studies have also shown that distributed practice is superior to massed practice in terms of retention; thus this aspect of LTP actually fits the behavioral literature reasonably well. LTP in neocortical synapses does not decay nearly as quickly as does LTP seen at hippocampal synapses (Teyler et al., 1990). This suggests that the properties of LTP may vary depending on the brain area under study. The extreme example of this is a form of synaptic plasticity seen in the cerebellum. The parallel fiber synapses to cerebellar Purkinje cells display a long-term depression (LTD) that shares a number of properties with LTP seen elsewhere (Ito, 1990).

LTP is not a cell-wide phenomenon; rather, it is limited to the synapses that have been activated (Andersen et al., 1977). This *input specificity* is an important contrast to the generalized increase in excitability which underlies pathological states such as seizure disorders. LTP also displays a *threshold* (sometimes called cooperativity; McNaughton et al., 1978) that results from the presence of a voltage-dependent block on the channels responsible for gating Ca^{2+} into the neuron. The Ca^{2+} flow into the postsynaptic neuron is responsible for initiating the changes underlying LTP and is regulated by a voltage-sensitive block of the N-methyl-D-aspartate (NMDA) receptor–gated Ca^{2+} channel whose relief requires a sufficient level of postsynaptic depolarization (Ascher and Nowak, 1988). The tetanus employed to initiate LTP provides the necessary postsynaptic depolarization to alleviate the magnesium block of the Ca^{2+} channels. A hallmark of behavioral memory, particularly in humans, is the ability to form *associations* between apparently tenuously related phenomena. LTP too displays associativity such that a weak stimulus (one insufficiently intense to induce LTP), when paired with a strong stimulus (one sufficient to produce LTP by itself), results in LTP on the weak pathway when both are presented simultaneously. Thus, the ability to associate a weak and a strong input at the cellular level would seem to be a key requirement for behavioral associative memory. Associative LTP has received some attention, and it has been determined that the rules linking the various inputs to be associated can be quite complex (Sastry et al., 1986; Stanton and Sejnowski, 1989). Some inputs strengthen, others weaken depending on the patterning of input and the level of membrane depolarization/hyperpolarization the inputs induce (some patterns of input are effective at activating a large GABAergic inhibitory influence). Thus, the machinery exists for not only strengthening some associations but for weakening other, perhaps inappropriate or conflicting, associations.

3   INDUCTION OF LTP: THE ROLE OF CALCIUM

The induction of LTP requires Ca^{2+} influx into the postsynaptic cell as an initiating event. The NMDA subtype of glutamate receptor has been found to be largely responsible for the induction of LTP in hippocampus and elsewhere. The NMDA receptor is coupled to a channel that gates Ca^{2+} into the cell when activated. This NMDA receptor-linked channel is normally blocked by magnesium in a voltage dependent manner. Ca^{2+} will enter the postsynaptic cell only when the cell is sufficiently depolarized to relieve the magnesium block of the Ca^{2+} channel (Collingridge et al., 1983) (figure 4.1). In experimental situations this occurs when the cells is sufficiently depolarized by a tetanus, and in nature probably occurs when sufficient convergence takes place onto the postsynaptic cell to again reach the depolarization threshold necessary for Ca^{2+} gating into the cell. Thus, Ca^{2+} entry is critical for the induction of LTP. The precise role of Ca^{2+} in initiating LTP remains unresolved. There are ample Ca^{2+} targets in the postsynaptic cell, many of which have been shown to be activated during LTP, including protein kinase C (Malenka et al., 1989),

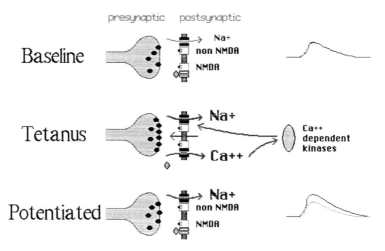

Figure 4.1 Cartoon illustrating the role of NMDA receptors in LTP. Under baseline conditions (single pulse afferent stimulation) EPSPs are evoked via non-NMDA glutamate (K/AMPA) receptors that gate Na^+. During tetanic afferent stimulation the voltage dependent Mg^{2+} block of the $NMDA_R$-linked calcium channel is relieved, allowing Ca^{2+} to enter the postsynaptic cell where it acts on Ca^{2+}-dependent kinases to ultimately facilitate Na^+ flux through the K/AMPA-linked channels. The potentiated synapse retains this facilitated Na^+ flux as is reflected in larger EPSPs. The $NMDA_R$-linked channel is again blocked by Mg^{2+}.

calcium-calmodulin kinase (Malinow et al., 1989), and proteases (Lynch and Baudry, 1984). As of yet, it is not possible to specify the precise roles of these agents in LTP induction and expression. The initial change in cell physiology, however, is reasonably well understood. The net result of the Ca^{2+} influx is to alter the baseline properties of Na^+/K^+ conductance mediated by non-NMDA glutamate receptors (and NMDA receptors to a lesser extent), making these receptor/channel complexes more effective in depolarizing the postsynaptic cell (e.g., larger EPSPs).

The presynaptic terminal has also been implicated in LTP through two different mechanisms. Over the short time course, nitric oxide (NO) has been shown to be generated postsynaptically and diffuse out of the cell to affect the presynaptic terminal, resulting in augmented neurotransmitter release (Schuman and Madison, 1991). Over a longer time course, the retrograde messenger arachidonic acid has also been implicated as a presynaptic signal resulting in enhanced transmitter release (Bliss et al., 1986). These changes, both presynaptic and postsynaptic, are believed to be responsible for the immediate and medium term events of LTP. Are they also responsible for changes seen at hours, days, weeks, or months later? This period of time, known as the period of *maintenance* of potentiation, is associated with protein synthesis (Duffy et al., 1981) and can be disrupted by protein synthesis inhibitors (Krug et al., 1984). This suggests that the processes set in motion by the entering Ca^+ eventually results in the expression of mRNA and the synthesis of new proteins. These structural changes may alter the cell over the long term. The maintenance phase of LTP has been relatively neglected with respect to isolating the proteins that are synthesized, their functions, and their fate and regulation. There has been considerable interest in the possibility that the conditions giving rise to LTP are also suitable for the initiation of events leading to gene expression in the postsynaptic neuron. There are a number of early intermediate genes such as c-*fos* and *jun* that have been studied with respect to their involvement in LTP (Cole et al., 1989) Whether these or similar genes are capable of ultimately triggering protein synthesis of specific proteins related to altered synaptic transmission remains to be determined.

Elevated postsynaptic Ca^{2+} thus appears to be the key controlling the expression of LTP. There are primarily three ways that Ca^{2+} levels can be elevated in neurons. The first is via the Ca^{2+} channel associated with the NMDA receptor. The second is via voltage-sensitive calcium channels. The third is by releasing Ca^{2+} from intracellular stores such as endoplasmic reticulum. There is now reason to believe that the LTP resulting from Ca^{2+} entry via these mechanisms is not the same. Experiments in our laboratory have selectively induced LTP by activating either the NMDA-linked Ca^{2+} channels or the voltage-dependent calcium channels. These experiments have shown that differences exist in the kinetics of LTP induction and decay, as well as its expression and properties. Some of these properties and differences will be reviewed in more depth in the next section.

4 NMDA$_R$ and NON-NMDA$_R$ LONG-TERM POTENTIATION

4.1 Induction of non-NMDA$_R$ LTP

Non-NMDA$_R$ LTP is induced by a subset of the stimulus patterns that are capable of inducing NMDA$_R$ LTP. The important characteristic of these stimulus patterns seems to be the frequency of the tetanic stimulation and the resultant level of postsynaptic depolarization used to induce the LTP. Lower frequency tetani (25–100 Hz) appear to induce only NMDA$_R$ LTP. Higher frequency tetani (> 150 Hz; we routinely use 200 Hz) are capable of inducing non-NMDA$_R$ LTP in addition to NMDA$_R$ LTP (Grover and Teyler, 1990).

4.2 Calcium Dependence

A necessary first step in LTP induction for both NMDA$_R$ and non-NMDA$_R$ LTP is Ca^{2+} influx into the postsynaptic neuron. This was demonstrated by injecting the Ca^{2+} chelator EGTA into postsynaptic neurons through an intracellular recording electrode for NMDA$_R$ LTP (Lynch et al., 1983) and the faster acting chelator BAPTA for non-NMDA$_R$ (Grover and Teyler, 1990). In both cases, the presence of the chelator prevented the induction of LTP. In this respect, the two LTPs appear identical. The difference is in the route for Ca^{2+} influx. We found that non-NMDA$_R$ LTP was sensitive to the dihydropyridine Ca^{2+} channel antagonist, nifedipine, suggesting that in this case Ca^{2+} influx is through voltage-dependent calcium channels (VDCC) instead of the NMDA receptor gated channel. It is not known if the Ca^{2+} activates the same processes leading to the expression of LTP in both cases. The delayed time course of non-NMDA$_R$ LTP expression suggests that there may be differences, but this is not compelling evidence.

4.3 Delayed LTP Onset

A second feature of non-NMDA$_R$ LTP is a delayed onset for expression of potentiation. We have been unable as yet to completely and unambiguously describe the precise time course for non-NMDA$_R$ LTP expression due to short-term synaptic modifications by other processes induced by the same tetani that are necessary to induce the LTP. These processes include post-tetanic potentiation (PTP) and a short duration heterosynaptic depression. Our best efforts to separate these processes suggest the following time courses: (1) PTP is induced immediately by tetanization, but decays very quickly (within 1–2 min); (2) depression is most likely also induced immediately, but decays over a longer time course (5 min) and is heterosynaptic; (3) non-NMDA$_R$ LTP may or may not be induced immediately (it is difficult to tell, because of the immediate presence of PTP and depression), but clearly does not reach a peak until about 10–15 min post tetanus. This delay in expression of non-NMDA$_R$ LTP contrasts with the expression of NMDA$_R$ LTP, which appears at peak amplitude within a minute or so of tetanization, and immediately begins to decay (Gustafsson and Wigstrom, 1988).

4.3 Input Specificity

The expression of non-NMDA$_R$ LTP, like that of NMDA$_R$ LTP, is specific to the input pathway that is tetanized. We demonstrated this by delivering test stimuli to two independent pathways while the NMDA$_R$ was inactivated. Tetanizing one pathway (TET S$_1$) led to LTP of responses evoked by test stimuli to that pathway, while the control (nontetanized pathway) showed no LTP (figure 4.2; Grover and Teyler, 1992).

4.4 Preclusion

Figure 4.2 illustrates a curious feature of non-NMDA$_R$ LTP. Following establishment of non-NMDA$_R$ LTP in the tetanized pathway, the control pathway was subsequently tetanized (TET S$_2$), but non-NMDA$_R$ LTP was *not* expressed. We have termed this effect preclusion. The mechanisms which underlie non-NMDA$_R$ LTP induction seem to be related to preclusion, since we found that preclusion only occurred when non-NMDA$_R$ LTP was first successfully induced in one input pathway. If non-NMDA$_R$ LTP induction failed in the first input (the failure rate for non-NMDA$_R$ LTP appears to be higher than the failure rate for NMDA$_R$ LTP, about 20–25% failure), then preclusion was not observed in the second input, while preclusion was observed in at least five or six slices where non-NMDA$_R$ LTP was induced in the first input. The input specificity of non-NMDA$_R$ LTP has previously been shown to be a

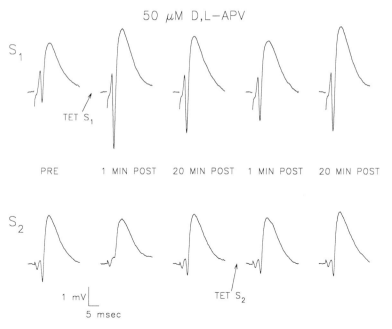

Figure 4.2 Non-NMDA$_R$ LTP is induced only in a tetanized pathway. Once induced, non-NMDA$_R$ LTP precludes later induction in an independent pathway. In this experiment, two independent pathways (S_1, S_2) were stimulated alternately. Tetanization of the first input pathway (TET S_1) produced non-NMDA$_R$ LTP. This LTP was present only for responses evoked by stimulating S_1, responses to S2 stimulation showed an initial depression (1 min posttetanus) but showed no potentiation. Twenty minuter after non-NMDA$_R$ LTP induction in the first input pathway, the second input pathway was tetanized (TET S_2). Non-NMDA$_R$ LTP induction failed in the second pathway, an effect we have called preclusion. APV was present throughout this experiment to prevent NMDA$_R$ LTP induction.

characteristic feature of NMDA$_R$ LTP, but we have never observed preclusion of NMDA$_R$ LTP, nor does preclusion of non-NMDA$_R$ LTP extend to NMDA$_R$ LTP. Our finding of a preclusion effect for non-NMDA$_R$ LTP suggests, but again does not compel, differences in mechanisms of expression for these two varieties of LTP.

4.5 NMDA$_R$ Blockade during the Tetanus

We typically induce non-NMDA$_R$ LTP by tetanizing at high frequency in the presence of moderate concentrations of the NMDA receptor antagonist, APV. Since APV is a competitive antagonist, it is conceivable that the large amount of glutamate released during a tetanus might successfully compete with APV for the receptor site, leading to a partial unblocking of NMDA receptors during tetanization. If this were the case, then we would observe an apparent APV-insensitive component of LTP that was in fact mediated by NMDA receptors.

The most convincing evidence against this possibility came from an examination of responses recorded from CA1 pyramidal cells during the tetanus.

We recorded from cells in which non-NMDA$_R$ LTP had been first induced. We then separated and measured the NMDA receptor mediated portion of the response during tetanic stimulation (blocking the kainate/AMPA receptors with CNQX/DNQX and GABA$_A$ receptors with bicuculline), and found that during the same tetani used to induce LTP, the NMDA receptor–mediated response was completely blocked by the same concentration of APV used during LTP induction (Grover and Teyler, 1990). Thus we are confident that non-NMDA$_R$ LTP is not an artifact of inadequately controlling for NMDA$_R$ activation during the tetanus.

4.6   Locus of non-NMDA$_R$ LTP

Previous studies of NMDA$_R$ LTP have demonstrated that the locus of change is the excitatory synapse onto pyramidal cells. That is, neither an increase in presynaptic excitability nor an increase in postsynaptic excitability is the basis for LTP expression (Andersen et al. 1980). The possibility of a decreased efficacy of inhibitory neurotransmission has been examined, but there is no evidence that such an effect exists (however, LTP of the excitatory input to interneurons seems to occur; Buszaki and Eidelberg, 1982; Taube and Schwartzkroin, 1987), nor is it a likely explanation of the synaptic potentiation. One way to assess the locus of change in LTP is to examine input/output functions and compare results obtained before and after LTP induction. This has been done by many investigators for NMDA$_R$ LTP. Typically there is no change in the stimulus intensity/presynaptic fiber volley function (ruling out an increase in presynaptic excitability), but increases are observed in the fiber volley/EPSP function (synaptic enhancement), and in the EPSP/spike function (spike potentiation). We have performed an analysis of input/output functions for non-NMDA$_R$ LTP (figure 4.3). We found two consistent effects: (1) no change in the stimulus intensity/fiber volley function, and (2) an increase in the fiber volley/EPSP function. In contrast, we observed variable results in the EPSP/spike function. In some slices, there was evidence of spike potentiation (an example is shown in figure 4.3D), while some slices showed no change in this function, and others showed no change in the slope of the function, but did show apparent changes in the maximum spike size. This pattern of change is similar to that seen in NMDA$_R$ LTP—both varieties of LTP show no change in presynaptic excitability, and both show a synaptic enhancement. It remains to be determined if spike potentiation can be reliably induced in some proportion of slices during non-NMDA$_R$ LTP.

Synaptic enhancement could occur due to either a presynptic or a postsynaptic mechanism (e.g., increased release of neurotransmitter vs. increased number of glutamate receptors). There are results supporting both possibilities (Bliss et al., 1986; Davies et al., 1989; Dolphin et al., 1982). Theoretically, this issue can be settled by a quantal analysis of neurotransmission at these synapses. With the advent of low-noise, whole-cell recording in slices, it seemed possible that this issue might finally be resolved. Unfortunately, results of quantal analyses of LTP at these synapses have not generated consistent

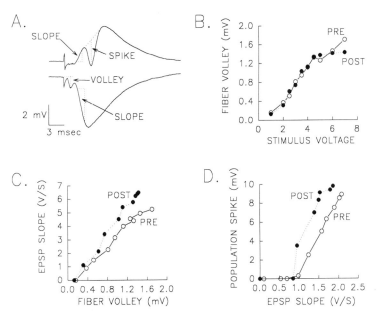

Figure 4.3 Input/output functions for one slice, before and after non-NMDA$_R$ LTP was induced. (A) Measurements of the presynaptic fiber volley, population EPSP slope, and population spike are illustrated here. (B) Induction of non-NMDA$_R$ LTP had no effect on the stimulus intensity/fiber volley relationship. (C) An increase in the relationship between fiber volley and EPSP followed non-NMDA$_R$ LTP induction, indicating a synaptic enhancement during expression of non-NMDA$_R$ LTP. (D) In this slice, there was also a leftward shift in the relationship between the EPSP and the population spike, demonstrating spike potentiation during non-NMDA$_R$ LTP expression. The changes illustrated in (B) and (C) were consistently seen in all slices examined, but spike potentiation (D) was variable.

conclusions (Bekkers and Stevens, 1990; Foster and McNaughton, 1991; Malinow and Tsien, 1990; Manabe, et al., 1992). The controversy surrounding these differences seems to be a direct consequence of the assumptions made and the techniques used by different groups (Korn and Faber, 1991). Until these issues can be resolved, there seems to be little point in attempting a quantal analysis of non-NMDA$_R$ LTP. Once these issues are resolved, it will be interesting to see if the two forms of LTP are expressed at the same site or at different sites.

4.7 Both NMDA and non-NMDA Receptor-mediated Responses Contribute to LTP

To study the two forms of LTP requires that they be isolated from one another. However, given the appropriate stimulus conditions (a high-frequency tetanus or substantial depolarization), both processes can be elicited simultaneously. The cartoon in figure 4.4 (top) illustrates the result of activating NMDA receptors at a low tetanus frequency. Here Ca^{2+} enters only through NMDA$_R$ channels because the tetanus-induced depolarization is insufficient to activate the non-NMDA$_R$ voltage-dependent calcium channels (VDCC). The

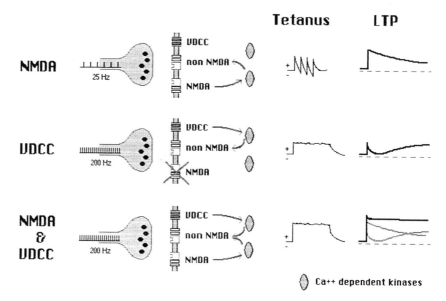

Figure 4.4 Cartoon depicting the differences between $NMDA_R$ and non-$NMDA_R$ LTP. (Top) Stimulating afferents at a low tetanus frequency activates only NMDA receptors. Under these conditions Ca^{2+} enters only through $NMDA_R$ channels because the tetanus-induced depolarization is insufficient to activate the non-$NMDA_R$ voltage-dependent calcium channels (VDCC). The resultant LTP peaks, quickly followed by a slow decline toward baseline. (Middle) The $NMDA_R$ channels are pharmacologically blocked but the afferent stimulation is frequent enough to activate the non-$NMDA_R$ channels. The resulting depolarization is greater and induces a slowly developing form of LTP. (Bottom) Both channel types are activated by the tetanus (no blockers present) and the resulting LTP is the sum of both $NMDA_R$ and non-$NMDA_R$ contributions. Whether the Ca^{2+} entering via the two routes acts on different targets (as depicted here) or on common targets is unknown.

resultant LTP peaks, quickly followed by a slow decline toward baseline. In the middle panel the $NMDA_R$ channels are pharmacologically blocked, but the tetanus is intense enough to activate the non-$NMDA_R$ channels. The resultant depolarization induces a slowly developing form of LTP. In the bottom panel, both sets of channels are activated by the tetanus (no blockers present), and the resulting LTP is the sum of both $NMDA_R$ and non-$NMDA_R$ contributions. Whether Ca^{2+} entering via the two routes acts on different targets (as depicted here) or on common targets is unknown.

4.8 Do $NMDA_R$ LTP and non-$NMDA_R$ LTP Share the Same Mechanism?

It is important to know if non-$NMDA_R$ LTP shares common mechanisms of expression with $NMDA_R$ LTP. It seems clear that the inducing conditions are different for the two forms of LTP and that the Ca^{2+} enters via different routes, but it is possible that subsequent steps leading to expression of LTP converge for both non-$NMDA_R$ LTP and $NMDA_R$ LTP. The traditional technique used to determine if potentiation induced by two different treatments share a common mechanism is the occlusion experiment. In this experiment, a maximal LTP is induced by one treatment. If the second treatment, delivered subsequently, induces additional potentiation, then the mechanisms must be different. If subsequent potentiation is occluded by the first treatment, then a common mechanism is implied (although this need only be one common but obligatory step in two largely different multistep processes). Since this is such an important question, we have begun the occlusion experiment for non-NMDA$_R$ and NMDA$_R$ LTP. Results to date have been equivocal. In some slices, complete occlusion has appeared to be the case, whereas in other slices occlusion has not occurred. Hopefully, continued experimentation will reveal a more consistent picture. Other evidence discussed above, including the different time courses for LTP expression and the preclusion effect, suggests some difference in mechanism beyond the initial induction event. Since it is likely that the process leading from tetanization to LTP expression is composed of multiple steps, and since both LTPs depend on increases in postsynaptic intracellular Ca^{2+} concentration, it would be surprising if at least one of these steps leading to LTP expression was not shared.

4.9   What Mechanisms Might Be Responsible for These Qualitative Differences?

Several possibilities come to mind. First, there may be differences in the amount of postsynaptic Ca^{2+} entry under the two conditions. The differential expression of LTP may reflect the effect of postsynaptic Ca^{2+} concentration on a common target. Calcium flux into the postsynaptic cell is a function of the distribution, concentration, conductance, activation and inactivation kinetics, and number of active channels. It is unlikely that these parameters are identical for calcium entry via NMDA and non-NMDA receptor activation. Calcium imaging has shown APV-antagonized Ca^{2+} accumulation in dendritic spines of CA3 neurons (Conner and Muller, 1991). The differences in NMDA$_R$ and non-NMDA$_R$ LTP may, then, be a Ca^{2+} concentration–dependent effect, limited to specific compartments of the postsynaptic cell. The delayed expression of non-NMDA$_R$ LTP cannot simply be attributed to low postsynaptic Ca^{2+} concentrations for two reasons. First, the tetanus conditions required to induce non-NMDA$_R$ LTP are associated with postsynaptic depolarization levels that can be expected to flux high levels of Ca^{2+}. Second, minimally activating NMDA receptors does not lead to a slowly developing LTP, but rather results in a more rapidly decaying potentiation.

Second, there may be high- and low-affinity Ca^{2+} binding targets in the postsynaptic cell. Such targets would be differentially affected by NMDA$_R$ and non-NMDA$_R$ activity. This possibility, like the former one, does not account for preclusion or one direction of occlusion. Third, the influx via the two types of channels may act on different targets, leading to their different expression of LTP. One can imagine different Ca^{2+}-dependent enzymes located on or near the cytoplasmic side of the NMDA$_R$-affiliated Ca^{2+} channel and the L-type Ca^{2+} channel. The enzymes may then initiate different cascades resulting in the differential expression of the two components of LTP. Fourth, the slow kinetics of non-NMDA$_R$ LTP raise the possibility that the expression of this component of LTP may be dependent on a slowly developing process—such as protein synthesis, which has been found to be elevated following LTP (Duffy et al., 1981)—although the time course of non-NMDA$_R$ LTP may be too rapid for this possibility. While protein synthesis inhibitors have little effect on the induction or initial expression of LTP in the dentate, they have been shown to block later phases (Krug et al., 1984; but see Stanton and Sarvey, 1984, for CA1). And fifth, since the levels of depolarizing current and Ca^{2+} required to induce the two components are likely to differ, it is possible that processes such as the chemical- or voltage-dependent release of Ca^{2+} from intracellular stores might be involved.

5 SUMMARY AND CONCLUSIONS

Both NMDA$_R$ and non-NMDA$_R$ components of LTP share several features. First, both are Ca^{2+}-dependent phenomena. Second, both can be elicited by tetanic activation of afferents. Third, both rely on voltage-dependent processes to increase Ca^{2+} flux. Fourth, both result in increases in the magnitude of the postsynaptic EPSP and population spike. Fifth, both are input-specific.

There are also several differences between NMDA$_R$ and non-NMDA$_R$ LTP. First, there are differences in the tetanus parameters required for their induction. This may reflect differences in the voltage dependencies of the two components, with the NMDA$_R$ LTP being engaged at lower levels of postsynaptic depolarization. Second, the kinetics differ. The kinetics of LTP expression of the potentiated response are considerably delayed and prolonged when induction is mediated via non-NMDA$_R$'s. NMDA$_R$ LTP peaks at 5 min (or less) post tetanus and declines slowly thereafter. Non-NMDA$_R$ LTP requires 10–20 min to peak expression. Third, non-NMDA$_R$ LTP displays preclusion.

The available data do not allow us to determine if both phenomena are mediated by the same cellular mechanisms, or if different means of expression are involved. The functional role of these two components of LTP remains to be determined. Since the non-NMDA$_R$ component is only induced by high-frequency afferent input, it may be a means to encode the intensity of potentiating synaptic inputs. Beyond the immediate comparison of two forms of hippocampal LTP, one possibility these experiments suggest is that LTP exists as a family of synaptic plasticities, each having somewhat different induction properties, each having different expression and maintenance properties, each occurring in different neural circuits, and perhaps each having different consequences for behavioral memory.

ACKNOWLEDGMENT

Supported by grant NS 28698 from the NIH.

REFERENCES

Andersen, P., Sundberg, S. H., Sveen, O., and Wigstrom, H. (1977) Specific long-lasting potentiation of synaptic transmission in hippocampal slices. *Nature* 266:736–737.

Andersen, P., Sundberg, S. H., Sveen, O., Swann, J. W., and Wigstrom, H. (1980) Possible mechanisms for long-lasting potentiation of synaptic transmission in hippocampal slices from guinea-pigs. *J. Physiol.* 302:463–482.

Ascher, P. and Nowak, L. (1988) The role of divalent cations in the N-methyl-D-aspartate responses of mouse central neurones in culture. *J. Physiol.* 399:247–266.

Bekkers, J. M., and Stevens, C. F. (1990) Presynaptic mechanism for long-term potentiation in the hippocampus. *Nature* 346:724–729.

Berger, T. (1984) Long-term potentiation of hippocampal synaptic transmission affects rate of behavioral learning. *Science* 224:627–630.

Bliss, T. V. P., Douglas, R. M., Errington, M. L., and Lynch, M. A. (1986) Correlation between long-term potentiation and release of endogenous amino acids from dentate gyrus of anaesthetised rats. *J. Physiol.* 377:391–408.

Buzsaki, G., and Eidelberg, E. (1982) Direct afferent excitation on long-term potentiation of hippocampal interneurons. *J. Neurophysiol.* 48:597–607.

Cole, A. J., Saffen, D. W., Baraban, J. M., and Worley, P. F. (1989) Rapid increase of an immediate early gene messenger RNA in hippocampal neurons by synaptic NMDA receptor activation. *Nature* 340:474–476.

Collingridge, G. L., Kehl, S., and McLennan, H. (1983) Excitatory amino acids in synaptic transmission in the Schaffer-commissural pathway of the rat hippocampus. *J. Physiol. (Lond.)* 334:33–46.

Conner, J. A., and Muller, W. (1991) Primary and secondary Ca^{2+} concentration changes resulting from transmitter stimulation in dendrites of neurons from the mammalian hippocampus. *Ann. N.Y. Acad. Sci.* 635:100–113.

Davies, S. N., Lester, R. A., Reymann, K. G., and Collingridge, G. L. (1989) Temporally distinct pre- and post-synaptic mechanisms maintain long-term potentiation. *Nature* 338:500–503.

Dolphin, A. C., Errington, M.L., and Bliss, T. V. P. (1982) Long-term potentiation of the perforant path in vivo is associated with increased glutamate release. *Nature* 297:496–497.

Duffy, C., Teyler, T. J., and Shashoua, V. E. (1981) Long-term potentiation in the hippocampal slice: Evidence for stimulated secretion of newly synthesized proteins. *Science* 212:1148–1151.

Foster, T. C., and McNaughton, B. L. (1991) Long-term enhancement of CA1 synaptic transmission is due to increased quantal size, not quantal content. *Hippocampus* 1:77–91.

Grover, L. M., and Teyler, T. J. (1990) Two components of LTP induced by different patterns of afferent activation. *Nature* 347:477–479.

Grover, L. M. and Teyler, T. J. (1992) N-methyl-D-aspartate receptor–independent long-term potentiation in area CA1 of rat hippocampus: Input specific induction and preclusion in a nontetanized pathway. *Neuroscience* 49:7–11.

Gustafsson, B., and Wigström, H. (1988) Physiological mechanisms underlying long-term potentiation. *Trends Neurosci.* 11:156–162.

Ito, M. (1990) Long-term depression in the cerebellum. *Semin. Neurosci.* 2:381–390.

Korn, H., and Faber, D. S. (1991) Quantal analysis and synaptic efficacy in the CNS. *Trends Neurosci.* 14:439–445.

Krug, M., Lossner, B., and Ott, T. (1984) Anisomycin blocks the late phase of long-term potentiation in the dentate gyrus of freely moving rats. *Brain Res. Bull.* 13:39–42.

Lynch, G. S., and Baudry, M. (1984) The biochemistry of memory: A new and specific hypothesis. *Science* 224:1057–1063.

Lynch, G. S., Larson, J., Kelso, S., Barrionuevo, G., and Schottler, F. (1983) Intracellular injections of EGTA block induction of hippocampal long-term potentiation. *Nature* 305:719–721.

Malenka, R. C., Kauer, J. A., Perkel, D. J., Mauk, M. D., Kelly, P. T., Nicol, R.A., and Waxham, M. N. (1989) An essential role for postsynaptic calmodulin and protein kinase activity in long-term potentiation. *Nature* 340:554–557

Malinow, R., and Tsien, R. W. (1990) Presynaptic enhancement shown by whole-cell recordings of long-term potentiation in hippocampal slices. *Nature* 346:177–181.

Malinow, R., Schulman, H., and Tsien, R. W. (1989) Inhibition of postsynaptic PKC or CaMKII blocks induction but not expression of LTP. *Science* 245:862–866.

Manabe, T., Renner, P., and Nicoll, R. S. (1992) Postsynaptic contribution to long-term potentiation revealed by the analysis of miniature synaptic currents. *Nature* 355:50–55.

McNaughton, B. L., Douglas, R. M., and Goddard, G. V. (1978) Synaptic enhancement in fascia dentata: Cooperativity among coactive elements. *Brain Res.* 157:277–293.

Morris, R. G. M., Anderson, E., Lynch, G. S., and Baudry, M. (1986) Selective impairment of learning and blockade of long-term potentiation by an N-methyl-D-aspartate receptor antagonist, AP5. *Nature* 319:774–776.

Sastry, B. R., Goh, J. W., and Auyeng, A. (1986) Associative induction of posttetanic and long-term potentiation in CA1 neurons of rat hippocampus. *Science* 232:998–990.

Schuman, E. M., and Madison, D. V. (1991) A requirement for the intercellular messenger nitric oxide in long-term potentiation. *Science* 254:1503–1506.

Sharp, P. E., McNaughton, B. L., and Barnes, C. A. (1985) Enhancement of hippocampal field potentials in rats exposed to a novel complex environment. *Brain. Res.* 339:361–365.

Stanton, P. K., and Sarvey, J. M. (1984) Blockade of long-term potentiation in rat hippocampal CA1 region hy inhibitors of protein synthesis. *J. Neurosci.* 4:3080–3088.

Stanton, P. K., and Sejnowski, T. J. (1989) Associative long-term depression in the hippocampus induced by Hebbian covariance. *Nature* 339:215–218.

Taube. J. S., and Schwartzkroin, P. A. (1987) Intracellular recording form hippocampal CA_1 interneuorns before and after development of long-term potentiation. *Brain Res.* 419:32–38.

Teyler, T. J., and DiScenna, P. (1984) Long-term potentiation as a candidate mnemonic device. *Brain Res. Rev.* 7:15–28.

Teyler, T. J., and DiScenna, P. (1987) Long-term potentiation. *Annu. Rev. Neurosci.* 10:131–161.

Teyler, T. J., Aroniadou, V., Berry, R. L., Borroni, A., DiScenna, P., Grover, L., and Lambert, N. (1990) LTP in neocortex. *Semin. Neurosci.* 2:365–380.

5　Long-term Potentiation: Biochemical Mechanisms

Michel Baudry and Gary Lynch

1　INTRODUCTION

The phenomenon of long-term potentiation (LTP) has in the past several years generated much excitement and controversy (Baudry and Davis, 1991; Landfield and Deadwyler, 1988). There are several reasons for this. First, this period witnessed an explosion of information about excitatory amino acids and their receptors (Mayer and Westbrook, 1987; Monaghan et al., 1989). Not surprisingly, after the successful cloning and sequencing of the acetylcholine, GABA, dopamine, and other neurotransmitter receptors, multiple families of glutamate receptors have been cloned, providing detailed information on their structures and properties. At the same time, a near consensus pharmacology of these receptors emerged and numerous drugs became available to tease out the relative contributions of different glutamate receptors in various experimental conditions. These events opened the way to the formulating and testing of hypotheses regarding the synaptic changes responsible for LTP. Second, a steady increase in the understanding of second messenger systems and of the complex interactions between them occurred during this period (Berridge and Irvine, 1984). This information, generated from studies on a wide array of biological systems, strengthened the notion that brain cells use regulatory devices shared with other cell types to perform operations unique to the synaptic environment. This general idea led to several concepts and tools that have been applied to the search for the cellular processes responsible for producing LTP. Finally, a major factor in the rapid progress over the last years has been a remarkable increase in the number of laboratories from molecular, cellular, organism, and cognitive neurosciences engaged in the analysis of LTP. Although numerous and excellent reviews of LTP have appeared recently (Baudry and Davis, 1991; Collingridge and Singer,1990; Kuba and Kumamoto, 1990; Teyler and DiScenna, 1987), we believe that the rapid progress in this field warrants an effort to provide an up-dated summary of the major findings as well as the theses and antitheses which have been generated to account for LTP. The chapter will start with a review of the characteristics of glutamatergic synapses with an emphasis on the properties of the glutamate receptors, which (as will become obvious later) are essential components of the mechanisms involved in triggering and maintaining LTP. This will be followed by a description of the mechanisms involved in LTP induction. A section will be devoted to the question of the time required for the establishment of a stable and permanent LTP, as several lines of evidence have demonstrated the role of a number of transient events in LTP formation. The problem of the mechanisms involved in LTP expression, a subject of intense controversy, will be addressed next. Finally, we will review data relevant to an issue not often discussed in the LTP literature, namely, the mechanisms that participate in the long-term maintenance of the modifications underlying the potentiation effect.

2 GLUTAMATERGIC TRANSMISSION

2.1 Glutamate as a Neurotransmitter

There is now little doubt that glutamate satisfies the criteria for a neurotransmitter. The major important advances that have been recently accomplished concern two of these criteria. The characterization of different classes of glutamate receptors and the identification of pharmacological compounds that compete with agonist binding to the receptors led to demonstrations that the receptors generate fast and slow excitatory postsynaptic currents in response to released neurotransmitter at identified synapses in many telencephalic loci (Mayer and Westbrook, 1987; Muller et al., 1988a; Sah et al., 1990). Second, the characteristics of glutamate release and transport have been partially clarified and these studies provided an answer to a question which had remained extremely difficult to resolve, whether glutamate or aspartate or a combination of both acidic amino acids is the neurotransmitter at excitatory synapses. It was found that, although both glutamate and aspartate share the same Na-dependent high-affinity transport system in plasma membranes, only glutamate is transported in synaptic vesicles by a Na-independent, ATP-driven transporter (Nicholls and Attwell, 1990). If one assumes that a vesicular localization is an additional criterion for a neurotransmitter candidate, this finding would strongly support the view that glutamate, but not aspartate, is the major excitatory neurotransmitter in the CNS.

2.2 Glutamate Receptors

At least three families of glutamate receptors have been identified by molecular, pharmacological, and physiological approaches and although there does not exist a general agreement concerning their nomenclature, we will use the classification based on agonist specificity, i.e. a triad of NMDA, AMPA and quisqualate (Quis) metabotropic receptors.

NMDA Receptors Pharmacological and electrophysiological studies have shown that the NMDA receptors exhibit a number of pharmacologically distinct domains (Watkins and Collingridge, 1989):

• a glutamate recognition site. This site is inhibited by several aminopho-sphono derivatives including amino-phosphono-pentanoate (AP-5) and acti-vated by several glutamate analogs including *N*-methyl-D-aspartate (NMDA) (Collingridge et al., 1983a, b; Lanthorn and Cotman, 1983).

• a glycine site. Increasing evidence indicates that glycine is a co-agonist of the receptors (Johnson and Ascher, 1987; Kleckner and Dingledine, 1988; Thomson, 1990); in particular, antagonists of glycine at this site, such as chlorokynurenate, block NMDA receptor function (Bashir et al., 1990; Kessler et al., 1989; Oliver et al., 1990), and it appears that the glycine and glutamate sites interact allosterically to control the opening of the NMDA receptor channel.

• a domain located within the channel that binds channel blockers such as phencyclidine and MK-801 (Foster and Wong, 1987; Huettner and Bean, 1988).

• a voltage-dependent Mg^{2+}-binding site that confers voltage dependency to the functioning of the NMDA receptor (Mayer et al., 1984; Nowack et al., 1984).

• one or more polyamine binding sites that regulate in part the rate of receptor desensitization (Lerma, 1992; Williams et al., 1991).

• a Zn^{2+} binding site (Westbrook and Mayer, 1987).

Furthermore, the channel gated by the NMDA receptor is permeant to calcium, adding yet another, but critical, feature to a remarkably complex entity (McDermott et al., 1986). The molecular characteristics of the receptor have been greatly clarified by the recent cloning of a cDNA which, after transcription and translation in oocytes, provided a functional NMDA recep-tor exhibiting most of the above characteristics (Moriyoshi et al., 1991). This suggests that a receptor is produced by a single polypeptidic chain, which contains the diverse domains described above. Analysis of the nucleotide sequence indicates that the NMDA R_1 receptor has some homology (overall 22−26%) with the AMPA receptors, and possesses a large extracellular do-main at the amino terminal, 4 transmembrane domains and a small intracellular domain at the carboxy terminal. Moreover, several phosphorylation sites for both protein kinase C (PKC) and calcium calmodulin kinase are located in the putative intracellular domains. More recently, three other members of an NMDA receptor family have been identified and in all likelihood others will be discovered shortly. Variants identified so far differ in terms of glycine regulation, Mg^{2+} blockade and cellular localization (Monyer et al., 1992).

AMPA Receptors   This receptor belongs to the class of ligand-gated chan-nels and is responsible for the fast EPSPs at excitatory synapses at many sites in mammalian brain. Important advances in the characterization of the AMPA receptor have resulted from the identification of a class of molecules, quinoxa-line derivatives, that are potent and relatively selective antagonists (Honore et al., 1988) as well as from the cloning of glutamate receptor subunits (Bettler et al., 1990; Boulter et al., 1990; Keinanen et al., 1990; Sommer et al., 1990). Pharmacological studies have not so far provided evidence for different subtypes of receptors except for the identification of a variant with high affinity for kainate (Monaghan et al., 1983; Patel et al., 1986; Represa et al., 1987). Binding studies detect a small number of high-affinity sites and a large number of low-affinity sites for AMPA in synaptic membrane fractions (Nielsen et al., 1990; Olsen et al., 1987; Terramani et al., 1988). Recent experiments indicate that these sites are likely to represent two states of the same receptors, with their affinity regulated by the local environment in synaptic membranes (Hall et al., 1992). Similarly, electrophysiological studies have revealed the existence of two groups of receptors, one with low conductance, slow desensitization, and activation at low concentrations of agonists (i.e., with a high affinity), and a second with high conductance, rapid desensitization, and a low affinity for agonists (Tang et al., 1989; Thio et al., 1991). The nootropic compound aniracetam decreases the rate of desensitization of the high conductance receptor (Isaacson and Nicoll, 1991; Tang et al., 1991) and comparisons of the drug's effect on single channels vs. excitatory postsynaptic currents indicates that synaptic receptors are high-conductance-state receptors and that the rate of desensitization determines the time course of the synaptic response (Tang et al., 1991).

Molecular approaches have shown the existence of a collection of related proteins that constitute a family of AMPA receptors. Six subunits have been cloned and designated as $GluR_{1-6}$; moreover, several of these subunits exist in two variants, designated as flip and flop, generated by alternate splicing of their encoding genes (Bettler et al., 1990; Boulter et al., 1990; Egebjerg et al., 1991; Keinanen et al., 1990; Monyer et al., 1911; Sommer et al., 1990; Werner et al., 1991). Each of the subunits is capable of forming homomeric ion channels with different characteristics, and receptors formed by the combination of different subunits exhibit properties that resemble those of AMPA receptors. Some combinations also exhibit calcium permeability of the ionic channel (Hollmann et al., 1991), and the functional properties of the receptors can be regulated by phosphorylation mediated by protein kinase A (Greengard et al., 1991). It has been hypothesized that the synaptic receptors are heteromeric proteins formed by a variety of combination of the subunits and that changes in the composition of the receptors might underlie various physiologically or pathologically related modifications of excitatory synapses (Monyer et al., 1991).

Quis Metabotropic Receptors   This receptor was first identified as a result of the stimulation by quisqualate of the inositol phosphate/Ca^{2+} pathway (Nicoletti et al., 1986; Palmer et al., 1988; Recasens et al., 1987; Sladeczek et al., 1985). This receptor ($mGluR_1$) is expressed abundantly in neonatal hippocampus and cortex and it has been proposed to participate in synapse formation. It is also present in glial cells where it may play important roles in neuron-glia signaling (Teichberg, 1991). Recently, molecular techniques have indicated the existence of a family of metabotropic glutamate receptors, which are coupled to G proteins but produce different signal transduction responses (Houamed et al., 1991; Masu et al., 1991; Tanabe et al., 1992). Although they have been implicated in the phenomenon of long-term depression in cerebellum (Ito, 1989), the lack of selective antagonists has hindered the efforts to understand the properties and functions of these receptors.

3 TRIGGERING MECHANISMS

In order to describe the cascade of events involved in LTP formation it is convenient to distinguish several different steps leading from triggering patterns of afferent activity to the establishment of stable potentiation.

3.1 Priming

One of the major advances of the last 5 years has been the realization that LTP is tightly linked with the theta rhythm, a prominent EEG pattern that appears in mammals engaged in exploratory behavior and that has long been suspected to be important in learning (Klemm, 1976; Landfield, 1976; Whishaw and Vanderwolf, 1973; Winson, 1990). This 5–7 Hz rhythm is readily apparent in much of the olfactory and limbic systems (Bland, 1986; Fox et al., 1986) and a rhythm of similar frequency is found in neocortex. Stimulation with short bursts that mimic a common discharge pattern of hippocampal neurons produces a robust and extremely stable LTP when the bursts are spaced apart by the period of the theta wave (Larson et al., 1986). Chronic recording studies have confirmed that cell activity patterns corresponding to the theta stimulation paradigm occur in hippocampus in rats during learning (Otto et al., 1991). Theta is related to LTP via its effects on inhibitory interneurons. IPSPs recorded in CA1 pyramidal neurons exhibit two components, a fast IPSP resulting from the activation of $GABA_A$ receptors and a slow IPSP produced by the activation of $GABA_B$ receptors coupled through a G protein to potassium channels. The fast IPSP normally prevents temporal summation of depolarization occuring during a short burst of stimulation. However, the fast IPSP is markedly reduced 200 msec following the activation of the feedforward interneurons, therefore allowing the temporal summation of depolarization if a burst occurs 200 msec later. This phenomenon has been called priming (Diamond et al., 1988; Larson and Lynch, 1986) and is due to the existence of $GABA_B$ receptors located on the presynaptic terminals of inhibitory interneurons which, when activated, mediate an inhibition of GABA release, and therefore a decreased postsynaptic inhibition of pyramidal cells (Davies et al., 1991; Mott and Lewis, 1991). The discovery of the priming phenomenon and of its underlying mechanisms provided a description of how brain activity related to learning can result in synaptic changes of the type assumed to encode memory.

3.2 NMDA Receptors

It is now clearly established that, at a variety of excitatory synapses, activation of NMDA receptors is a necessary and sufficient condition to trigger LTP. The priming mechanism, by allowing temporal summation of depolarization, relieves the NMDA receptor/channel from its voltage-dependent magnesium blockade. NMDA receptor antagonists do not modify EPSPs generated by low-frequency stimulation in the presence of magnesium at most glutamatergic synapses, but they decrease the burst response evoked following priming and prevent LTP triggered by stimulation with short, high-frequency bursts delivered at theta rhythm (Larson and Lynch, 1988). Conversely, the same pattern of stimulation performed in the presence of an antagonist of the AMPA receptor, such as DNQX, results in LTP once the antagonist is washed out (Kauer et al., 1988; Muller et al., 1988a). In vivo experiments have also shown that NMDA receptor antagonists totally blocked LTP induction without affecting basal synaptic transmission (Morris et al., 1986). In addition, antagonists of the glycine site of the NMDA receptors also block LTP induction in vitro as well as in vivo (Bashir et al., 1990; Oliver et al., 1990; Thiels et al., 1992). This result has been taken as evidence that glycine is a co-agonist with glutamate at the NMDA receptors.

3.3 Non-NMDA Receptor Mechanisms

Quis Metabotropic Receptor A number of reports have implicated the quis metabotropic receptor in the induction of LTP (Goh and Pennefather, 1989; Ito et al., 1988; Izumi et al., 1991). This is based mainly on the observation that a putative antagonist of the receptor, amino-phosphono-propionate (AP-3) blocks LTP induction in hippocampal slices. In addition, other experiments have linked metabotropic receptor activation to an increase in NMDA receptor-mediated response as a result of activation of protein kinase C (Aniksztejn et al., 1992). However, it is clear that AP-3 is not selective for the metabotropic receptors, and therefore the evidence connecting this receptor to LTP must be regarded as tentative.

Voltage-dependent Ca^{2+} Channels Teyler and colleagues (Grover and Teyler, 1990) have shown that LTP-like effects can be elicited by relatively long trains of high-frequency stimulation even in the presence of NMDA receptor antagonists. This effect is dependent on postsynaptic calcium, suggesting that a voltage-dependent channel can in some circumstances produce calcium elevations sufficient to activate the LTP-producing machinery. It needs to be noted that there are few agreed-upon descriptors of LTP and thus not all of the physiologically or pharmacologically induced increases in synaptic responses referred to as LTP are necessarily the same phenomenon. For example, the extreme stability that is the hallmark of LTP has only been tested in a small number of experiments (Staubli and Lynch, 1987) and cannot be assumed to be present when unusual stimulation conditions or experimental conditions are employed. The existence of non-LTP forms of facilitation lasting for at least a few hours is strikingly illustrated by studies on mossy fiber synapses. Potentiation in this system does not involve NMDA receptors (Harris and Cotman, 1986) or postsynaptic calcium (Zalutsky and Nicoll, 1990) and is associated with a reduction of paired-pulse facilitation (Staubli et al., 1990b), something that is not seen with LTP. Mossy fiber potentiation is thus likely to be a novel form of synaptic enhancement that superficially resembles LTP but in fact is unrelated to it. The possibility of confusing LTP with other phenomena is also raised by McNaughton and co-workers, who have suggested that at least some examples of potentiation induced in slices maintained at room temperature are reflections of processes not operative at body temperature (McNaughton et al., 1993). The issue of whether a given effect is LTP may prove to have been a serious problem in efforts to develop and test hypotheses regarding the substrates of the potentiation effect.

4   Development of LTP

4.1   Increase in Intracellular Ca^{2+}

It is now general agreed that an increase in the intracellular concentration of Ca^{2+} in postsynaptic structures is a critical factor to produce LTP. In particular intracellular injections of calcium chelators in CA1 pyramidal cells prevent LTP induction (Lynch et al., 1983), while intracellular release of Ca^{2+}, through photoactivation of a caged calcium complex, produces synaptic potentiation (Malenka et al., 1988). As the NMDA receptor/channel is permeant to calcium, it has generally been assumed that the rise in intracellular calcium concentration was provided by NMDA receptor activation. Recently, supplementary mechanisms have been proposed. First, some combinations of AMPA receptor subunits provide Ca^{2+} permeability in addition to the traditional Na^{+}/K^{+} permeability (Hollmann et al., 1991), suggesting that AMPA receptor activation could also lead to increased influx of calcium. However, the observation that blockers of AMPA receptors do not prevent LTP induction (Muller et al., 1988a) indicates that calcium entry through the AMPA receptor/channel is probably not critical for LTP induction. Second, activation of the quis metabotropic receptor, by increasing the synthesis of inositol-triphosphate (IP_3), might also elevate intracellular calcium via release of calcium from intracellular stores. As noted, available antagonists are not sufficiently selective to indicate whether the metabotropic receptor participates in LTP induction.

The duration and amplitude of the calcium signal is a question of great importance with regard to the nature of the Ca-dependent processes involved in the development of LTP. Direct visualization of calcium has recently been achieved using fluorescent techniques and indicates that calcium concentration remains elevated for several minutes in individual dendritic spines as a result of tetanic stimulation (Muller and Connor, 1991). Similar techniques show that the spine is relatively well isolated from calcium fluctuations taking place in dendrites possibly because of the spine apparatus (Fifkova, 1985; Guthrie et al., 1991). The question of the concentration of calcium reached as a result of repetitive stimulation is more difficult to answer. Although the visualization techniques demonstrate that an average calcium concentration in the low micromolar range is possible, they are not sensitive enough to allow an accurate determination of local concentrations, especially in submembrane domains. Computer simulations using realistic parameters for calcium pumps and channels have indicated the possibility that Ca^{2+} could reach much higher concentrations, although for very short periods of time (Holmes and Levy, 1990; Koch et al., 1992). It should also be noted that tests for calcium changes following the minimal stimulation needed to induce LTP have not been reported.

4.2   Role of Platelet-activating Factors and Phospholipase A_2

In cultured neurons, NMDA receptor stimulation and with it an influx of calcium activate phospholipase A_2 (PLA_2), the hydrolysis of membrane phospholipids, and the formation and release of arachidonic acid and its metabolites (Dumuis et al., 1988). Although the direct pathway leading from arachidonic acid to the platelet-activating factor (PAF) does not exist in the brain, alternate synthesis pathways beginning with PLA_2 exist, and thus NMDA receptor activation could lead to the synthesis and release of PAF. PAF causes a rapid and pronounced increase in calcium levels in hippocampal neurons via release from intracellular stores and perhaps an effect on membrane channels (Marcheselli et al., 1990; Shukla, 1992). One type of PAF receptor is extremely abundant in synaptic membranes and thus well positioned to elevate calcium concentrations in spines, an event that would activate the calcium sensitive PLA_2 and hence further synthesis of PAF. This positive feedback loop could represent one mechanism by which a brief activation of NMDA receptors could produce a long lasting increase in intracellular calcium (conceivably the several minutes revealed by fluorescent techniques). Recent pharmacological studies have provided evidence that PAF receptors do participate in formation of stable LTP (del Cerro et al., 1990a).

Is the duration of this signaling mechanism compatible with the time-course of LTP development? A number of approaches have been used to evaluate the necessary time to produce the nondecremental form of LTP observed in CA1 for instance (Gustafsson and Wigström, 1990; McNaughton, 1982) A general agreement is that it takes probably 1–5 min to produce stable LTP, and that events taking place during this period might interfere with LTP formation. In particular, when an hypoxic episode is applied within 1 to 2 min after tetanization, LTP was reversed (Arai et al., 1990). Applying the hypoxic episode later, while transiently depressing synaptic responses, did not reverse LTP. Although it is tempting to make analogies between the vulnerable phase of LTP development with the consolidation period defined by behavioral experiments, there are not enough data at this point to make definite conclusions.

4.3 Ca^{2+}-dependent Enzymes

A variety of Ca-dependent enzymes has been postulated to be implicated in the formation of LTP. As was discussed above, elevated levels of calcium are likely to be maintained possibly for minutes in postsynaptic structures and it is reasonable to assume that a wide range of Ca-dependent processes participate in the formation of LTP.

Ca^{2+}-dependent Proteases   In 1984, we proposed that the activation of calpain was an important step in the formation of LTP (Lynch and Baudry, 1984). Since then, additional evidence implicating calpain in the potentiation effect has emerged. First, calpain and one if its preferred substrates, the cytoskeletal spectrin, are localized in postsynaptic structures (Carlin et al., 1983; Perlmutter et al., 1988; Siman et al., 1985); thus, changes in calcium concentrations in dendritic spines to values greater than 1 μM are likely to trigger the protease. Second, stimulation of NMDA receptors produces a rapid proteolysis of spectrin, as evidenced by the accumulation of spectrin breakdown products with characteristics identical to those generated by calpain-mediated degradation of purified spectrin (Seubert et al., 1988). Finally, several calpain inhibitors have been shown by different laboratories to prevent LTP both in vivo and in vitro (del Cerro et al., 1900b; Denny et al., 1990; Oliver et al., 1989; Staubli et al., 1984) Protein kinase C is also a substrate of calpain, and the calpain-mediated partial proteolysis generates a constitutively active kinase, kinase M (Kajikawa et al., 1983). Although such a mechanism has been postulated to participate in LTP (Lovinger et al., 1987), more recent evidence does not support this hypothesis (Muller et al., 1990). In any event, by partially degrading cytoskeletal and cross-linking proteins, calpain is ideally suited to participate in the remodeling of postsynaptic structures that might contribute to the stability of LTP (see below).

Ca^{2+}-dependent Phospholipases   As noted, NMDA receptor activation results in the formation and release of arachidonic acid, a metabolite of phospholipids generated by a calcium-dependent phospholipase, phospholipase A$_2$. PLA$_2$ inhibitors have also been found to inhibit LTP both in vivo and in vitro (Lynch et al., 1989; Massicotte et al., 1900; Williams and Bliss, 1988, 1989) and PLA$_2$ has been linked to the regulation of the properties of the AMPA receptors. In particular, treatment of synaptic membranes from adult rat brain with PLA$_2$ results in an increased affinity for agonists to the AMPA receptors (Massicotte and Baudry, 1990). Furthermore, PLA$_2$-induced modification of AMPA receptors is not present in tissues in which LTP cannot be induced, such as after seizure activity or in the neonatal period (Baudry et al., 1991a; Massicotte et al., 1991) The effects of phospholipase treatment of synaptic membranes on the characteristics of the AMPA receptors are probably due to modifications of the lipid environment of the receptors, rather than to the formation of phospholipid metabolites, such as arachidonic acid. This interpretation is supported by the observation that incorporation of phosphatidylserine (PS) in synaptic membranes also results in an increased affinity of agonists for the AMPA receptors (Baudry et al., 1991b).

Ca^{2+}-dependent Kinases   The calcium–calmodulin-dependent protein kinase type II (CaM II kinase) is one of the most abundant proteins in postsynaptic membranes and as such its participation in mechanisms of synaptic plasticity has been widely discussed (Kennedy, 1989). Moreover, it exhibits some interesting and complex regulations of its properties through autophosphorylation that confers this enzyme characteristics of a biochemical switch. Inhibitors of the kinase are reported to inhibit LTP formation (Malenka et al., 1989; Malinow et al., 1988) and there is some evidence that its activity is increased for some period of time following LTP induction. Two recent publications reporting the results of studies using transgenic mice lacking the alpha subunit of CaM II kinase also support the idea that this kinase plays a critical role in LTP and learning (Silva et al., 1992a,b). How increases in kinase activity might increase synaptic activity is rarely discussed but it is likely to be part of a coordinated pattern of enzymatic events. Defining the nature of this pattern constitutes the essential challenge facing attempts to develop formal hypotheses of LTP induction. Considerable attention has also been given to the phospholipid-dependent calcium-dependent protein kinase, referred to as kinase C, and the question of its participation in LTP induction and/or maintenance has been a matter of intense controversy. The initial observation that LTP was accompanied by an increased phosphorylation of protein F$_1$, a substrate of PKC (Routtenberg, 1985), prompted speculation that PKC activation was a critical step in LTP formation (Routtenberg, 1991). Dramatic evidence for this idea came with reports that phorbol esters, compounds that activate PKC, produce LTP and that inhibitors of PKC reverse LTP without affecting control responses (Malenka et al., 1986; Malinow et al., 1989). These data were taken to indicate that PKC remains activated for long periods of time and in this way produces and maintains potentiation (Malinow et al., 1988). However, subsequent work showed that the response facilitation produced by phorbol esters reverses upon washout of the compounds (Muller et al., 1988b) and in critical regards is qualitatively distinct from LTP (Muller et al., 1990). Indeed, phorbol ester-induced potentiation does not interact with physiologically induced LTP, a result which strongly suggests that the mechanisms whereby PKC and LTP increase synaptic responses are orthogonal. Attempts to confirm that inhibitors of PKC have selective effects on potentiated responses have also proven negative. In all, it seems unlikely that PKC activity contributes to LTP expression. A direct role of the enzyme in inducing LTP is also questionable in light of evidence that activators and inhibitors of PKC depress the burst responses that trigger potentiation; however, a modulatory role through the phosphorylation of the NMDA receptor is not excluded. Finally, other Ca-dependent enzymes such as Ca-dependent transglutaminases (Friedrich et al., 1991) have also been proposed to participate in LTP formation.

5 EXPRESSION OF LTP

The mechanisms underlying LTP expression are usually discussed in terms of (1) presynaptic mechanisms resulting in increased transmitter release, (2) structural modifications producing changes in current flow through the spine complex and (3) postsynaptic mechanisms that could modify the properties of the neurotransmitter receptors.

5.1 Presynaptic Mechanisms

Several lines of arguments and experimentation have been used to support or oppose the idea that LTP expression is due to alterations in properties of presynaptic factors involved in regulating transmitter release. We have previously discussed certain of these arguments (Lynch and Baudry, 1991), and only a brief summary of the critical points will be made here.

Increased Transmitter Release   Bliss and colleagues have reported a series of experimental results, obtained primarily in the dentate gyrus, indicating that LTP is accompanied by an increase in the amount of glutamate release (Bliss and Lynch, 1988; Bliss et al., 1986, 1990; Dolphin et al., 1982). Evaluation of this conclusion has been hampered by uncertainties regarding the nature and localization of the pool of sampled glutamate. Furthermore, similar experiments performed in field CA1 found only a transient increase in glutamate release following LTP induction (Aniksztejn et al., 1989). Thus, attempts to directly measure transmitter release have failed to provide compelling evidence for a long-lasting change in presynaptic mechanisms.

Quantal Analysis   Over the years, numerous attempts have been made to apply physiological techniques and mathematical analyses (i.e., quantal analysis) for evaluating parameters describing transmitter release at the neuromuscular junction to central synapses and the problem of LTP. Experiments performed under different conditions yielded opposite results, with some indicating an increased quantal content (suggesting that LTP was associated with modification of transmitter release) (Bekkers and Stevens, 1990; Malinow and Tsien, 1990) while others indicated an increased quantal size (suggesting postsynaptic modifications) (Foster and McNaughton, 1991). The debate has now been enlarged to the question of whether traditional quantal analysis and models of transmitter release are appropriate for studies of central synapses.

Retrograde Messengers   The notion that LTP expression is due to a presynaptic modification while LTP induction requires the postsynaptic activation of NMDA receptors and a change in intracellular calcium concentration raised the issue of the existence of a retrograde messenger that would be released from postsynaptic sites and act presynaptically to produce a long-lasting modification of transmitter release. Two candidates have been proposed to play such a role, arachidonic acid and nitric oxide (NO). Evidence supporting a retrograde messenger role for arachidonic acid include the fact that, as was previously discussed, increased calcium concentration stimulates the activity of PLA_2, thus producing the hydrolysis of phospholipids and the release of arachidonic acid. In turn, arachidonic acid was shown to produce a slowly developing increase in EPSPs when applied exogenously in hippocampus in vitro or in vivo (Bliss et al., 1990; Williams et al., 1989). PLA_2 inhibitors such as nordihydroguaiaretic acid (NDGA) were also found to prevent LTP formation and to reverse LTP, suggesting the continuous need for arachidonic acid release in order to maintain LTP (Williams and Bliss, 1989). However, similar experiments using a different PLA_2 inhibitor, bromophenacyl bromide (BPB) did not produce the same results (Massicotte et al., 1990). More recently, NO has been proposed to be the retrograde messenger in both dentate gyrus and CA1 pyramidal cells (Bohme et al., 1991; Bredt and Snyder, 1992; O'Dell et al., 1991; Schuman and Madison, 1991). This idea was based on the fact that nitric oxide synthase (NOS), the enzyme synthesizing nitric oxide from the precursor arginine, is stimulated by calcium-calmodulin. In addition, inhibitors of NOS such as L-nitro-arginine, and NO scavengers, such as hemoglobin, have been reported to prevent LTP formation in hippocampal slices. Moreover, sodium nitroprusside and hydroxylamine, compounds that release NO, induce an LTP-like increase in EPSPs which occluded tetanus-induced LTP. However, this hypothesis faces a number of difficulties. First, NOS is not found in pyramidal cells and an enzyme with similar properties, NADPH diaphorase, is only found in scattered interneurons in CA1 (Bredt et al., 1991; Vincent and Kimura, 1992). Several laboratories have failed to reproduce the effects of inhibitors, and there is evidence that the drugs used to support the role of NO have effects unrelated to NO synthesis or availability (Fujimori and Pan-Hou, 1991; Kiedrowski et al., 1992). In all, the experimental evidence regarding contributions by NO and arachidonic acid to LTP is confusing and in any event cannot be interpreted as indicating the existence of retrograde messengers; that is, any postsynaptically generated messenger is as likely to act postsynaptically as presynaptically.

Evidence that LTP Is Not Expressed by Enhanced Transmitter Release
A variety of manipulations are known that increase release including paired-pulse facilitation, post-tetanic potentiation, compounds that prolong presynaptic calcium influx, drugs likely to influence calcium processing in the terminal, and changes in extracellullar calcium concentrations. These treatments interact with each other (i.e., they are not multiplicative in their effects, most likely because they act on the probability of a release event). Accordingly, if LTP increased the probability parameter of the release equation, it too should interact with the above manipulations. This does not occur (Muller and Lynch, 1989). Stronger evidence against a release explanation came with experiments in which the effects of LTP on the AMPA receptor-mediated component of the synaptic response were compared with those on the NMDA receptor-generated component (Kauer et al., 1988; Muller and Lynch, 1988; Muller et al., 1989). Since the receptors are localized in synapses, enhanced

release should stimulate greater populations of both NMDA and AMPA receptors. This point was confirmed in experiments showing that treatments that enhance release have larger effects on NMDA receptor-dependent vs. AMPA receptor-dependent components of the synaptic response (Muller and Lynch, 1989). In sharp contrast to this result, LTP enhances the AMPA receptor component with little or no effect on the NMDA receptor component. The above experiments did show that a measurable degree of potentiation could be induced in synaptic responses recorded under conditions in which AMPA receptors were blocked and NMDA receptor function enhanced. Subsequent studies confirmed this and demonstrated that intense stimulation enhances the effect (Bashir et al., 1991). Recent observations have called into question the extent to which the potentiation seen under these conditions corresponds to LTP. In any event, the very different effects of LTP on the two groups of postsynaptic glutamate receptors argue strongly that increased release is not involved.

5.2 Structural Modifications

Several laboratories have reported that LTP is accompanied by a variety of structural modifications affecting existing synapses as well as related to the formation of new synaptic contacts. These studies have been extensively reviewed recently (Wallace et al., 1991), and we will only briefly underline the major conclusions. Separate studies in field CA1 are in agreement that LTP does not cause detectable presynaptic alterations but does modify the numerical balance of synaptic types found on dendrites (Chang and Greenough, 1984; Lee et al., 1980). Morphological changes in spines have also been reported to occur in association with LTP in the dentate gyrus (Desmond and Levy, 1990). An essential question left unanswered by the electron microscopic studies is whether the observed effects are due to transformation of extant spines from one configuration to another vs. the formation of new contacts. Spine transformations, by reducing neck resistance, could possibly increase the flow of current from the synapse to the parent dendrite. However, this should work for both NMDA and AMPA receptor-mediated synaptic currents and, as described above, LTP has very different effects on these currents. Biophysical modeling studies have raised the possibility that neck resistance changes could differentially affect the driving force on fast vs. slow synaptic currents (Wilson, 1984). Experimental tests of this idea with regard to LTP have proven negative (Jung et al., 1991; Larson and Lynch, 1991). New contacts as an explanation for LTP could account for the differential effects of the potentiation effect on AMPA vs. NMDA receptor-mediated response components only if the added synapses were greatly deficient in NMDA receptors. Additional difficulties for the new synapse argument are descibed in the following section.

In summary, changes in the anatomy of the postsynaptic region appear to accompany LTP but are not likely to directly (i.e., via biophysical variables) potentiate synaptic currents. What role might they play in LTP? Spine configuration presumably reflects the organization of the spine cytoskeleton, and it is not unreasonable to assume that this latter variable affects the physiology/chemistry of the postsynaptic zone. Thus, the morphological alterations seen with LTP may be reflections of membrane cytoskeletal factors that indirectly influence the synaptic response.

5.3   Receptor Modifications

The selectivity of the increases in postsynaptic currents found with LTP is most easily explained by modifications selective to the AMPA receptor. Evidence supporting this idea (see Lynch and Baudry, 1984, for an early formulation) has been steadily accumulating over the last several years. First, recordings carried out under conditions in which inhibitory potentials and postsynaptic spiking were blocked revealed that LTP distorted the waveform of the synaptic responses and in particular changed its decay time constant (decay τ) (Ambros-Ingerson et al., 1991). The decay τ of synaptic currents is directly related to the mean open time of the receptor population (Magelby and Stevens, 1972), and this was confirmed for hippocampal synapses using a drug that slows the closing rate of AMPA receptor channels (Tang et al., 1991). Moreover, increasing the size of the responses by stimulating more synapses or enhancing release did not affect the decay τ, as expected for a variable dependent on the voltage-independent AMPA receptor ionophore. Thus, the observed change in decay τ with LTP provides direct evidence that potentiation influences the kinetic properties of the AMPA receptor channel. However, biophysical changes due to spine reconfiguration remain an alternative, if unlikely, explanation. Tests of this idea and of predictions from the receptor kinetic argument are in progress. Second, quantitative autoradiographic analyses of ligand binding to the receptors have indicated an increase in agonist binding in hippocampus following LTP induction in the perforant path to dentate gyrus pathway in anesthetized animals (Tocco et al., 1992). Moreover, when care was taken to restrict the extent of depolarization during the tetanus to the ipsilateral side of the hippocampus, the increase in binding in the molecular layer was well correlated with the magnitude of LTP (Maren et al., 1993). It should be noted that earlier attempts to demonstrate increased binding in slices of hippocampus following induction of LTP were not successful (Kessler et al., 1991). Tissue processing was different in these later studies vs. the above noted positive experiments and this is likely the source of the discrepancy. Nonetheless, these points need to be explored in detail before strong conclusions can be reached. Third, if LTP changes the properties of the receptors, then it would be expected to interact with at least some sets of non-LTP manipulations that also affect receptor functioning (i.e., LTP, by changing the receptor protein, should alter the physiological effects of at least some treatments directly targeted at the receptor). This prediction has been verified. Aniracetam is a nootropic drug that selectively increases currents mediated by AMPA receptors (Ito et al., 1990) by slowing the desensitization of the receptor channel (Isaacson and Nicoll, 1991; Tang et al., 1991). As expected from this, it increases the amplitude and prolongs the duration of synaptic currents mediated by the AMPA receptors. The effects of aniracetam on the amplitude and waveform of synaptic responses are quite different on potentiated vs. control responses (Staubli et al., 1990a). Changing the size of synaptic potentials by increasing release or partially blocking postsynaptic receptors does not alter the effects of aniracetam on synaptic responses or its interaction with expressed LTP (Xiao et al., 1991b). Results qualitatively similar to these have recently been reported using chaotropic ions which increase the affinity of AMPA receptors for various agonists (Shahi and Baudry, 1992). These ions increase the slope and amplitude of synaptic responses and have smaller effects on potentiated vs. control potentials.

In all, LTP changes response parameters dependent upon receptor channel kinetics, increases agonist binding in some circumstances, and alters the effects of drugs targeted at the AMPA receptor. Combined with the selective changes in postsynaptic currents produced by LTP, these data leave little doubt that expression of potentiation involves the AMPA receptor. Assembling these various observations into a unitary hypothesis of the precise type of receptor change underlying LTP remains a critical problem.

6 LONG-TERM MAINTENANCE

In addition to identifying the mechanisms responsible for LTP expression, an understanding of LTP requires the elucidation of the mechanisms involved in its long-term maintenance as LTP has been reported to least for several weeks in CA1 (Staubli and Lynch, 1987). This aspect of LTP is clearly the least understood one at present, although a few hypotheses have started to be explored.

6.1 Biochemical Switches

Several reports have developed the notion that certain enzymatic cascades exhibit properties of biochemical switches and could therefore provide potential mechanisms for LTP expression (Crick, 1984; Lisman and Goldring, 1988). The most extensively discussed of these enzyme cascades consists of the CaM II kinase which undergoes autophosphorylation and in its phosphorylated form does not require Ca^{2+} for activation (Miller and Kennedy, 1986). There is therefore the possibility, at least theoretically, that once autophosphorylated as a result of an influx of calcium, the CaM kinase remains activated for long periods of time and, by phosphorylating new enzyme copies, maintains the cascade beyond the time course of protein turnover. Kinases could potentially enhance synaptic responses by a direct or indirect (i.e., via other enzymes) action on AMPA receptors (Greengard et al., 1991) but there is little evidence for this in situ. That is, it has yet to be shown that kinase inhibitors reduce synaptic potentials or reverse LTP except as part of a generalized change in cell physiology. Moreover, it might be expected that conditions which transiently deplete ATP would break the circular kinase cascade and thus reverse fully expressed LTP. Against this is the observation that even prolonged episodes of anoxia applied 10 min or more after the induction of LTP do not reduce the potentiation found after slices have recovered from the anoxic episode (Arai et al., 1990). There is, however, good experimental evidence that PKC modulates NMDA receptor function and that such regulation might be important to adjust the threshold for LTP induction (Ben-Ari et al., 1992). Furthermore, since PLA$_2$ activity is subjected to inhibition by CaM II Kinase (Piomelli and Greengard, 1991), there is a link, even though indirect, between CaM II kinase and AMPA receptors.

6.2 Gene Expression and Protein Synthesis

Studies of synaptic plasticity in invertebrates have rejuvenated the notion that long-term changes in synaptic efficacy require modification of gene expression and that the triggering events are linked to the genomic apparatus and produce the induction (or possibly the repression) of genes (Goelet et al., 1986). Protein synthesis inhibitors have been reported to interfere with LTP (Deadwyler et al., 1987), but the specificity of these drugs is questionable. Moreover, the results could be taken as evidence that some background level proteins with rapid turnover (e.g., ornithine decarboxylase) are needed for LTP to occur. Newly synthesized proteins also appear to be released into the extracellular space following high-frequency stimulation (Fazeli et al., 1988; Otani et al., 1992); whether this is related to LTP as opposed to intense depolarization (a general problem for the studies of the biochemical correlates of LTP) remains to be determined. Steward as well as Greenough have observed that polyribosomes are often found at the base of dendritic spines in the dentate gyrus and suggested that these produce a means whereby localized protein synthesis might in some way contribute to LTP (Greenough et al., 1985; Steward and Levy, 1982). In support of this idea, high-frequency stimulation of the perforant path was found to change the aggregation state of polyribosomes in the molecular (dendritic) layer of the dentate gyrus (Desmond and Levy, 1990). It is not clear what contribution enhanced protein synthesis, even in regions proximal to activated synapses, might make to LTP. Given the rapidity with which LTP is expressed and made resistant to disruption, it is unlikely that new proteins contribute to events related to initial consolidation. The hypothesis that calcium-driven proteolysis is an essential step in the formation of stable LTP raises the possibility that replacement copies for digested and partially cleaved proteins are needed to "normalize" a potentiated configuration of the spine/synapse complex. Thus one could hypothesize the existence of a secondary stabilization period during which cytoskeletal and other such proteins are needed to anchor LTP.

Recent work using in situ hybridization and other molecular techniques has shown that intense physiological activity alters the expression of a variety of genes including those for neuroactive peptides and members of the neuro-trophin family (Gall et al., 1990, 1991; Isackson et al., 1991). In the latter case, stimulation conditions not far removed from those used to induce LTP were found to be sufficient. Other work indicates that high-frequency stimulation of the perforant path triggers a rapid and pronounced increase in the expression of certain immediate early genes (IEGs) and that this effect is blocked by NMDA receptor antagonists (Cole et al., 1989; Wisden et al., 1990). However, it appears that the IEG effect does not correlate with potentiation (Schreiber et al., 1991), casting doubt on its possible contribution to LTP.

While it is tempting to speculate that a gene cascade involving IEGs and growth factors contributes to the stabilization of LTP, enthusiasm for such suggestions has to be tempered by the synapse specificity of the potentiation effect. That is, it is difficult to envision how changes in gene expression could produce proteins that would selectively affect the tiny percentage of synapses on a given neuron that are involved in a single LTP episode. In all, physiologically induced changes in translation and transcription seem more likely to contribute to the general status of neurons rather than to individual episodes of synaptic plasticity.

6.3 Structural Modifications

The changes in spine number and spine shape that were discussed earlier could possibly participate in LTP maintenance as long as they are tied in with other mechanisms such as the change in AMPA receptor properties. For example, it is conceivable that a sessile-shape spine favors a certain configuration of the AMPA receptors as opposed to the mushroom-shape spine, which would confer a greater responsiveness to the receptor. We have previously discussed the possibility that the initial influx of calcium and the resulting activation of several calcium-dependent enzymes (proteases, phospholipases, kinases, etc.) play a critical role in the structural modifications of dendritic spines as these enzymes interact with cytoskeletal proteins, membrane phospholipids, and possibly membrane proteins (Baudry et al., 1987; Lynch and Baudry, 1987; Massicotte and Baudry, 1991). Thus, we argued that the structural modifications coupled with the change in receptor properties could be responsible for the maintenance and expression of LTP respectively.

6.4 Cell-adhesion Mechanisms

It has started to be recognized that cell-adhesion mechanisms could play important roles in adult systems as well as during development (Edelman, 1984; Schubert, 1991; Seki and Arai, 1991). The first evidence that such mechanisms could be involved in LTP came from experiments using the tripeptide arginine-glycine-glycine (RGG), which has been shown in several systems to inhibit the binding of extracellular matrix proteins (ECMs) to integrins. RGG was found to prevent LTP formation in adult hippocampal slices (Xiao et al.,

1991a). Since then it has been shown that synaptic membranes express high amounts of an RGG-binding protein which belongs to the family of integrin proteins (Bahr and Lynch, 1992; Bahr et al., 1991). These cell-adhesion molecules (N-CAMs) have been proposed to stabilize the changes in configuration produced during the initial phase of LTP and to maintain the new configuration. Moreover, it has also been found that N-CAMs are substrates of calcium-dependent proteases and that calpain actually removes the intracellular domain (Sheppard et al., 1991). Interestingly, proteins analog to N-CAM have recently been implicated in the mechanisms of synaptic plasticity in *Aplysia* (Mayford et al., 1992) and thus there is the possibility that cell-adhesion mechanisms play a ubiquitous role in mechanisms of synaptic plasticity.

7 CONCLUSION

It should be clear at this point that, although no definite answer has yet been proposed which could account for a full understanding of the molecular and cellular mechanisms involved in LTP, key elements of the answer have been identified. In particular, the mechanisms involved in LTP induction are fairly well understood. Although there still remains the possibility that some presynaptic mechanisms participate in LTP expression, there is overwhelming evidence that changes in some properties of the AMPA receptors contribute significantly to the increase in synaptic efficacy, and the next few years should provide a clearer identification of the nature of the changes in AMPA receptors. When this is achieved, it should be possible to propose a plausible mechanism incorporating the numerous enzymatic cascades that have been identified so far as playing some roles in LTP and thus in linking the initial change in intracellular calcium to the changes in AMPA receptors. Likewise, the coming years should provide important information concerning the mechanisms involved in the stabilization of LTP and in particular in the roles of adhesion molecules and of extracellular matrix proteins and their integrin receptors. There is thus the real possibility that the Decade of the Brain will indeed be characterized by the understanding of one of the greatest challenge for neuroscience, the mechanisms used by the brain to store information.

REFERENCES

Ambros-Ingerson, J., Larson, J., Xiao, P., and Lynch, G. (1991) LTP changes the waveform of synaptic responses. *Synapse* 9:314–316.

Aniksztejn, L., Roisin M. O., Amsellem, R., and Ben-Ari, Y. (1989) Long-term potentiation in the hippocampus of the anesthetized rat is not associated with a sustained enhanced release of endogenous excitatory amino acids. *Neuroscience* 28:387–92.

Aniksztejn, A., Otani, S., and Ben-Ari, Y. (1992) Quisqualate metabotropic receptors modulate NMDA currents and facilitate induction of long-term potentiation through protein kinase C. *Europ. J. Neurosci.* 4:500–505.

Arai, A., Larson, J., and Lynch, G. (1990) Anoxia reveals a vulnerable period in the development of long-term potentiation. *Brain Res.* 511:353–7.

Bahr, B., and Lynch, G. (1992) Purification of an Arg-Gly-Asp selective matrix receptor from brain synaptic plasma membranes. *Biochem. J.* 281:137–142.

Bahr, B., Sheppard, A., and Lynch, G. (1991) Fibronectin binding by brain synaptosomal membranes may not involve conventional integrins. *Neuro Report* 2:13–16.

Bashir, Z. I., Tam, B., and Collingridge, G. L. (1990) Activation of the glycine site in the NMDA receptor is necessary for the induction of LTP. *Neurosci. Lett.* 180:261–266.

Bashir, Z. I., Alford, S., Davies, S. N., Randall, A. D., and Collingridge, G. L. (1991) Long-term potentiation of NMDA receptor-mediated synaptic transmission in the hipposcampus. *Nature* 349:146–148.

Baudry, M. and Davis, J. L. (eds) (1991) *Long-Term Potentiation: A Debate of Current Issues.* MIT Press, Cambridge.

Baudry, M., Seubert, P. and Lynch, G. (1987) A possible second messenger system for the production of long-term changes in synapses. *Adv. Exp. Med. Biol.* 221:291–311.

Baudry, M., Massicotte, G., and Hauge, S. (1991a) Opposite effects of PLA_2 on ^3H-AMPA binding in adult and neonatal membranes. *Develop. Brain Res.* 61:265–267.

Baudry, M., Massicotte, G. and Hauge, S. (1991b) Phosphatidylserine increases the affinity of the AMPA/quisqualate receptor in rat brain membranes. *Behav. Neural Biol.* 55:137–140.

Bekkers, J. M., and Stevens, C. F. (1990) Presynaptic mechanism for long-term potentiation in the hippocampus. *Nature* 346:724–729.

Ben-Ari, Y., Aniksztejn, L., and Bregetovski, P. (1992) Protein kinase C modulation of NMDA currents: an important link for LTP induction. *Trends Neurosci.* 15:333–339.

Berridge, M. J., and Irvine, R. F. (1984) Inositol triphosphate, a second messenger in cellular signal transduction. *Nature* 312:315–21.

Bettler, B., Boulter, J., Hermans-Borgmeyer, I., O'Shea-Greenfield, A., Deneris, E. S., Moll, C., Borgmeyer, U., Hollmann, M., and Heinenmann, S. (1990) Cloning of a novel glutamate receptor subunit, Glu R5: Expression in the nervous system during development. *Neuron* 5:583–595.

Bland, B. H. (1986) The physiology and pharmacology of hippocampal formation theta rhytm. *Prog. Neurobiol.* 26:1–54.

Bliss, T. V. P., and Lynch, M. A. (1988). Long-term potentiation: mechanisms and properties. In P. W. Landfield and S. A. Deadwyler (eds)., *Long-Term Potentiation: From Biophysics to Behavior.* Alan Liss, New York, pp. 3–72.

Bliss, T. V. P., Douglas, R. M., Errington, M. L., and Lynch, M. A. (1986) Correlation between long-term potentiation and release of endogenous amino acids from dentate gyrus of anesthetized rats. *J. Physiol. (Lond.)* 337:391–408.

Bliss, T. V. P., Clements, M. P., Errington, M. L., Lynch, M. A., and Williams, J. (1990) Presynaptic changes associated with long-term potentiation in the dentate gyrus. *Semin. Neurosci.* 2:345–354.

Bohme, G. A., Bon, C., Stutzman, J. M., Doble, A., and Blanchard, A. (1991) Possible involvement of nitric oxide in long-term potentiation. *Europ. J. Pharmacol.* 199:379–381.

Boulter, J., Hollmann, M., O'Shea-Greenfield, A., Hartley, M., Deneris, E., Maron, C., and Heinemann, S. (1990) Molecular cloning and functional expression of glutamate receptor subunit genes. *Science* 249:1033–1037.

Bredt, D. S., and Snyder, S. H. (1992) Nitric oxide, a novel neuronal messenger. *Neuron* 8:3–11.

Bredt, D. S., Glatt, C. E., Hwang, P. M., Fotuhi, M., Dawson, T. M., and Snyder, S. H. (1991) Nitric oxide synthase protein and mRNA are discretely localized in neuronal populations of the mammalian CNS together with NADPH diaphorase. *Neuron* 7:615–624.

Carlin, R. K., Bartelt, D. C., and Siekevitz, P. (1983) Identification of fodrin as a major calmodulin-binding protein in postsynaptic density preparations. *J. Cell Biol.* 96:443–448.

Chang, F., and Greenough, W. T. (1984) Transient and enduring morphological correlates of synaptic activity and efficacy change in the rat hippocampal slice. *Brain Res.* 309:35–46.

Cole, A. J., Saffen, D. W., Baraban, J. M., and Worley, P. F. (1989) Rapid increase of an immediate early gene messenger RNA in hippocampal neurons by synaptic NMDA receptor activation. *Nature* 340:474–476.

Collingridge, G. L. and Singer, W. (1990) Excitatory amino acid receptors and synaptic plasticity. *Trends Pharmacol. Sci.* 11:290–296.

Collingridge, G. L., Kehl, S. J., and McLennan, H. (1983a) The antagonism of amino acid–induced excitations of rat hippocampal CA1 neurones in vitro. *J. Physiol. (Lond.)* 334:19–31.

Collingridge, G. L., Kehl, S. J. and McLennan, H. (1983b) Excitatory amino acids in synaptic transmission in the Schaffer collateral-commissural pathway of the rat hippocampus. *J. Physiol. (Lond.)* 334:33–46.

Crick, F. (1984) Memory and molecular turn-over. *Nature* 312:101.

Davies, C. H., Starkey, S. J., Pozza, M. F., and Collingridge, G. L. (1991) $GABA_B$ autoreceptors regulate the induction of LTP. *Nature* 349:609–611.

Deadwyler, S. A., Dunwiddie, T., and Lynch, G. (1987) A critical level of protein synthesis is required for long-term potentiation. *Synapse* 1:90–95.

del Cerro, S., Arai, A., and Lynch, G. (1990a) Inhibition of long-term potentiation by an antagonist of platelet-activating factor receptors. *Behav. Neural Biol.* 54:213–217.

del Cerro, S., Larson, J., Oliver, M. W. and Lynch, G. (1990b) Development of hippocampal long-term potentiation is reduced by recently introduced calpain inhibitors. *Brain Res.* 530:91–95.

Denny, J. B., Polan-Curtain, J., Ghuman, A., Wayner, M. J., and Armstrong, D. L. (1990) Calpain inhibitors block long-term potentiation. *Brain Res.* 534:317–320.

Desmond, N. L., and Levy, W. B. (1990) Morphological correlates of long-term potentiation imply the modification of existing synapses, not synaptogenesis, in the hippocampal dentate gyrus. *Synapse* 5:139–43.

Diamond, D. M., Dunwiddie, T. V., and Rose, G. M. (1988) Characteristics of hippocampal primed burst potentiation in vitro and in the awake rat. *J. Neurosci.* 8:4079–4088.

Dolphin, A. C., Errington, M. L., and Bliss, T. V. (1982) Long-term potentiation of the perforant path in vivo is associated with increased glutamate release. *Nature* 297:496–498.

Dumuis, A., Sebben, M., Haynes, L., Pin, J. P., and Bockaert, J. (1988) NMDA receptors activate the arachidonic acid cascade system in striatal neurons. *Nature* 336:69–70.

Edelman, G. M. (1984) Modulation of cell adhesion during induction, histogenesis, and perinatal development of the nervous system. *Annu. Rev. Neurosci.* 7:339–377.

Egebjerg, J., Bettler, B., Hermans, B. I., and Heinemann, S. (1991) Cloning of a cDNA for a glutamate receptor subunit activated by kainate but not AMPA. *Nature* 351:745–748.

Fazeli, M. S., Errington, M. L., Dolphin, A. C., and Bliss, T. V. (1988) Long-term potentiation in the dentate gyrus of the anaesthetized rat is accompanied by an increase in protein efflux into push-pull cannula perfusates. *Brain Res.* 473:51–59.

Fifkova, E. (1985) Possible mechanism of morphometric changes in dendritic spines induced by stimulation. *Cell Mol. Neurobiol.* 5:47–63.

Foster, A. C., and Wong, E. H. F. (1987) The novel anticonvulsant MK-801 binds to the activated state of the N-methyl-D-aspartate receptor in rat brain. *Br. J. Pharmacol.* 91:403–409.

Foster, T. C., and McNaughton, B. L. (1991) Long-term synaptic enhancement in CA1 is due to increased quantal size, not quantal content. *Hippocampus* 1:79–91.

Fox, S. E., Wolfson, S., and Ranck, J. B. (1986) Hippocampal theta rhythm and the firing of neurons in walking and urethane-anesthetized rats. *Exp. Brain Res.* 62:495–508.

Friedrich, P., Fesus, L., Tarcsa, E., and Czeh, G. (1991) Protein cross-linking by transglutaminase induced in long-term potentiation in the CA1 region of hippocampal slices. *Neuroscience* 43:331–334.

Fujimori, H., and Pan-Hou, H. (1991) Effect of nitric oxide on L-[^{3}H]glutamate binding to rat brain synaptic membranes. *Brain Res.* 554:355–357.

Gall, C. M., Lauterborn, J., Isackson, P., and White, J. (1990) Seizures, neuropeptide regulation, and mRNA expression in the hippocampus. *Prog. Brain Res.* 83:371–390.

Gall, C. M., Murray, K., and Isackson, P. (1991) Kainic acid-induced seizures stimulate increased expression of nerve growth factor mRNA in rat hippocampus. *Mol. Brain Res.* 9:113–123.

Goelet, P., Castellucci, V. F., Schcher, S., and Kandel, E. R. (1986) The long and the short of long-term memory—a molecular framework. *Nature* 322:419–422.

Goh, J. W., and Pennefather, P. S. (1989) A pertussis toxin-sensitive G protein in hippocampal long-term potentiation. *Science* 244:980–983.

Greengard, P., Jen, J., Nairn, A. C., and Stevens, C. F. (1991) Enhancement of the glutamate receptor response by cAMP dependent protein kinase in hippocampal neurons. *Science* 253:1135–1138.

Greenough, W. T., Larson, J., and Withers, G. (1985) Effects of unilateral and bilateral training in a teaching task on dendritic branching of neurons in the rat somato-sensory forelimb cortex. *Behav. Neural Biol.* 44:301–314.

Grover, L. M., and Teyler, T. (1990) Two components of long-term potentiation induced by different patterns of afferent activation. *Nature* 347:477–479.

Gustafsson, B., and Wigström, H. (1990) Long-term potentiation in the hippocampal CA1 region: Its induction and early temporal development. *Prog. Brain Res.* 83:223–232.

Guthrie, P. B., Segal, M., and Kater, S. B. (1991) Independent regulation of calcium revealed by imaging dendritic spines. *Nature* 354:76–80.

Hall, R., Kessler, M., and Lynch, G. (1992) Evidence that high and low affinity AMPA binding sites reflect membrane-dependent states of a single receptor. *J. Neurochem.* 59:1997–2004.

Harris, E. W. and Cotman, C. W. (1986) Long-term potentiation of guinea pig mossy fiber responses is not blocked by N-methyl-D-aspartate receptor antagonists. *Neurosci. Lett.* 70:132–137.

Hollmann, M., Hartley, M., and Heinemann, S. (1991) Ca^{2+} permeability of KA-AMPA–gated glutamate receptor channels depends on subunit composition. *Science* 252:851–853.

Holmes, W. R., and Levy, W. B. (1990) Insights into associative long-term potentiation from computational models of NMDA receptor-mediated calcium influx and intracellular calcium concentration changes. *J. Neurophysiol.* 6:1148–1168.

Honore, T., Davies, S. N., Drejer, J., Fletcher, E. J., Jacobsen, P., Lodge, D., and Nielsen, F. E. (1988) Quinoxalinediones: Potent competitive non-NMDA glutamate antagonists. *Science* 241:701–703.

Houamed, K. M., Kuijper, J. L., Gilbert, T. L., Haldeman, B. A., O'Hara, P. J., Mulvihill, E. R., Almers, W., and Hagen, F. S. (1991) Cloning, expression, and gene structure of a G-protein–coupled glutamate receptor from rat brain. *Science* 252:1318–1321.

Huettner, J. E., and Bean, B. P. (1988) Block of *N*-methyl-D-aspartate-activated current by the anticonvulsant MK-801: Selective binding to open channels. *Proc. Natl. Acad. Sci. USA* 85:1307–1311.

Isaacson, J. S., and Nicoll, R. A. (1991) Aniracetam reduces glutamate receptor desensitization and slows the decay of fast excitatory synaptic currents in the hippocampus. *Proc. Natl. Acad. Sci. USA* 88:10936–10940.

Isackson, P., Huntsman, M. M., Murray, K. D., and Gall, C. M. (1991) BDNF mRNA expression is increased in adult rat forebrain after limbic seizures: Temporal patterns of induction distinct from NGF. *Neuron* 6:937–948.

Ito, I., Okada, D., and Sugiyama, H. (1988) Pertussis toxin supresses long-term potentiation of hippocampal mossy fiber synapses. *Neurosci. Lett.* 90:181–185.

Ito, I., Tanabe, S., Khoda, A., and Sugiyama, H. (1990) Allosteric potentiation of quisqualate receptors by a nootropic drug aniracetam. *J. Physiol.* 424:533–543.

Ito, M. (1989) Long-term depression. *Annu. Rev. Neurosci.* 12:85–102.

Izumi, Y., Clifford, D. B., and Zorumski, C. F. (1991) 2-Amino-3-phosphonoprionate blocks the induction and maintenance of long-term potentiation in rat hippocampal slices. *Neurosci. Lett.* 122:187–190.

Johnson, J. W., and Ascher, P. (1987) Glycine potentiates the NMDA response in cultured mouse brain neurons. *Nature* 325:529–531.

Jung, M. W., Larson, J., and Lynch, G. (1991) Evidence that changes in spine neck resistance are not responsible for expression of LTP. *Synapse* 7:216–220.

Kajikawa, N., Kishimoto, A., Shiota, M., and Nishizuka, Y. (1983) Ca^{2+}-dependent neutral protease and proteolytic activation of Ca^{2+}-activated, phospholipid-dependent protein kinase. *Methods Enzymol.* 102:279–290.

Kauer, J. A., Malenka, R. C., and Nicoll, R. A. (1988) A persistent postsynaptic modification mediates long-term potentiation in the hippocampus. *Neuron* 1:911–917.

Keinanen, K., Wisden, W., Sommer, B., Werner, P., Herb, A., Verdoorn, T. A., Sakmann, B., and Seeburg, P. H. (1990) A family of AMPA-selective glutamate receptors. *Science* 249:556–560.

Kennedy, M. B. (1989) Regulation of synaptic transmission in the central nervous system: Long-term potentiation. *Cell* 59:777–787.

Kessler, M., Terramani, T., Lynch, G., and Baudry, M. (1989) A glycine site associated with *N*-methyl-D-aspartic acid receptors: Characterization and identification of a new class of antagonists. *J. Neurochem.* 52:1319–1328.

Kessler, M., Arai, A., Vanderklish, P., and Lynch, G. (1991) Failure to detect changes in AMPA receptor binding after long-term potentiation. *Brain Res.* 560:337–341.

Kiedrowski, L., Costa, E., and Wroblewski, J. T. (1992) Sodium nitroprusside inhibits *N*-methyl-D-aspartate–evoked calcium influx via a nitric oxide- and cGMP-independent mechanism. *Mol. Pharmacol.* 41:779–784.

Kleckner, N. W., and Dingledine, R. (1988) Requirement for glycine in activation of NMDA receptors expressed in *Xenopus* oocytes. *Science* 241:835–837.

Klemm, W. R. (1976) Hippocampal EEG and information processing: A special role for theta rhythm. *Prog. Neurobiol.* 7:197–214.

Koch, C., Zador, A., and Brown, T. H. (1992) Dendritic spines: Convergence of theory and experiments. *Science* 256:973–974.

Kuba, K., and Kumamoto, E. (1990) Long-term potentiation in vertebrate synapses: A variety of cascades with common subprocesses. *Prog. Neurobiol.* 34:197–269.

Kumar, K.-N., Tilakaratne, N., Johnson, P.-S., Allen, A.-E., and Michaelis, E.-K. (1991) Cloning of cDNA for the glutamate-binding subunit of an NMDA receptor complex. *Nature* 354:70–73.

Landfield, P. W. (1976). Synchronous EEG rhythms: Their nature and possible function in memory. In W. H. Gispen (ed.), *Molecular and Functional Neurobiology*. Elsevier, Amsterdam.

Landfield, P. W., and Deadwyler, S. A. (eds.) (1988) *Long-Term Potentiation: From Biophysics to Behavior*. Alan Liss, New York.

Lanthorn, T. H., and Cotman, C. W. (1983) Relative potency of analogues of excitatory amino acids on hippocampal CA1 neurons. *Neuropharmacology* 22:1343–1348.

Larson, J., and Lynch, G. (1986) Induction of synaptic potentiation in hippocampus by patterned stimulation involves two events. *Science* 232:985–988.

Larson, J., and Lynch, G. (1988) Role of N-methyl-D-aspartate receptors in the induction of synaptic potentiation by burst stimulation patterned after the hippocampal theta rhythm. *Brain Res.* 441:111–118.

Larson, J., and Lynch, G. (1991) A test of the spine resistance hypothesis for LTP expression. *Brain Res.* 538:347–350.

Larson, J., Wong, D., and Lynch, G. (1986) Patterned stimulation at the theta frequency is optimal for induction of long-term potentiation. *Brain Res.* 368:347–350.

Lee, K., Schottler, F., Oliver, M., and Lynch, G. (1980) Brief bursts of high frequency stimulation produce two types of structural changes in rat hippocampus. *J. Neurophysiol.* 44:247–258.

Lerma, J. (1992) Spermine regulates N-methyl-D-aspartate receptor desensitization. *Neuron* 8:343–352.

Lisman, J. E., and Goldring, M. A. (1988) Feasibility of long-term storage of graded information by the Ca^{++}/calmodulin dependent protein kinase molecules of the post-synaptic density. *Proc. Natl. Acad. Sci. USA* 83:5320–5324.

Lovinger, D. M., Wong, K. L., Murakami, K., and Routtenberg, A. (1987) Protein kinase C inhibitors eliminate hippocampal long-term potentiation. *Brain Res.* 436:177–183.

Lynch, G., and Baudry, M. (1984) The biochemical basis of learning and memory: A new and specific hypothesis. *Science* 224:1057–1063.

Lynch, G., and Baudry, M. (1987) Brain spectrin, calpain and long-term changes in synaptic efficacy. *Brain Res. Bull.* 18:809–815.

Lynch, G., and Baudry, M. (1991) Re-evaluating the constraints on hypothesis regarding LTP expression. *Hippocampus* 1:9–14.

Lynch, G., Larson, J., Kelso, S., Barrionuevo, G., and Schottler, F. (1983) Intracellular injections of EGTA block induction of hippocampal long-term potentiation. *Nature* 305:20–26.

Lynch, M. A., Errington, M. L., and Bliss, T. V. (1989) Nordihydroguaiaretic acid blocks the synaptic component of long-term potentiation and the associated increases in release of glutamate and arachidonate: An in vivo study in the dentate gyrus of the rat. *Neuroscience* 30:693–701.

Magelby, K. L., and Stevens, C. F. (1972) A quantitative description of end-plate currents. *J. Physiol.* 223:173–197.

Malenka, R. C., Madison, D. B., and Nicoll, R. A. (1986) Potentiation of synaptic transmission in the hippocampus by phorbol esters. *Nature* 321:175–177.

Malenka, R. C., Kauer, J. A., Zucker, R. S., and Nicoll, R. A. (1988) Postsynaptic calcium is sufficient for potentiation of hippocampal synaptic transmission. *Science* 242:81–84.

Malenha, R. C., Kauer, J. A., Perkel, D. J., Mauk, M. D., Kelly, P. T., Nicoll, R. A., and Waxham, M. N. (1989) An essential role for postsynaptic calmodulin and protein kinase activity in long-term potentiation. *Nature* 340:554–557.

Malinow, R., and Tsien, R. W. (1990) Presynaptic enhancement shown by whole-cell recordings of long-term potentiation in hippocampal slices. *Nature* 346:177–180.

Malinow, R., Madison, D. V., and Tsien, R. W. (1988) Persistent protein kinase activity underlying long-term potentiation. *Nature* 335:820–824.

Malinow, R., Schulman, H., and Tsien, R. W. (1989) Inhibition of postsynaptic PKC or CaMKII blocks induction but not expression of LTP. *Science* 245:862–866.

Marcheselli, V. L., Rossowska, M. J., Domingo, M. T., Braquet, P., and Bazan, N. G. (1990) Distinct platelet-activating factor binding sites in synaptic endings and in intracellular membranes of rat cerebral cortex. *J. Biol. Chem.* 265:9140–9145.

Maren, S., Tocco, G., Standley, S., Baudry, M., and Thompson, R. F. (1993) Postsynaptic factors in the expression of long-term potentiation (LTP): Increased glutamate receptor binding following LTP induction in vivo. *Proc. Natl. Acad. Sci. USA*, in press.

Massicotte, G., and Baudry, M. (1990) Modulation of AMPA/quisqualate receptors by phospholipase A2 treatment. *Neurosci. Lett.* 118:245–248.

Massicotte, G., and Baudry, M. (1991) Triggers and substrates of hippocampal synaptic plasticity. *Neuro. Biobehav. Rev.* 15:415–423.

Massicotte, G., Oliver, M. W., Lynch, G., and Baudry, M. (1990) Effect of bromophenacylbromide, a phospholipase A_2 inhibitor, on the induction and maintenance of LTP in hippocampal slices. *Brain Res.* 537:49–53.

Massicotte, G., Vanderklish, P., Lynch, G., and Baudry, M. (1991) Modulation of AMPA/quisqualate receptors by phospholipase A_2: A necessary step in long-term potentiation. *Proc. Natl. Acad. Sci. USA* 88:1893–1897.

Masu, M., Tanabe, Y., Tsuchida, K., Shigemoto, R., and Nakanishi, S. (1991) Sequence and expression of a metabotropic glutamate receptor. *Nature* 349:760–765.

Mayer, M. L., and Westbrook, G. L. (1987) The physiology of excitatory amino acids in the vertebrate central nervous system. *Prog. Neurobiol.* 28:197–276.

Mayer, M. L., Westbrook, G. L., and Guthrie, P. B. (1984) Voltage-dependent block by Mg^{++} of NMDA responses in spinal cord neurones. *Nature* 309:261–263.

Mayford, M., Barzilai, A., Keller, F., Schacher, S., and Kandel, E. R. (1992) Modulation of an N-CAM-related adhesion molecule with log-term synaptic plasticity in *Aplysia*. *Science* 256:638–644.

McDermott, A. B., Mayer, M. L., Westbrook, G. L., Smith, S. J., and Barker, J. L. (1986) NMDA-receptor activation increases cytoplasmic calcium concentration in cultured spinal cord neurons. *Nature* 321:519–522.

McNaughton, B. L. (1982) Long-term synaptic enhancement and short-term potentiation in rat fascia dentata act through different mechanisms. *J. Physiol. (Lond.)* 324:249–262.

McNaughton, B. L., Shen, J., Rao, G., Foster, T. C., and Barnes, C. A. (1993) Increased CA1 axon terminal excitability following repetitive electrical stimulation: Dependence on NMDA receptor activity, nitric oxide synthase, and temperature. *Proc. Natl. Acad. Sci. USA*, in press.

Miller, S., G., and Kennedy, M. B. (1986) Regulation of brain type II Ca^{++}/calmodulin–dependent protein kinase by autophosphorylation: A Ca^{++} triggered molecular switch. *Cell* 44:861–870.

Monaghan, D. T., Holets, V. R., Toy, D. W., and Cotman, C. W. (1983) Anatomical distributions of four pharmacologically distinct ^{3}H-L-glutamate binding sites. *Nature* 306:10–16.

Monaghan, D. T., Bridges, R. J., and Cotman, C. W. (1989). The excitatory amino acid receptors: Their classes, pharmacology, and distinct properties in the function of the central nervous system. *Annu. Rev. Pharmacol. Toxicol.* 29:365–402.

Monyer, H., Seeburg, P. H., and Wisden, W. (1991) Glutamate-operated channels: Developmentally early and mature forms arise by alternative splicing. *Neuron* 6:799–810.

Monyer, H., Sprengel, R., Schoepfer, R., Herb, A., Higuchi, M., Lomeli, H., Burnashev, N., Sakmann, B., and Seeburg, P. H. (1992) Heteromeric NMDA receptors: Molecular and functional distinction of subtypes. *Science* 256:1217–1221.

Moriyoshi, K., Masu, M., Ishii, T., Shigemoto, R., Mizuno, N., and Nakanishi, S. (1991) Molecular cloning and characterization of the NMDA receptor. *Nature* 354:31–37.

Morris, R. G. M., Anderson, E., Lynch, G. S., and Baudry, M. (1986) Selective impairment of learning and blockade of long-term potentiation by the N-methyl-D-aspartate receptor antagonist, AP-5. *Nature* 319:774–776.

Mott, D. D., and Lewis, D. V. (1991) Facilitation of the induction of long-term potentiation by $GABA_B$ receptors. *Science* 252:1718–1720.

Muller, D., and Lynch, G. (1988) Long-term potentiation differentially affects two components of synaptic responses in hippocampus. *Proc. Natl. Acad. Sci. USA* 85:9346–9350.

Muller, D., and Lynch, G. (1989) Evidence that changes in presynaptic calcium currents are not responsible for long-term potentiation in hippocampus. *Brain Res.* 479:290–299.

Muller, D., Joly, M., and Lynch, G. (1988a) Contributions of quisqualate and NMDA receptors to the induction and expression of LTP. *Science* 242:1694–1697.

Muller, D., Turnbull, J., Baudry, M., and Lynch, G. (1988b) Phorbol ester-induced synaptic facilitation is different than long-term potentiation. *Proc. Natl. Acad. Sci. USA* 85:6997–7000.

Muller, D., Larson, J., and Lynch, G. (1989) The NMDA receptor-mediated components of responses evoked by patterned stimulation are not increased by long-term potentiation. *Brain Res.* 477:1–2.

Muller, D., Buchs, P.-A., Dunant, Y., and Lynch, G. (1990) Protein kinase C activity is not responsible for the expression of long-term potentiation in hippocampus. *Proc. Natl. Acad. Sci. USA* 87:4073–4077.

Muller, W., and Connor, J. A. (1991) Dendritic spines as individual neuronal compartments for synaptic Ca^{++} responses. *Nature* 354:73–76.

Nicholls, D., and Attwell, D. (1990) The release and uptake of excitatory amino acids. *Trends Pharmacol. Sci.* 11:462–468.

Nicoletti, F., Iadarola, J. J., Wroblewski, J. T., and Costa, E. (1986) Excitatory amino acid recognition sites coupled with inositol phospholipid metabolism: Developmental changes and interaction with α-adrenoreceptors. *Proc. Natl. Acad. Sci. USA* 83:1931–1935.

Nielsen, E. O., Drejer, J., Cha, J. H., Young, A. B., and Honore, T. (1990) Autoradiographic characterization and localization of quisqualate binding sites in rat brain using the antagonist [^{3}H]6-cyano-7-nitroquinoxaline-2,3-dione: Comparison with (R,S)-[^{3}H]alpha-amino-3-hydroxy-5-methyl-4-isoxazolepropionic acid binding sites. *J. Neurochem.* 54:686–695.

Nowack, L., Bregestovski, P., Ascher, P., Herbert, A., and Prochiantz, A. (1984) Magnesium gates glutamate-activated channels in mouse central neurones. *Nature* 307:462–465.

O'Dell, T. J., Hawkins, R. D., Kandel, E. R., and Arancio, O. (1991) Tests of the roles of two diffusible substances in long-term potentiation: Evidence for nitric oxide as a possible early retrograde messenger. *Proc. Natl. Acad. Sci. USA* 88:11285–11289.

Oliver, M. W., Baudry, M., and Lynch, G. (1989) The protease inhibitor leupeptin interferes with the development of LTP in hippocampal slices. *Brain Res.* 505:233–238.

Oliver, M. W., Kessler, M., Larson, J., Schottler, F., and Lynch, G. (1990) Glycine site associated with the NMDA receptor modulates long-term potentiation. *Synapse* 5:265–270.

Olsen, R. W., Szamraj, O., and Houser, C. R. (1987) [^{3}H]AMPA binding to glutamate receptor subpopulations in rat brain. *Brain Res.* 402:243–254.

Otani, S., Roisin-Lallemand, M. P., and Ben-Ari, Y. (1992) Enhancement of extracellular protein concentrations during long-term potentiation in the rat hippocampal slice. *Neuroscience* 47:265–272.

Otto, T., Eichenbaum, H., Wiener, S., and Wible, C. (1991) Learning-related patterns of CA1 spike trains parallel stimulation parameters optimal for inducing long-term potentiation. *Hippocampus* 1:181–192.

Palmer, E., Monaghan, D. T., and Cotman, C. W. (1988) Glutamate receptors and phosphoinositide metabolism/stimulation via quisqualate receptors is inhibited by *N*-methyl-D-aspartate receptor activation. *Mol. Brain Res.* 4:161–165.

Patel, S., Meldrum, B. S., and Collins, J. F. (1986) Distribution of ^{3}H-kainic acid binding sites in the rat brain: In vivo and in vitro receptor autoradiography. *Neurosci. Lett.* 70:301–307.

Perlmutter, L. S., Siman, R., Gall, C., Seubert, P., Baudry, M., and Lynch, G. (1988) The ultrastructural localization of calcium-activated protease "calpain" in rat brain. *Synapse* 2:79–88.

Piomelli, D., and Greengard, P. (1991) Bidirectional control of phospholipase A2 activity by Ca^{++}/calmodulin-dependent protein kinase II, cAMP-dependent protein kinase, and casein kinase II. *Proc. Natl. Acad. Sci. USA* 88:6770–6774.

Recasens, M., Sassetti, I., Nourigat, A., Sladeczek, F., and Bockaert, J. (1987) Characterization of subtypes of excitatory amino acid receptors involved in the stimulation of inositol phosphate synthesis in rat brain synaptoneurosomes. *Europ. J. Pharmacol.* 141:87–93.

Represa, A., Tremblay, E., and Ben-Ari, Y. (1987) Kainate binding sites in the hippocampal mossy fibers: Localization and plasticity. *Neuroscience* 20:739–748.

Routtenberg, A. (1985) Protein kinase C activation leading to protein F1 phosphorylation may regulate synaptic plasticity by presynaptic terminal growth. *Behav. Neural Biol.* 44:186–200.

Routtenberg, A. (1991). Trans-synaptophobia revisited. In M. Baudry and J. L. Davis (eds.), *Long-Term Potentiation: A Debate of Current Issues*. MIT Press, Cambridge, pp. 155–167.

Sah, P., Hestrin, S., and Nicoll, R. A. (1990) Properties of excitatory postsynaptic currents recorded in vitro from rat hippocampal interneurones. *J. Physiol. (Lond.)* 430:605–616.

Schreiber, S. S., Maren, S., Tocco, G., Shors, T. J., and Thompson, R. F. (1991) A negative correlation between the induction of long-term potentiation and activation of immediate early genes. *Mol. Brain Res.* 11:89–91.

Schubert, D. (1991) The possible role of adhesion in synaptic modification. *Trends Neurosci.* 14:127–130.

Schuman, E., and Madison, D. V. (1991) A requirement for the intercellular messenger nitric oxide in long-term potentiation. *Science* 254:1503–1506.

Seki, T., and Arai, Y. (1991) The persistent expression of a highly polysialylated NCAM in the dentate gyrus of the adult rat. *Neurosci. Res.* 12:503–513.

Seubert, P., Larson, J., Oliver, M., Jung, M. W., Baudry, M., and Lynch, G. (1988) Stimulation of NMDA receptors induces proteolysis of spectrin in hippocampus. *Brain Res.* 460:189–194.

Shahi, K., and Baudry, M. (1992) Increasing binding affinity of agonists to glutamate receptors increases synaptic responses at glutamatergic synapses. *Proc. Natl. Acad. Sci. USA* 89:6881–6885.

Sheppard, A., Wu, J., Rutishauser, U., and Lynch, G. (1991) Proteolytic modification of neural cell adhesion molecule (NCAM) by the intracellular proteinase calpain. *Biochim. Biophys. Acta* 1076:156–160.

Shukla, S. D. (1992) Platelet-activating factor receptor and signal transduction mechanisms. *FASEB J.* 6:2296–2301.

Silva, A. J., Stevens, C. F., Tonegawa, S., and Wang, Y. (1992a) Deficient hippocampal long-term potentiation in a-calcium-calmodulin kinase II mutant mice. *Science* 257:201–206.

Silva, A. J., Paylor, R., Wehner, J. M., and Tonegawa, S. (1992b) Impaired spatial learning in a calcium-calmodulin kinase II mutant mice. *Science* 257:206–211.

Siman, R., Gall, C., Perlmutter, L. S., Christian, C., Baudry, M., and Lynch, G. (1985) Distribution of calpain I, an enzyme associated with degenerative activity, in rat brain. *Brain Res.* 347:399–403.

Sladeczek, F., Pin, J. P., Recasens, M., Bockaert, J., and Weiss, S. (1985) Glutamate stimulates inositol phosphate formation in striatal neurones. *Nature* 317:24–30.

Solis, J.-M., and Nicoll, R.-A. (1992) Pharmacological characterization of GABAB-mediated responses in the CA1 region of the rat hippocampal slice. *J. Neurosci.* 12:3466–3472.

Sommer, B., Keinanen, K., Verdoorn, T. A., Wisden, W., Burnashev, N., Herb, A., Kohler, M., Takagi, T., Sakmann, B., and Seeburg, P. H. (1990) Flip and flop: A cell-specific functional switch in glutamate-operated channels of the CNS. *Science* 249:1580–1585.

Staubli, U., and Lynch, G. (1987) Stable hippocampal long-term potentiation elicited by "theta" pattern stimulation. *Brain Res.* 435:1–2.

Staubli, U., Baudry, M., and Lynch, G. (1984) Leupeptin, a thiol-proteinase inhibitor, causes a selective impairment of maze performance in rats. *Behav. Neurol Biol.* 40:58–69.

Staubli, U., Kessler, M., and Lynch, G. (1990a) Aniracetam has proportionately smaller effects on synapses expressing long-term potentiation: Evidence that receptor changes subserve LTP. *Psychobiology* 18:377–381.

Staubli, U., Larson, J., and Lynch, G. (1990b) Mossy fiber potentiation and long-term potentiation involve different expression mechanisms. *Synapse* 5:333–335.

Steward, O., and Levy, W. B. (1982) Preferential localization of polyribosomes under the base cells of dentate gyrus. *J. Neurosci.* 2:284–291.

Tanabe, Y., Masu, M., Ishii, T., Shigemoto, R., and Nakanishi, S. (1992) A family of metabotropic glutamate receptors. *Neuron* 8:169–179.

Tang, C. M., Dichter, M., and Morad, M. (1989) Quisqualate activates a rapidly inactivating high conductance ionic channel in hippocampal neurons. *Science* 243:1474–1477.

Tang, C. M., Shi, Q. Y., Katchman, A., and Lynch, G. (1991) Modulation of the time-course of fast EPSCs and glutamate channel kinetics by aniracetam. *Science* 254:288–290.

Teichberg, V. I. (1991) Glial glutamate receptors: Likely actors in brain signaling. *FASEB J.* 5:3086–3091.

Terramani, T., Kessler, M., Lynch, G., and Baudry, M. (1988) Effects of thiol reagents on ^{3}H-AMPA binding to rat relencephalic membranes. *Mol. Pharmacol.* 34:117–123.

Teyler, T. J., and DiScenna, P. (1987) Long-term potentiation. *Annu. Rev. Neurosci.* 10:131–161.

Thiels, E., Weisz, D. J., and Berger, T. W. (1992) In vivo modulation of N-methyl-D-aspartate receptor–dependent long-term potentiation by the glycine modulatory site. *Neuroscience* 46: 501–509.

Thio, L. L., Clifford, D. B., and Zorumski, C. F. (1991) Characterization of quisqualate receptor desensitization in cultured postnatal rat hippocampal neurons. *J. Neurosci.* 11:3430–3441.

Thomson, A. M. (1990) Glycine is a coagonist at the NMDA receptor/channel complex. *Prog. Neurobiol.* 35:53–74.

Tocco, G., Maren, S., Shors, T., Baudry, M., and Thompson, R. F. (1992) Long-term potentiation is associated with increased ^{3}H-AMPA binding in rat hippocampus. *Brain Res.* 573:228–234.

Vincent, S. R., and Kimura, H. (1992) Histochemical mapping of nitric oxide sunthase in the rat brain. *Neuroscience* 46:755–784.

Wallace, C. S., Hawrylak, N., and Greenough, W. T. (1991). Studies of synaptic structural modifications after long-term potentiation and kindling: context for a molecular morphology. In M. Baudry and J. L. Davis (eds.), *Long-Term Potentiation: A Debate of Current Issues.* MIT Press, Cambridge, pp. 189–232.

Watkins, J. C., and Collingridge, G. L. (eds.) (1989). *The NMDA Receptor.* Oxford University Press, Oxford.

Werner, P., Voigt, M., Keinanen, K., Wisden, W., and Seeburg, P. H. (1991) Cloning of a putative high affinity kainate receptor expressed predominantly in hippocampal CA3 cells. *Nature* 351:742–744.

Westbrook, G. L., and Mayer, M. L. (1987) Micromolar concentrations of Zn^{++} antagonize NMDA and GABA responses of hippocampal neurons. *Nature* 328:640–643.

Whishaw, I. Q., and Vanderwolf, C. H. (1973) Hippocampal EEG and behaviour: Changes in amplitude and frequency of RSA (theta rhythm) associated with spontaneous and learned movement patterns in rats and cats. *Behav. Biol.* 8:461–484.

Williams, J. H., and Bliss, T. V. (1988) Induction but not maintenance of calcium-induced long-term potentiation in dentate gyrus and area CA1 of the hippocampal slice is blocked by nordihydroguaiaretic acid. *Neurosci. Lett.* 88:81–85.

Williams, J. H., and Bliss, T. V. (1989) An in vitro study of the effect of lipoxygenase and cyclo-oxygenase inhibitors of arachidonic acid on the induction and maintenance of long-term potentiation in the hippocampus. *Neurosci. Lett.* 107:1–3.

Williams, J. H., Errington, M. L., Lynch, M. A., and Bliss, T. V. (1989) Arachidonic acid induces a long-term activity-dependent enhancement of synaptic transmission in the hippocampus. *Nature* 341:739–742.

Williams, K., Romano, C., Dichter, M., and Molinoff, P. (1991) Modulation of the NMDA receptor by polyamines. *Life Sci.* 48:469–498.

Wilson, C. J. (1984) Passive cable properties of dendritic spines and spiny neurons. *J. Neurosci.* 4:281–297.

Winson, J. (1990) The meaning of dreams. *Sci. Am.* 263:86–96.

Wisden, W., Errington, M. L., Williams, S., Dunnett, S. B., Waters, C., Hitchcock, D., Evan, G. Bliss, T. V., and Hunt, S. P. (1990) Differential expression of immediate early genes in the hippocampus and spinal cord. *Neuron* 4:603–614.

Xiao, P., Bahr, B. A., Staubli, U., Vanderklish, P. W., and Lynch, G. (1991a) Evidence that matrix recognition contributes to stabilization but not induction of LTP. *Neuroreport* 2:461–464.

Xiao, P., Staubli, U., Kessler, M., and Lynch, G. (1991b) Selective effects of aniracetam across receptor types and forms of synaptic facilitation in hippocampus. *Hippocampus* 1:373–380.

Zalutsky, R. A., and Nicoll, R. A. (1990) Comparison of two forms of long-term potentiation in the single hippocampal neurons. *Science* 248:1619–1624.

6 Cerebellar Mechanisms of Long-term Depression

Masao Ito

1 INTRODUCTION

If the cerebellum is an organ for motor learning, as has long been assumed, neuronal circuitry of the cerebellum must contain synaptic plasticity as a memory element and thereby be able to perform activity-dependent self-organization. In accordance with this theoretical expectation (Albus, 1971; Marr, 1969), long-term depression (LTD) was found to occur in Purkinie cells of the cerebellar cortex (Ito et al., 1982).

Purkinje cells receive two distinct excitatory inputs, one from climbing fibers, axons of inferior olive neurons in the medulla oblongata, and the other from parallel fibers, axons of granule cells (figure 6.1). LTD is the persistent reduction of transmission efficacy of parallel fiber synapses which follows repeated conjunctive activation of the parallel fiber synapses with climbing fiber synapses, not repeated activation of parallel fibers or climbing fibers alone (Ekerot and Kano, 1985; Ito and Kano, 1982).

The occurrence of LTD has been confirmed using various materials and recording and stimulating techniques. LTD was reproduced in slice preparations in vitro (Crepel and Krupa, 1988; Sakurai, 1987) and tissue-cultured Purkinje cells on which both granule cells and olivary neurons formed synapses (Hirano, 1990a). Besides conventional intracellular and extracellular recording, the patch clamp technique proved to be useful in revealing LTD (Konnerth et al., 1992). Monitoring of extracellular potassium concentration in cerebellar slices also reflects LTD (Shibuki and Okada, 1991).

The final event that accounts for the LTD has been shown to be sustained desensitization of glutamate receptors mediating parallel fiber synapses on Purkinje cells (Crepel and Krupa, 1988; Ito et al., 1982; Kano and Kato, 1987). In order to reveal molecular mechanisms underlying LTD, recent efforts have been devoted to inducing sustained desensitization of glutamate receptors in Purkinje cells by applying glutamate or its agonists in place of parallel fiber stimulation, by depolarizing Purkinje cell membrane in place of climbing fiber stimulation which produces large depolarization of Purkinje cell membrane, or by combination of these two processes (Crepel and Krupa, 1988; Hirano, 1990b; Linden et al., 1991). Further bypassing of intracellular processes lead-

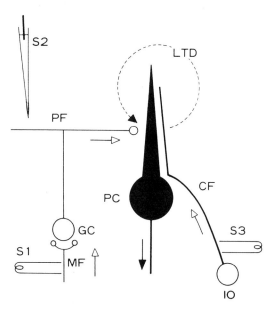

Figure 6.1 The site of long-term depression (LTD) PC, Purkinje cell; PF, parallel fiber; CF, climbing fiber; GC, granule cell; MF, mossy fiber; S_1, S_2, S_3, stimulating electrodes; IO, inferior olive.

ing to sustained desensitization of glutamate receptors has been attempted (Ito and Karachot, 1989, 1990a,b; Shibuki and Okada 1991).

This chapter summarizes recent research into molecular processes of LTD and learning mechanisms of the cerebellum based on LTD.

2 EVENTS IN PARALLEL FIBER SYNAPSES

Parallel fiber synapses are the site where LTD takes place. Accumulated evidence indicates that parallel fibers release L-glutamate as a neurotransmitter, which acts on a particular subtype of glutamate receptors selective to AMPA. The transmission is effectively blocked by specific non-NMDA antagonists, CNQX (Hirano, 1990c; Konnerth et al., 1990), and also by a synthetic analog of Joro spider toxin, 1-acetylnaphthyl sperimin (Ajima et al., 1991).

The question of whether or not LTD is due to depression at the presynaptic or postsynaptic side of parallel fiber synapses has been answered by demonstration of prominent postsynaptic desensitization (Ito et al., 1982) and by an analysis of quantal-transmission in tissue-cultured Purkinje cells (Hirano, 1991). Hirano's quantal analysis revealed that the quantal size for the parallel fiber neurotransmitter representing postsynaptic receptor sensitivity was reduced during LTD, while the quantal content, indicating the number of quantal units of the transmitter released from parallel fibers, remained unchanged.

Since LTD occurs only when parallel fiber synapses are activated in conjunction with climbing fiber synapses, it is likely that LTD is due to sustained desensitization of AMPA receptors facilitated under the influence of climbing fiber synapses. By definition, desensitization should be induced by prolonged activation of a receptor by its agonist and should not refer to deterioration of the receptor, which could be induced by various causes. Desensitization thus explains well the dependence of LTD on the activity of parallel fibers.

It has been found that AMPA receptors of Purkinje cells are persistently desensitized when a rat cerebellar slice was exposed to quisqualate (Ito and Karachot, 1989). The desensitization was followed for 10 hr with no sign of recovery (Ito and Karachot, 1990a). Since no such desensitization was induced by exposure to AMPA, metabotropic glutamate receptors, which are also activated by quisqualate, are likely to be involved in inducing the desensitization. In fact, the desensitization of AMPA receptors was induced by combined application of AMPA and t-ACPD, an agonist of metabotropic glutamate receptors (Ito and Karachot, 1990b). Thus, the quisqualate-induced desensitization is effected by activation of metabotropic glutamate receptors, differing from the Ca^{2+} entry through voltage-dependent channels that leads to LTD (see below). Yet, the quisqualate-induced desensitization seems to share a major part of the molecular processes underlying LTD.

3   EVENTS IN CLIMBING FIBER SYNAPSES

L-Aspartate has been proposed as a likely neurotransmitter for climbing fiber synapses, but more recent evidence does not favor this possibility. L-Aspartate-like immunoreactivity is in fact sparse in climbing fiber terminals (Zhang et al., 1990). Instead, L-homocysteate has drawn attention because K^+-induced Ca^{2+}-dependent release from L-homocysteate from cerebellar slices is abolished by destruction of climbing fibers (Vollenweider et al., 1990). L-Homocysteate has therefore been proposed as a putative neurotransmitter of climbing fibers; however, a recent immunohistochemical study has revealed localization of L-homocysteate in Bergmann glia fibers, but not in climbing fibers (Cuénod et al., 1990). The suggestion is, then, that L-homocysteate is released from glial cells under the influence of a messenger substance produced in Purkinje cells activated via climbing fiber synapses, so as to intensify action of a climbing fiber neurotransmitter (yet unknown) on Purkinje cells.

Pharmacological tests revealed that climbing fiber transmission is effectively blocked by CNQX (Knöpfelo et al., 1990a) but not by APV (Perkel et al., 1990). A synthetic analog of Joro spider toxin that blocks parallel fiber–Purkinje cell synapses does not affect climbing fiber synapses (Ajima et al., 1991). Hence. postsynaptic receptors in climbing fiber synapses cannot be defined as either NMDA or non-NMDA glutamate receptors.

Climbing fiber–evoked EPSPs lead to generation of Ca^{2+}-dependent spikes and plateau potentials in Purkinje cell dendrites. Climbing fiber-induced enhancement of intracellular Ca^{2+} concentration has been demonstrated with microfluorometric measurements (Knöpfel et al., 1990b; Konnerth et al., 1992; Ross et al., 1990b). Enhanced Ca^{2+} concentration has been observed even in the periphery of Purkinje cell dendrites where climbing fiber synapses are absent, suggesting that Ca^{2+} spikes conduct along dendrites.

Intradendritic injection of a Ca^{2+} chelator, EGTA or BAPTA, abolished LTD (Konnerth et al., 1992; Sakurai, 1990). Perfusion of a cerebellar slice with membrane-soluble Ca^{2+} chelator, BAPTA-AM, effectively abolishes quisqualate-induced desensitization of AMPA receptors (Ito and Karachot, 1990b). Ca^{2+} spikes induced directly by depolarizing membrane of a Purkinje cell effectively induce LTD when paired with parallel fiber stimulation (Crepel and Krupa, 1988). These observations clearly indicate the role of Ca^{2+} in the induction of LTD.

4 INTERMEDIATE PROCESSES FOR LTD

Recent investigations suggest roles for NO, cyclic GMP (cGMP), and cGMP-dependent protein kinase in LTD. These would constitute a chain reaction as illustrated in figure 6.2. Further, the involvement of protein kinase C and Protein phosphatase 1 is indicated by recent data.

4.1 Nitric Oxide

NO has recently drawn attention as a novel neuronal messenger (Bredt and Snyder, 1992). NO acts to stimulate guanylate cyclase (Garthwaite et al., 1988). Stimulation of white matter in a cerebellar slice causes a transient elevation of NO concentration (Shibuki and Okada, 1991). Since this NO

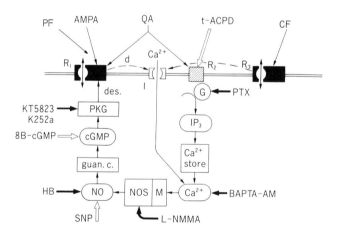

Figure 6.2 Schematic diagram showing signal transduction processes presumed to underlie LTD. R_1, glutamate receptor mediating parallel fiber-Purkinje cell synapses and responsive to QA and AMPA; R_2, metabotropic glutamate receptor sensitive to t-ACPD; R_3, receptor for the unknown neurotransmitter of climbing fibers. R_1 and R_3 are associated with a cation-selective channel. I, voltage-sensitive Ca^{2+} ion channel; G, G protein; M, calmodulin; NOS, nitric oxide synthase; guan. c., guanylate cyclase; d, depolarization; des., desensitization. Agents that either block (solid arrows) or drive (open arrows) the chain reaction are indicated. PTX, pertussis toxin; HB, hemoglobin; 8B-cGMP, 8 bromo-cyclic GMP; BAPTA-AM, membrane-soluble Ca^{2+} chelator; L-NMMA, inhibitor of NOS; SNP, sodium nitroprusside, which releases NO in solution; K252a and KT5823, nonspecific and specific inhibitors of PKG. (Modified from Ito and Karachot, 1990b.)

response is largely diminished after 3-acetylpyridine destruction of climbing fibers, it is likely to be caused by climbing fiber impulses. A similar conclusion was reached by measurement of cGMP production, which NO stimulates (Southam and Garthwaite, 1991). Since NO synthase requires Ca^{2+}-activated calmodulin, it is natural to suppose that climbing fiber impulses activate NO production in Purkinje cells via elevation of intradendritic Ca^{2+} concentration. In accordance with this view, LTD as well as quisqualate-induced desensitization is abolished by hemoglobin, which absorbs NO, and also by L-NMMA, which inhibits production of NO (Ito and Karachot, 1990b; Shibuki and Okada, 1991). Further. sodium nitroprusside, which releases NO in solution, induces LTD when combined with parallel fiber activation (Shibuki and Okada, 1991). It also produces sustained desensitization of AMPA receptors when combined with AMPA application (Ito and Karachot, 1990b).

However, NO synthase isolated from a cytosolic fraction of cerebellar tissues and cloned has been located immunohistochemically in a granule cell layer (Bredt and Snyder, 1992; Bredt et al., 1991; Ross et al., 1990a). Basket cells and some mossy fibers have been labeled. No evidence is available to support the presence of NO synthase in climbing fibers or Purkinje cells. This negative finding creates a difficulty in explaining the role of NO in LTD unless we assume a remote interaction between Purkinje cells and other types of cells via a messenger going out of the cell membrane (for example, arachidonic acid). Nevertheless, the possibility remains that a particulate fraction of cerebellar tissues contains another type of NO synthase. The cytochrome P450 reductase exists in Purkinje cells (Bredt et al., 1991), which produces CO instead of NO. Like NO, CO activates guanylate cyclase, but it is insensitive to L-NMMA, inhibitor of NO synthase.

Another complication is that there is no evidence that NO plays a role in the LTD induced in tissue-cultured Purkinje cells (Linden and Connor, 1992). The LTD was induced by combined application of AMPA and membrane depolarization even under hemoglobin or L-NMMA. Thus, the current state of research pertaining to NO in the cerebellum is complicated. Further information is required before a conclusion can be reached as to the site of NO production and the role in LTD.

4.2 Guanylate Cyclase and cGMP

Guanylate cyclase is located in Purkinje cells, especially in primary dendrites (Ariano et al., 1982). It may be expected that climbing fiber impulses act to enhance the cGMP level in Purkinje cells via elevation of Ca^{2+} and subsequently of NO. Indeed, application of membrane-soluble cGMP derivatives induces LTD when combined with parallel fiber stimulation (Shibuki and Okada, 1991) or it causes sustained desensitization of AMPA receptors when combined with AMPA application (Ito and Karachot, 1990b).

Although earlier studies indicated the presence of cGMP in Purkinje cells, a recent immunohistochemical labeling revealed the abundance of cGMP in

Bergmann glia fibers, Purkinje cell somata lacking cGMP (De Vente et al., 1990). Nevertheless, a low level of cGMP has been found also in Purkinje cells (Garthwaite, personal communication).

4.3 cGMP-dependent Kinase and Protein Phosphatase

cGMP-dependent kinase (PKG) has been isolated and cloned (Scott, 1991). The abundance of PKG in Purkinje cells has been revealed immunohistochemically (Lohman et al., 1981). A specific inhibitor of cytosolic PKG, KT5823, effectively blocks the quisqualate-induced desensitization of AMPA receptors (Ito and Karachot, 1990b).

Purkinje cells also contain the substrate specific to PKG, namely, G-substrate (Detre et al., 1984; Nairn et al., 1985). When phosphorylated by PKG, G-substrate acts to inhibit protein phosphatases 1 and 2_A (see Cohen, 1989). The phosphorylated G-substrate shares some chemical properties with protein phosphatase 1 in other neural tissues. Involvement of G-substrate in LTD is suggested because inhibitors of protein phosphatases, okadaic acid (Tachibana et al., 1981) and calyculin A (Kato et al., 1986) induce desensitization of AMPA receptors when combined with AMPA (Ito and Karachot, 1992). Since calyculin A is more potent than okadaic acid, protein phosphatase 1 but not 2_A is likely to be involved, in accordance with the chemical properties of G-substrate.

Thus, it seems that climbing fiber impulses eventually influence AMPA receptors through inhibition of protein phosphatase, as illustrated in figure 6.3, thus shifting the balance between phosphorylation and dephosphorylation of AMPA receptors to phosphorylation. However, the possibility remains that PKG acts also to directly phosphorylate AMPA receptors (figure 6.3).

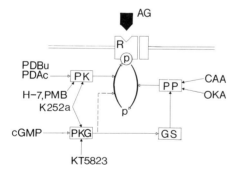

Figure 6.3 Schematic diagram illustrating possible chemical processes underlying long-term desensitization of AMPA receptors in cerebellar Purkinie cells. K, AMPA receptor; AG, agonist; GS, G-substrate; PK, protein kinase, which is probably a Ca^{2+}-insensitive PKC; PP, protein phophatase, presumably of type 1; CAA, calyculin A; OKA, okadaic acid; PBM, polymyxin B; PDBu and PDAc, phorbol 12, 13-dibutyrate and diacetate. Open arrowheads indicate facilitation and solid arrow heads inhibition. (From Ito and Karachot, 1992.)

4.4 Protein Kinase C

Purkinje cells are rich in protein kinase C (PKC) (Kose et al., 1988). Phorbol esters which activate PKC induce desensitization of AMPA receptors and a PKC inhibitor stops LTD (Crepel and Jaillard, 1990; Crepel and Krupa, 1988; Linden and Connor, 1991). PKC inhibitors also antagonize calyculin A in inducing sustained desensitization of AMPA receptors (Ito and Karachot, 1992).

PKC could interact with guanylate cyclase by phosphorylation (Crepel and Ardinat, 1991). However, since PKC inhibitors antagonize calyculin A in inducing desensitization of AMPA receptors (Ito and Karachot, 1992), it is probable that PKC acts to phosphorylate AMPA receptors, counterbalancing the dephosphorylating action of protein phosphatases (figure 6.3). In fact, phorbol esters act to desensitize AMPA receptors when combined with AMPA. It is still unclear how PKC is activated in normal situations producing LTD.

4.5 Metabotropic Glutamate Receptors and IP$_3$ Metabolism

Purkinje cells are equipped with a metabotropic subtype of glutamate receptors (Sugiyama et al., 1987) that have been cloned (Masu et al., 1991). These metabotropic glutamate receptors are coupled through activation of G proteins with an inositolphospholipid metabolism which synthesizes IP$_3$ compound (see figure 6.2). Receptors for IP$_3$ are abundant in Purkinje cells, especially in the endoplasmic reticulum which stores Ca^{2+} ions (Furuichi et al., 1989; Ross et al., 1989). Application of a metabotropic glutamate receptor agonist, trans-D,L,-1-amino-1,3-cyclopentanedicarboxylic acid (t-ACPD) facilitates phosphoinositide turnover in the cerebellum (Hwang et al., 1990). Stimulation with glutamate or quisqualate leads to enhanced Ca^{2+} levels in the cerebellar cortex even in a Ca^{2+}-free medium (Llano et al., 1991). Quisqualate stimulates both metabotropic glutamate receptors and ionotropic AMPA receptors. t-ACPD raises Ca^{2+} levels primarily in the soma but also, to a lesser degree, in a restricted part of the dendrites of Purkinje cells, in contrast to climbing fiber impulses which induce elevation of Ca^{2+} levels confined to the dendrites (Vranesic et al. 1991).

Hence, activation of metabotropic glutamate receptors more or less mimics climbing fiber impulses in terms of enhanced Ca^{2+} levels. However, the recently cloned metabotropic glutamate receptor 1α has been immunohistochemically located in the postsynaptic membrane of dendritic spines of Purkinje cells (Görcs et al., 1993). By recording from Purkinje cells with a grease method, a slow depolarization followed by a hyperpolarization was shown to follow repetitive stimulation of parallel fibers (Bachelor and Garthwaite, 1993). These potentials were Ca^{2+}-dependent and were replicated by perfusion of an exogenous agonist of metabotropic glutamate receptors (1S, 3R-1-aminocyclopentate-1, 3-dicarboxylic acid; 1S, 3R-ACPD). Therefore, metabotropic glutamate receptors are more likely to be associated with parallel fibers. Since stimulation of parallel fiber does not induce LTD (see above), it is still an open question how metabotropic glutamate receptors are related to LTD.

5 INVOLVEMENT OF LTD IN MOTOR LEARNING

To constitute a nerve network capable of learning, not only LTD but also potentiation would be necessary. In theories of the cerebellum, it has been assumed that the product of discharge frequencies in parallel fibers and climbing fibers plays a key role in effecting LTD or potentiation (Fujita, 1982). If the product is larger than a certain value, LTD will occur, while if smaller, potentiation will occur. When climbing fibers convey signals that represent errors in motor performance (see Ito, 1989), LTD will lead to elimination of those synapses that are concurrently activated and that are responsible for the erroneous performance. By contrast, those parallel fiber synapses that are activated when no error signals are conveyed by climbing fibers would be recognized as competent. In this way, the cerebellar network will be reorganized to yield improved motor performance. Motor learning would thus be effected.

A counterpart of the theoretically postulated potentiation so far found is that when parallel fibers alone are stimulated repetitively (Sakurai, 1987), this potentiates parallel fiber–Purkinje cell transmission. An analysis in cultured Purkinje cells revealed an increased quantal content, which indicates an augmented release of parallel fiber neurotransmitters (Hirano, 1991). When LTD is abolished by injection of the Ca^{2+} chelator, combined parallel fiber and climbing fiber stimulation induces only the potentiation (Sakurai, 1990). Phorbol esters facilitate the release of parallel fiber neurotransmitter (Crepel and Jaillard, 1991), and hence it is possible that PKC is involved in the anti-LTD potentiation. Whether or not potentiation also occurs on the postsynaptic side in the form of sensitization of AMPA receptors is still unclear.

Involvement of LTD has been suggested in the adaptation of monkey's arm movement (Gilbert and Thach, 1977), adaptation of rabbit's and monkey's vestibulo-ocular reflex (VOR; Ito, 1989), and rabbit's classical conditioning of eye blink reflex (Thompson, 1986). These motor operations represent a simple form of learning. The above-described recent research on molecular mechanisms of LTD provides a new tool for proving the involvement of LTD in motor learning. In fact, subdural injection of 0.1 ml of 5 μM hemoglobin to the flocculus abolishes adaptation of VOR without affecting dynamic characteristics of the oculomotor system (Nagao and Ito, 1991).

Injection of a β-noradrenergic agonist, isoproterenol, into rabbit's flocculus facilitated adaptation of VOR, while that of a β-antagonist, sotalol, depressed the adaptation (van Neerven et al., 1990). Yet, it is unclear how these drugs interfere with LTD.

6 COMMENT

During the past decade, LTD has been established as one important type of synaptic plasticity which accounts for learning capability of the cerebellum, and its molecular mechanisms have been revealed in some detail. Thus, LTD appears to be due to the occurrence of persistent desensitization in phosphorylated AMPA receptors. The time now seems ripe for investigating gene regulation mechanisms linked with the phosphorylation processes of AMPA receptors. Such investigation would lead to understanding how LTD is related to permanent motor memory that may be stored in the cerebellar cortex.

Recently, it has been proposed that the cerebellum is involved not only in motor and autonomic functions, but also in certain mental activities (Leiner et al., 1986). This view has been supported by findings in human cerebellar studies (Fiez et al., 1992; Ingvar, 1990; Petersen et al., 1989). The author provided a system theory basis, suggesting the analogy between movement and thought (Ito, 1990). As we move limbs in movement, we manipulate concepts and ideas in thought. Even though the control objects are very different in these two instances, the same control principle may underlie both processes. Further investigation of LTD would thus lead to the understanding of learning even in a certain category of mental functions.

REFERENCES

Ajima. A., Hensch, T., Kado, R. T., and Ito, M. (1991) Differential blocking action of Joro spider toxin analog on parallel fiber and climbing fiber synapses in cerebellar Purkinje cells. *Neurosci. Res.* 12:281–286.

Albus, J. S. (1971) A theory of cerebellar function. *Math. Biosci.* 10:25–61.

Ariano, M. A., Lewicki, J. A., Brandwein, H. J., and Murad, F. (1982) Immunohistochemical localization of guanylate cyclase within neurons of rat brain. *Proc. Natl. Acad Sci. USA* 79: 1316–1320.

Bachelor, A. M., and Garthwaite, J. (1993) Novel synaptic potentials in cerebellar Purkinje cells: Probable mediation by metabotropic glutamate receptors. *Neuropharmacology* 32:11–20.

Bredt, D. S., and Snyder S. H. (1992) Nitric oxide, a novel neuronal messenger. *Neuron* 8:3–17.

Bredt, D. S., Hwang, P. M., Glatt, C. E., Lowenstein, C., Reed, R. R., and Snyder, S. H. (1991) Cloned and expressed nitric oxide synthase structurally resembles cytochrome P-450 reductase. *Nature* 351:714–718.

Cohen, P. (1989) The structure and regulation of protein phosphatases. *Annu. Rev. Biochem.* 58:453–508.

Crepel, F., and Audinat, E. (1991) Excitatory amino acid receptors of cerebellar Purkinje cells: Development and plasticity. *Prog. Biophys. Molec. Biol.* 55:31–46.

Crepel, F., and Jaillard, D. (1990) Protein kinases, nitric oxide and long-term depression of synapses in the cerebellum. *NeuroReport* 1:133–136.

Crepel, F., and Jaillard, D. (1991) Pairing of pre- and postsynaptic activities in cerebellar Purkinje cells induces long-term changes in synaptic efficacy. An in vitro study. *J. Physiol. (Lond.)* 432: 123–141.

Crepel, F., and Krupa, M. (1988) Activation of protein kinase C induces a long-term depression of glutamate sensitivity of cerebellar Purkinje cells. *Brain. Res.* 458:397–401.

Cuénod, M., Do, K. Q., and Streit, P. (1990) Homocysteic acid as an endogenous excitatory amino acid. *Trends Pharmacol. Sci.* 11:477–478.

Detre, J. A., Nairn, A. C., Aswad, D. W., and Greengard, P. (1984) Localization in mammalian brain of G-substrate, a specific substrate for guanosine 3′, 5′-cyclic monophosphate-dependent protein kinase. *J. Neurosci.* 4:1843–2849.

De Vente, J., Bol, J. G. J. M., Berkelmans, H. S., Schipper, J., and Steinbusch, H. M. W. (1990) Immunocytochemistry of cGMP in the cerebellum of the immature, adult, and aged rat: The involvement of nitric oxide. A micropharmacological study. *Eur. J. Neurosci.* 2:845–862.

Ekerot, C.-F., and Kano, M. (1985) Long-term depression parallel fibre synapses following stimulation of climbing fibres. *Brain Res.* 342:357–360.

Fiez, J. A., Petersen, S. E., Cheney, M. K., and Raichle, M. E. (1992) Impaired nonmotor learning and error detection associated with cerebellar damage; single-case study. Brain, in press.

Fujita, M. (1982) Adaptive filter model of the cerebellum. *Biol. Cybern.* 45:195–206.

Furuichi, T., Yoshikawa, S., Miyawaki, A., Wada, K., Maeda, N., and Mikoshiba, K. (1989) Primary structure and functional expression of the inositol 1, 4, 5-triphosphate-binding protein P_{400}. *Nature* 342:32–38.

Garthwaite, J., Charles, S. L., and Chess-Williums, R. (1988) Endothelium-derived relaxing factor release on activation of NMDA receptors suggests role as intracellular messenger in the brain. *Nature* 336:385–388.

Gilbert, P. F. C., and Thach, W. T. (1977) Purkinje cell activity during motor learning. *Brain Res.* 128:309–328.

Görcs, T. J., Penke, B., Böti, Z., Katarova, Z., and Hámori, J. (1993) Immunohistochemical visualization of a metabotropic glutamate receptor. *NeuroReport* 4:283–286.

Hirano, T. (1990a) Depression and potentiation of the synaptic transmission between a granule cell and a Purkinje cell in rat cerebellar culture. *Neurosci. Lett.* 119:141–144.

Hirano, T. (1990b) Effects of postsynaptic depolarization in the induction of synaptic depression between a granule cell and a Purkinje cell in rat cerebellar culture. *Neurosci. Lett.* 119:145–147.

Hirano, T. (1990c) Synaptic transmission between rat inferior olivary neurons and cerebellar Purkinje cells in culture. *J. Neurophysiol.* 63:181–189.

Hirano, T. (1991) Differential pre- and postsynaptic mechanisms for synaptic potentiation and depression between a granule cell and a Purkinje cell in rat cerebellar culture. *Synapse* 7:321–323.

Hwang, P. M., Bredt, D. S., and Snyder, S. H. (1990) Autoradiographic imaging of phosphoinositide turnover in the brain. *Science* 249:802–804.

Ingvar, P. (1990) On ideation and ideography. In *The Principles of Design and Operation of the Brain*, J. C. Eccles and O. Creutzfeldt (eds.). Springer-Verlag, Berlin, pp. 433–453.

Ito, M. (1989) Long-term depression. *Annu. Rev. Neurosci.* 12:85–102.

Ito, M. (1990) A new physiological concept of cerebellum. *Rev. Neurol. (Paris)* 146:564–569.

Ito, M., and Kano, M. (1982) Long-lasting depression of parallel fiber-Purkinje cell transmission induced by conjunctive stimulation of parallel fibers and climbing fibers in the cerebellar cortex. *Neurosci. Lett.* 33:253–258.

Ito, M., and Karachot, L. (1989) Long-term desensitization of quisqualate-specific glutamate receptors in Purkinje cells investigated with wedge recording from rat cerebellar slices. *Neurosci. Rev.* 7:168–171.

Ito, M., and Karachot, L. (1990a) Receptor subtype involved in, and time course of, the long-term desensitization of glutamate receptors in cerebellar Purkinje cells. *Neurosci. Res.* 8:303–307.

Ito, M., and Karachot, L. (1990b) Messengers mediating long-term desensitization in cerebellar Purkinje cells. *NeuroReport* 1:129–132.

Ito, M., and Karachot, L. (1992) Protein kinases and phosphatase inhibitors mediating long-term desensitization of glutamate receptors in cerebellar Purkinje cells. *Neurosci. Res.* 14: in press.

Ito, M., Sakurai, M., and Tongroach, P. (1982) Climbing fibre induced depression of both mossy fibre responsiveness and glutamate sensitivity of cerebellar Purkinje cells. *J. Physiol. (Lond.)* 324:113–134.

Kano, M., and Kato, M. (1987) Quisqualate receptors are specifically involved in cerebellar synaptic plasticity. *Nature* 325:276–279.

Kato, Y., Fusetani, N., Matsunaga, S., and Hashimoto, K. (1986) Calyculin A, a novel antitumor metabolite from the marine sponge *Discodermia* calyx, *J. Am. Chem. Soc.* 108:2780–2781.

Knöpfel, T., Audinat, E., and Gähwiler, B. H. (1990a) Climbing fibre responses in olivo-cerebellar slice cultures. I. Microelectrode recordings from Purkinje cells. *Eur. J. Neurosci.* 2:726–732.

Knöpfel, T., Staub, V. C., and Gähwiler, B. H. (1990b) Climbing fibre responses in olivo-cerebellar slice cultures. II. Dynamic of cytosolic calcium in Purkinje cells. *Eur. J. Neurosci.* 3:343–348.

Konnerth, A., Llano, I., and Armstrong, C. M. (1990) Synaptic currents in cerebellar Purkinje cells. *Proc. Natl. Acad. Sci. USA* 87:2662–2665.

Konnerth, A., Dreessen, J., and Augustine, J. (1992) Brief dendritic calcium signals initiate long-lasting synaptic depression in cerebellar Purkinje cells. *Proc. Natl. Acad. Sci. USA* 89:7051–7055.

Kose, A., Saito, N., Ito, H., Kikkawa, U., Nishizuka, Y., and Tanaka, C. (1988) Electron microscopic localization of type I protein kinase C in rat Purkinje cells. J. Neurosci. 8:4262–4268.

Leiner, H. C., Leiner, A. L., and Dow, R. S. (1986) Does the cerebellum contribute to mental skills? *Behav. Neurosci.* 100:443–454.

Linden, D. J., and Connor, J. A. (1991) Participation of postsynaptic OKC in cerebellar long-term depression in culture. *Science* 254:1656–1659.

Linden, D. J., and Connor, J. A. (1992) Long-term depression of glutamate currents in cultured cerebellar Purkinje neurons does not require nitric oxide. *Eur. J. Neurosci.* 4:10–15.

Linden, D. J., Dickinson, M. H., Smeyne, M., and Connor, J. A. (1991) A long-term depression of AMPA currents in cultured cerebellar Purkinje neurons. *Neuron* 7:81–89.

Llano, I., Dreesen, J., Kano, M., and Konnerth, A. 1991. Intradendritic release of calcium induced by glutamate in cerebellar Purkinje cells. *Neuron* 7:577–583.

Lohman, S. M., Walter, U., Miller, P. E., Greengard, P., and Camilli, P. D. (1981) Immunohistochemical localization of cyclic GMP-dependent protein kinase in mammalian brain. *Proc. Natl. Acad. Sci. USA* 78:653–657.

Marr, D. (1969) A theory of cerebellar cortex. *J. Physiol. (Lond.)* 202:437–470.

Masu, M., Tanabe, Y., Tsuchida, K., Shigemoto, R., and Nakanishi, S. (1991) Sequence and expression of a metabotropic glutamate receptor. *Nature* 349:760–765.

Nagao, S., and Ito, M. (1991) Subdural application of hemoglobin to the cerebellum blocks vestibulocular reflex adaptation. *NeuroReport* 2:193–196.

Nairn, A. C., Hemmings, H. C., Jr., and Greengard, P. (1985) Protein kinases in the brain. *Annu. Rev. Biochem.* 54:931–976.

Perkel, D. J., Hestrin, S., Sah, P., and Nicoll, R. A. (1990) Excitatory synaptic currents in Purkinje cells. *Proc. Roy. Soc. Lond. (Biol.)* 241:116–121.

Peterson, S. E., Fox, P. T., Posner, M. I. Mintun, M., and Raichle, M. E. (1989) Positron emission tomographic studies of the processing of single words. *J. Cog. Neurosci.* 1:153–170.

Ross, C. A., Meldolesi, J., Milner, T. A., Satoh, T., Supattapone, S., and Snyder, S. H. (1989) Inositol 1, 4, 5-triphosphate receptor localized to endoplasmic reticulum in cerebellar Purkinje neurons. *Nature* 339:460–470.

Ross, C. A., Bredt, D., and Snyder, S. H. (1990a) Messenger molecules in the cerebellum. *Trends Neurosci.* 13:216–222.

Ross, W. N., Lasse-Ross, N., and Werman, R. (1990b) Spatial and temporal analysis of calcium-dependent electrical activity in guinea pig Purkinje cell dendrites. *Proc. Roy. Soc. Lond. (Biol.)* 240:173–185.

Sakurai, M. (1987) Synaptic modification of parallel fibre-Purkinje cell transmission in in vitro guinea pig cerebellar slices. *J. Physiol. (Lond.)* 394:463–480.

Sakurai, M. (1990) Calcium is an intracellular mediator of the climbing fiber in induction of cerebellar long-term depression. *Proc. Natl. Acad. Sci. USA* 87:3383–3385.

Scott, J. D. (1991) Cyclic nucleotide-dependent protein kinases. *Pharmacol. Ther.* 50:123–145.

Shibuki, K., and Okada, D. (1991) Endogenous nitric oxide release required for long-term synaptic depression in the cerebellum. *Nature* 349:326–328.

Southam, E., and Garthwaite, J. (1991) Climbing fibrres as a source of nirtic oxide in the cerebellum. *Eur. J. Neurosci.* 3:379–382.

Sugiyama, H., Ito, I., and Hirono, C. (1987) A new type of glutamate receptor linked to inositol phospholipid metabolism. *Nature* 325:531–533.

Tachibana, K., Scheuer, P. J., Tsukitani, Y., Kikuchi, H., Engen, D. V., Clardy, J., Gopichand, Y., and Schmitz, F. J. (1981) Okadaic acid, a cytotoxic polyether from two marine sponges of the genus *Halichondria*. *J. Am. Chem. Soc.* 103:2469–2471.

Thompson, R. F. (1986) The neurobiology of learning and memory. *Science* 233:941–947.

van Neerven, J., Pompeiano, O., Collewijn, H., and van der Steen, J. (1990) Injections of β-noradrenergic substances in the flocculus of rabbits affect adaptation of the VOR gain. *Exp. Brain Res.* 79:249–260.

Vollenweider, F. X., Cuénod, M., and Do, K. Q. (1990) Effect of climbing fiber deprivation on release of endogenous aspartate, glutamate, and homocysteate in slices of rat cerebellar phemisphere and vermis. *J. Neurochem.* 54:1533–1540.

Vranesic, I., Bachelor, A., Gähwiller, B. H., Garthwaite, J., Staub, C., and Köpfel, T. (1991) Trans-ACPD-induced Ca^{2+} signals in cerebellar Purkinje cells. *NeroReport* 2:759–762.

Zhang, N., Walberg, F., Laake, J. H., Meldrum, B. S., and Ottersen, O. P. (1990) Aspartate-like and glutamate-like immunoreactivities in the inferior olive and climbing fiber system: A light microscopic and semiquantitative electron microscopic study in rat and baboon (*Papio anubis*). *Neuroscience* 38:61–80.

7

Long-term Depression: Related Mechanisms in Cerebellum, Neocortex, and Hippocampus

Alain Artola and Wolf Singer

1 INTRODUCTION

Use-dependent long-term changes of synaptic efficacy are thought to form a basis for learning and memory. Since the discovery of long-term potentiation (LTP) in the hippocampus (Bliss and Lømo, 1973) use-dependent enhancement of synaptic transmission has been observed in a variety of brain structures. In the majority of cases this potentiation has associative properties, that is, a synapse will potentiate if it is active at the time when the respective dendrite is sufficiently depolarized.

The large number of studies on LTP contrasts with the relative paucity of reports on long-term depression (LTD) of synaptic transmission. Two types of use-dependent LTD have been described: a weakening of inactive inputs to cells strongly activated by other inputs (heterosynaptic depression) and a weakening of the active inputs themselves (homosynaptic depression).

2 EVIDENCE FOR HETEROSYNAPTIC DEPRESSION

In the mammalian brain the phenomenon of heterosynaptic depression has been observed in the hippocampus and in the neocortex. Its discovery was a by-product of the attempt to verify the input specificity of tetanus-induced LTP in area CA1 of hippocampal slices. It was observed that following tetanic stimulation which led to LTP of the tetanized pathway other, nonstimulated inputs to the same neuron remained either unchanged (Andersen et al., 1977, 1980) or underwent a depression of synaptic transmission. This depression was reported to last for at least 15 min after the tetanus (Dunwiddie and Lynch, 1978; Lynch et al., 1977), while others described it as a transient phenomenon lasting less than 5 min (Alger et al., 1978). Later, in vivo studies in the dentate gyrus have provided evidence that heterosynaptic depression can actually be a long-lasting phenomenon (Abraham and Goddard, 1983). Tetanic stimulation of the lateral or the medial component of the perforant path induced depression of synaptic transmission in the respective other component which lasted for at least 3 hr. A similar LTD has been found for the sparse cross-projection from the contralateral entorhinal cortex to the dentate gyrus after tetanic stimulation of the ipsilateral projection (Levy and Steward,

1979, 1983; White et al., 1990). More recently, heterosynaptic LTD has been described in several in vitro preparations: (1) in hippocampal area (CA3) for mossy afferents after tetanic stimulation of non-mossy fibers, either Schaffer collateral/commissural or fimbrial fibers (Bradler and Barrionuevo, 1989, 1990), and (2) in visual cortex for tangential intracortical connections or white matter afferents to cells in layer III after tetanic stimulation of the respective other input (Artola and Singer, submitted).

As heterosynaptic LTD is defined as a depression of nonstimulated input systems it can in principle affect a variety of afferent pathways simultaneously. The initial observation in CA1 was that all nonstimulated inputs to a particular cell underwent LTD regardless of whether the stimulated input projected on apical or basal dendritic compartments (Dunwiddie and Lynch, 1978; Lynch et al, 1977). However, there are also examples for more selective interactions between different input systems. Reports on heterosynaptic LTD in the dentate gyrus have described spatial vicinity with respect to the stimulated input as a necessary requirement for the induction of heterosynaptic LTD (White et al., 1990). Moreover, in CA3, tetanization of non-mossy fiber afferents induces heterosynaptic LTD in mossy fiber afferents, but not vice versa. Tetanization of mossy fiber afferents actually induces heterosynaptic LTP rather than LTD in non-mossy fiber afferents (Bradler and Barrionuevo, 1989).

At present little is known about the mechanisms responsible for the depression of synaptic transmission in heterosynaptic LTD but available evidence suggests reduced sensitivity of the postsynaptic transmission mechanism. After induction of heterosynaptic LTD postsynaptic responses to iontophoretically applied glutamate were found to be decreased (Lynch et al., 1976).

3 REQUIREMENTS FOR THE INDUCTION OF HETEROSYNAPTIC LTD

The stimulation protocols that have been identified as effective for the induction of heterosynaptic LTD have in common that they lead to a strong activation and depolarization of the respective postsynaptic target cells. As strong postsynaptic depolarization is also a condition that facilitates the occurrence of LTP in the stimulated pathway, homosynaptic LTP and heterosynaptic LTD are often concomitant. But the two processes are not causally related. Heterosynaptic LTD can be induced in the absence of homosynaptic LTP (Abraham and Goddard, 1983; Artola and Singer, submitted; Bradler and Barrionuevo, 1989) and vice versa, homosynaptic LTP is not necessarily associated with heterosynaptic LTD.

The notion that induction of heterosynaptic depression requires strong postsynaptic depolarization is in line with the evidence that blockade of NMDA receptors prevents the induction of heterosynaptic LTD by tetanic stimulation (in CA1: Wickens and Abraham, 1991; in dentate gyrus: Desmond et al., 1991; in the visual cortex: Artola and Singer, submitted; but see in CA3: Bradler and Barrionuevo, 1990). Because of the voltage-dependence of the

NMDA receptor-mediated conductance (Mayer et al., 1984; Nowack et al., 1984) and because of the long duration of the NMDA receptor-mediated EPSP this transmission system is particularly effective in enhancing depolarizing responses to high-frequency stimulation (Collingridge et al., 1988). Without having access to this booster, tetanic stimuli are much less effective in producing strong and long-lasting plateau-depolarization of the postsynaptic neurons. Support for strong depolarization being a requirement for the induction of depression of inactive synaptic inputs comes also from the finding that the induction of heterosynaptic LTD is facilitated by concomitant reduction of GABAergic inhibition (in CA1: Abraham and Wickens, 1991; in CA3: Bradler and Barrionuevo, 1989, 1990; in neocortex: et al., Artola and Singer, submitted). Finally, depression of synaptic input was also obtained by high-frequency antidromic stimulation of CA1 pyramidal cells in hippocampal slices that were kept in high magnesium to block synaptic transmission (Pockett and Lippold, 1986; Pockett et al., 1990). This result, too, is compatible with the view that strong postsynaptic depolarization is required for the depression of inactive synapses.

In search for a messenger that could mediate such a voltage-dependent depression of unstimulated synapses, evidence has been obtained which suggests that heterosynaptic LTD requires a surge of intracellular free $[Ca^{2+}]$. Induction of heterosynaptic LTD could be prevented in CA1 by blocking voltage-gated Ca^{2+} channels (Sastry et al., 1984; Wickens and Abraham, 1991) and it could be facilitated by application of BAY-K8644, an agonist of L-type calcium channels (Wickens and Abraham, 1991). Finally, in slices of the rat visual cortex depression of both tangential intracortical afferents and white matter input to layer III cells could be induced by raising the concentration of extracellular $[Ca^{2+}]$ transiently to 4 mM. This Ca^{2+}-induced LTD was voltage-dependent and occurred only in the most depolarized of the recorded cells (Artola et al., 1992). This suggests that depression of nonstimulated synaptic inputs results from Ca^{2+} entry through voltage-gated Ca^{2+} channels.

4 EVIDENCE FOR HOMOSYNAPTIC LTD

Homosynaptic LTD is defined as a use-dependent, long-lasting depression affecting the activated synapses themselves. This phenomenon was first observed although not addressed as such by Dunwiddie and Lynch (1978) in the hippocampus. The first formal description of homosynaptic LTD goes back to in vivo studies in the cerebellum. It was found that simultaneous activation of climbing fibers (CFs) and parallel fibers (PFs), both of which converge onto Purkinje cells (PCs), leads to a lasting depression of the response to PF stimulation (Ito and Kano, 1982; Ito et al., 1982). Activation of the PF or CF input alone has no effect on synaptic transmission. This result has subsequently been confirmed in slices (Crepel and Krupa, 1988; Sakurai, 1987) and in tissue cultures. In the latter PCs were co-cultured with granular cells and olivary neurons which provided the PF and CF input, respectively (Hirano, 1990a).

Since then homosynaptic LTD has also been demonstrated in slices of the hippocampus and the neocortex. Subicular afferents to neurons in hippocampal area CA1 undergo LTD if they are activated with low-frequency, low-intensity stimuli in counterphase with high-frequency stimulation of Schaffer collaterals and commissural pathways (Stanton and Sejnowski, 1989). Likewise, in CA3, commissural/associational afferents become depressed if they are activated at low frequency out of phase with tetanic stimulation of mossy fibers. Interestingly, the reverse is not true. The mossy fiber input does not undergo LTD if activated out of phase with tetanic stimulation of the commissural input (Chattarji et al., 1989).

Finally, in the neocortex LTD of tetanized afferents has been observed without concomitant or out-of-phase activation of additional excitatory inputs. Both in the visual cortex (Artola et al., 1990) and in the prefrontal cortex (Hirsch and Crepel, 1990) LTD of the tetanized pathway was obtained whenever tetanic stimulation had caused a sufficient depolarization of the postsynaptic target cell. Recently, it has been reported that homosynaptic LTD can be induced in hippocampal CA1 also by activating a single afferent system (Dudek and Bear, 1992). This required a rather special stimulation protocol in that 900 pulses had to be given at a frequency of 1 Hz.

5   THE MECHANISM OF THE MAINTENANCE OF HOMOSYNAPTIC LTD

In contrast to hippocampal LTP, where evidence is available that the changes in synaptic transmission are due to both presynaptic and postsynaptic modifications (for review, see chapter 5) there is so far only evidence for postsynaptic changes after LTD induction. In the cerebellum the results of quantal analysis suggest that LTD is associated with a reduced sensitivity of the postsynaptic glutamate receptors on PCs (Hirano, 1991). This is supported by experiments in which PF activation was substituted by direct iontophoretic application of glutamate or quisqualate. It has been shown that repeated pairing of CF activation with application of the excitatory amino acids led to a strong and lasting decrease of the sensitivity to the iontophoretically applied amino acids (Crepel and Krupa, 1988; Ito et al., 1982; Kano and Kato, 1987). In another experiment on cultured PCs both CF and PF activation were substituted by direct depolarization of the PCs by current injection and iontophoretic administration of glutamate or quisqualate, respectively, and the results were similar (Linden et al., 1991). There was a marked and lasting reduction of the response to the excitatory amino acids after these had been applied repeatedly in conjunction with postsynaptic depolarization of the PC. Thus, activation conditions closely resembling those leading to LTD in vivo or in slice preparations are associated with postsynaptic modifications that reduce the sensitivity to the putative transmitter of PFs.

In the neocortex comparably detailed investigations of the site of the modification responsible for the maintenance of LTD are still lacking. The only result pertinent to this question is that paired pulse facilitation is unchanged after induction of LTD (Artola et al., 1992). This suggests that in the neo-cortex LTD is probably not associated with a major change in presynaptic release mechanisms. Evidence from the cerebellum indicates that if there is a change in release, it actually consists of an increase rather than a decrease. Tetanic stimulation of PFs leads to an enhancement of the PF response if measures are taken that prevent LTD. This occurs when PFs are activated in slices or co-cultures in the absence of CF stimulation (Crepel and Jaillard, 1991; Hirano, 1990a; Sakurai, 1987) or when PFs and CFs are activated in conjunction but PCs are loaded at the same time with EGTA (Sakurai, 1990) or are hyperpolarized by current injection (Hirano, 1990b). The evidence available so far suggests that this potentiation of PF responses is due to changes in transmitter release (Crepel and Jaillard, 1991; Hirano, 1991). It is thus conceivable that tetanic stimulation of PFs always leads to an enhanced transmitter release and that this effect is normally overcompensated by the reduction of post-synaptic sensitivity when the LTD inducing processes are not inhibited.

6 REQUIREMENTS FOR THE INDUCTION OF HOMOSYNAPTIC LTD

At first sight it appears as if the conditions required for the induction of homosynaptic LTD differ in the various structures: cerebellar LTD requires conjunctive activation of CFs and PFs, hippocampal LTD is obtained best with out-of-phase activation of two different inputs, and cortical LTD can be induced by tetanic stimulation of a single input. However, closer examination of the processes involved in the induction of homosynaptic LTD reveals a number of similarities suggesting that the processes leading to depression of synaptic transmission in the different structures share common features.

Both in the cerebellum (Crepel and Krupa, 1988; Hirano, 1990a) and in the neocortex (Artola et al., 1990) induction of LTD requires a critical level of postsynaptic depolarization. In both structures coactivation of GABAergic inhibitory inputs to the postsynaptic cells reduces the probability that active inputs to these cells undergo LTD (Artola et al., 1992; Ekerot and Kano, 1985) while pharmacological blockade of inhibition enhances this probability (Artola et al., 1990; Hirsch and Crepel, 1990). Likewise, LTD induction can be blocked by directly hyperpolarizing the postsynaptic cell with current injection. This has been shown for cerebellar cultures (Hirano, 1990b) and for slice preparations of the cerebellum (Crepel and Jaillard, 1991) and of the visual cortex (Artola et al., 1990). In the cerebellum evidence is also available that the concomitant CF activation normally required for the induction of LTD in PFs can be substituted by direct depolarization of PCs (in slices: Crepel and Krupa, 1988; Crepel and Jaillard, 1991; in culture: Linden et al., 1991). These results suggest that CF activation is primarily required to obtain a sufficiently strong depolarization of PCs during the interval at which PFs are active. As will be discussed below, the out-of-phase activation of additional inputs to hippocampal cells is likely to have a similar function, namely, the adjustment of an appropriate depolarization level of the postsynaptic target.

Another similarity between cerebellar and neocortical LTD is the dependence on intracellular Ca^{2+}. Injection of the Ca^{2+} chelators BABTA or EGTA into PCs (Sakurai, 1990) or into neocortical cells (Bröcher et al., 1992; Hirsch and Crepel, 1992) blocks the induction of LTD, suggesting that a minimum or even a surge of intracellular $[Ca^{2+}]$ is required for LTD induction in both cerebellum and neocortex. Evidence that LTD induction actually requires a surge of intracellular $[Ca^{2+}]$ above the normal resting level due to Ca^{2+} entry from extracellular space comes from two observations. In slices of the visual cortex an increase of extracellular $[Ca^{2+}]$ to 4 mM facilitates tetanus-induced LTD (Artola et al., 1992), and in cultured PCs reduction of extracellular Ca^{2+} to zero prevents the depression of responses to iontophoretically applied glutamate that would normally occur when PCs are strongly depolarized in the presence of glutamate (Linden et al., 1991). The interpretation that induction of homosynaptic LTD requires a surge of intracellular $[Ca^{2+}]$ agrees also with the known effect of CF activation. CF stimulation produces a compound depolarization of PCs (Ekerot and Oscarsson, 1981; Konnerth et al., 1990), activates voltage-gated Ca^{2+} conductances (Llinas and Sugimori, 1980), and leads to a massive increase of intracellular $[Ca^{2+}]$ (Ross and Werman, 1987).

Furthermore, evidence is available that in all structures investigated so far induction of homosynaptic LTD is facilitated by the activation of metabotropic glutamate receptors. In cultured PCs, in cerebellar wedges, and in slices of area CA1 combined application of AMPA and ACPD, an agonist of the metabotropic glutamate receptor, induced a persistent desensitization of AMPA receptors (Ito and Karachot, 1990; Linden et al., 1991; Stanton, personal communication). Conversely, blockade of metabotropic glutamate receptors by AP3 prevented the induction of LTD in hippocampus (Stanton et al., 1991), neocortex (Artola, unpublished observations; Crepel, personal communication) and cultured PCs (Linden et al., 1991).

Finally, neither cerebellar nor hippocampal and neocortical LTD appear to require activation of NMDA receptors. Both hippocampal and neocortical LTD can be induced in the presence of the NMDA receptor blocker AP5 (Artola et al., 1990; Hirsch and Crepel, 1991; Stanton and Sejnowski, 1989) and cerebellar PCs lack NMDA receptors altogether. However, under special circumstances a slight activation of NMDA receptors may actually facilitate the induction of LTD in the hippocampus (see below).

So far then, all available evidence indicates that the signals which lead to homosynaptic LTD are generated in the postsynaptic neuron following a surge of intracellular $[Ca^{2+}]$. The existence of a voltage-dependent threshold for LTD induction suggests further that this Ca^{2+} entry is at least in part mediated by voltage-gated Ca^{2+} channels. The finding that activation of metabotropic glutamate receptors facilitates LTD induction can be interpreted in two ways: As activation of metabotropic glutamate receptors leads to an increase of intracellular IP3 (Sladeczek et al., 1985) and as a consequence to release of Ca^{2+} from internal stores (Berridge and Irvine, 1989), this mechanism can contribute directly to the surge of intracellular $[Ca^{2+}]$ (in PCs: Llano et al., 1991). Alternatively or in addition, the reduction of K^+ conductances which has also been observed after activation of metabotropic glutamate receptors (Charpak et al., 1990; Charpak and Gähwhiler, 1991) could enhance the depolarizing response to afferent stimulation and thereby increase the activation of voltage-gated Ca^{2+} conductances.

The analysis of the signal cascades which eventually lead to the modifications responsible for homosynaptic LTD has so far been confined to the cerebellar preparation (see chapter 6). One of the messengers that have attracted considerable attention is nitric oxyde (NO). Blockade of NO synthesis by L-NMMA or of NO action by hemoglobin has been shown to prevent LTD induction (Crepel and Jaillard, 1991; Ito and Karachot, 1990; Shibuki and Okada, 1991). However, NO does not appear to be involved directly in mediating the desensitization of postsynapatic glutamate receptors, because the depression that results in cultured cerebellar PCs from pairing iontophoretically applied glutamate with direct postsynaptic depolarization persists after blockade of NO synthesis (Linden and Connor, 1992). It is thus possible that NO is only required as a messenger when LTD is induced by synaptic activation. A possible scenario is that NO is released as a consequence of strong local activation, diffuses into presynaptic terminals, and enhances transmitter release (O'Dell et al., 1991), which would in turn increase postsynaptic depolarization and raise the probability of reaching the activation threshold of the LTD-inducing process.

Another possible messenger in the cascade of events leading to LTD is protein kinase C (PKC). Phorbol esters, which are known to activate PKC, have been shown in the cerebellum to reduce the sensitivity of postsynaptic glutamate receptors in a similar way as has been shown for LTD (Crepel and Jaillard, 1991; Crepel and Krupa, 1988; Linden and Connor, 1991). Conversely, LTD is blocked by applying antagonists of PKC (Crepel and Jaillard, 1991; Linden and Connor, 1991). While these results suggest phosphorylation as a requirement for LTD induction, other evidence points toward an involvement of dephosphorylation. Protein phosphatase inhibitors such as okadaic acid or calyculin block the induction of glutamate desensitization in cerebellar wedges (Ito, personal communication).

7   COMPARISON BETWEEN HETEROSYNAPTIC AND HOMOSYNAPTIC LTD IN HIPPOCAMPUS AND IN NEOCORTEX

Homosynaptic and heterosynaptic depression appear to share a number of features both with respect to the conditions required for their induction and the mechanisms responsible for their maintenance. In both cases induction requires postsynaptic depolarization above a critical threshold and a rise of intracellular $[Ca^{2+}]$. Direct support for the possibility that induction of homosynaptic and heterosynaptic LTD depends on the same postsynaptic mechanism comes from a recent finding in visual cortex slices. The input-

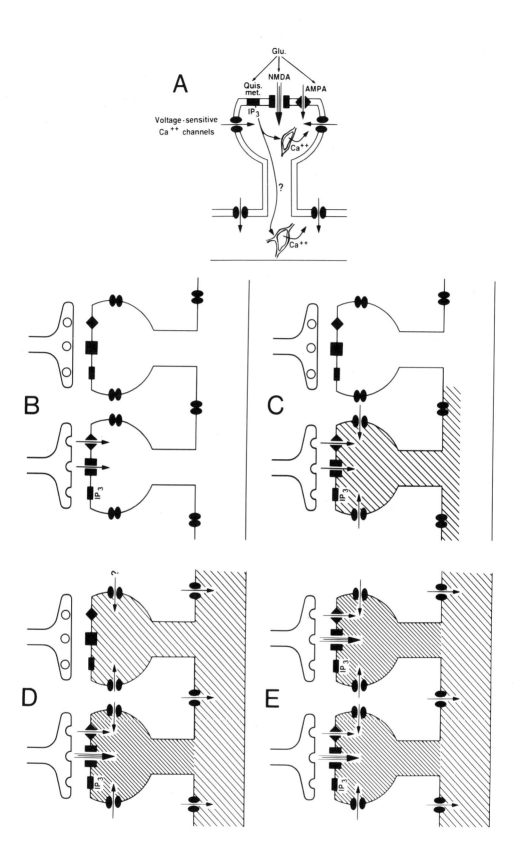

independent LTD that can be induced by raising extracellular [Ca^{2+}] occluded the input-specific tetanus-induced LTD (Artola et al., 1992). This suggests that the LTD-inducing mechanisms are the same in the two cases. The scenario that could account for a common mechanism of both homosynaptic and heterosynaptic depression is summarized in figure 7.1A. The assumption is that depression results whenever there is a sufficient accumulation of free Ca^{2+} in the vicinity of the synapses that are going to be depressed, irrespective of whether these synapses had been active or inactive during LTD induction.

During induction of heterosynaptic LTD, the modified synapses are inactive and cannot contribute to the postulated surge of [Ca^{2+}]. Hence, it must result from other excitatory inputs. One possibility is that the depolarization caused by the active inputs spreads electrotonically or through regenerative mechanisms and activates voltage-gated Ca^{2+} conductances in the vicinity of the postsynaptic domains of the synapses that undergo depression. This possibility would account for the fact that high-frequency antidromic activation can also produce input-independent LTD (Dunwiddie and Lynch, 1978; Pockett et al., 1990). Another possibility is that Ca^{2+} diffuses from the activated dendritic segments to the postsynaptic compartments of the synapses that undergo depression. The question here is whether sufficient Ca^{2+} can diffuse into the spine to reach the level required for LTD induction. Recent

Figure 7.1 Schematic representation of the suggested role of intracellular calcium in use-dependent synaptic modifications. (A) Summary of ligand- and voltage-gated mechanisms that modulate calcium concentration in the postsynaptic dendritic compartment. (B–E) Homosynaptic and heterosynaptic modifications of synaptic transmission for two inputs terminating on spines of the same dendritic segment. Mechanisms influencing intracellular calcium concentration are indicated by symbols as in (A). Arrows indicate calcium fluxes and their number the amplitude of the flux. The density of the hatching in the postsynaptic compartment reflects the expected concentration increase of intracellular calcium. In (B) to (D) only the lower input is assumed to be active, while in (E) both inputs are simultaneously active. The four conditions differ in addition by the amplitude of the depolarizing responses of the postsynaptic dendrite. It is assumed that this amplitude is determined both by the activity of the modifiable synapses and by the state of the many other excitatory, inhibitory and modulatory inputs to the same dendritic compartment (not shown). (B) AMPA, NMDA, and metabotropic quisqualate receptors are only moderately activated; voltage-gated calcium conductances are inactive. There is no substantial rise of intracellular calcium and no lasting modification of synaptic transmission at the active synapse. (C) In addition to the activation condition in (B), voltage-gated calcium conductances in the dendritic spine are also activated. Postsynaptic calcium rises to an intermediate level and induces long-term depression of the active synapse. There is only little spread of calcium from the active spine to other dendritic compartments. (D) Activation causes more postsynaptic depolarization as in (B) and (C) accordingly, NMDA receptor–gated conductances and voltage-gated calcium channels are strongly activated. The massive increase of calcium in the activated spine leads to long-term potentiation. Moreover, depolarization spreads to other compartments of the dendrite, where it activates voltage-gated calcium conductances. This leads to an intermediate rise of calcium also at the postsynaptic side of the inactive synapse which therefore undergoes heterosynaptic depression. (E) The second input is now activated as well. It no longer undergoes long-term depression but becomes potentiated because the rise of calcium in the postsynaptic compartment is now sufficient for the induction of LTP.

data from Ca^{2+} imaging have shown that the spine neck forms a barrier for the diffusion of high $[Ca^{2+}]$ from the dendritic shaft into spines (Guthrie et al., 1991). Nevertheless, both possibilities need to be considered, as both are compatible with the evidence that processes which enhance depolarization (NMDA receptor activation, disinhibition, closure of K^+ channels) and increase Ca^{2+} entry (NMDA receptor activation, high extracellular Ca^{2+}, enhanced depolarization) facilitate the occurrence of heterosynaptic LTD.

In this scenario homosynaptic LTD differs from heterosynaptic LTD only with respect to the input causing the required postsynaptic activation and the rise of $[Ca^{2+}]$. In the case of homosynaptic LTD, activation is caused by the same afferents that are going to be depressed. Hence, transmitter is released at the synapses that undergo modification, and Ca^{2+} can be provided not only by voltage-gated but also by ligand-gated Ca^{2+} conductances and by metabotropic glutamate receptors. This agrees with the evidence that activation of metabotropic glutamate receptors and, under certain conditions, activation of NMDA receptor–gated conductances (see below) facilitate induction of homosynaptic LTD.

Viewed in this way both the homosynaptic LTD observed in the cerebellum after conjunctive stimulation of PFs and CFs and also the depression observed in the hippocampus in pathways activated out of phase with another strongly activated input (Chattarji et al., 1989; Stanton and Sejnowski, 1989) would have to be considered as a mixture of homosynaptic and heterosynaptic LTD. In both cases, only activation of the pathway that is going to be depressed is not sufficient to induce depression but requires the coactivation of other excitatory inputs. In the case of the cerebellum, it is easy to see how activation of CFs can contribute to raise intracellular $[Ca^{2+}]$ to the level required for LTD induction. It is more difficult to explain why the out-of-phase activation of strongly activated inputs in the hippocampus should promote homosynaptic LTD of other weakly activated afferents. There are two possibilities: Synaptic inputs to hippocampal cells are very susceptible to undergoing LTP if they activate NMDA receptor-gated conductances. Thus, the priming input, by generating inhibition, could prevent the input system that is going to be depressed from activating its NMDA receptor-gated conductances. Another possibility is that the priming input preloads the cells with Ca^{2+}, which then adds to the Ca^{2+} influx caused by the activation of the input that will be depressed. Both interpretations are compatible with the fact that LTD induction in the hippocampus depends critically on a precise adjustment of the stimulus parameters and the timing of the priming and the test input. LTD is expected to occur only if the test input does not cause strong NMDA receptor activation—as this would induce LTP—but despite this triggers sufficient Ca^{2+} entry to reach the LTD threshold. In the neocortex, LTD induction requires a less critical adjustment of stimulation parameters. The activated input depresses whenever it produces a sufficient depolarization of the postsynaptic target and concomitant Ca^{2+} entry without simultaneously activating NMDA receptor–gated conductances.

8 COMPARISON OF LTD AND LTP IN HIPPOCAMPUS AND IN NEOCORTEX

The requirements for LTD induction, strong postsynaptic depolarization associated with a rise of intracellular $[Ca^{2+}]$, closely resemble those required for the induction of associative LTP (for review see chapter 5). The only major difference appears to be that LTP induction requires a stronger postsynaptic depolarization. This is particularly clear in the neocortex, where LTD and LTP can be induced in alternation in the same pathway solely by varying the level of postsynaptic depolarization. These results have led to the notion of two voltage-dependent thresholds for LTD and LTP induction, respectively. If the first is reached, the activated synapses depress, and if the second is reached, which requires stronger depolarization, the activated synapses potentiate (Artola et al., 1990). The observation in CA1 that low-frequency (around 1 Hz) stimulation induces LTD (Dudeck and Bear, 1992; Dunwiddie and Lynch, 1978) while high-frequency stimulation (above 1 Hz) with the same number of pulses induces LTP is consistent with the above conclusion if one assumes that postsynaptic depolarization increases with stimulation frequency.

The evidence that LTP induction requires stronger depolarization than LTD induction suggests the possibility that the former requires a greater surge of intracellular Ca^{2+} than the latter. This hypothesis is supported by several observations: First, in neocortex, incomplete buffering of intracellular Ca^{2+} by EGTA or BAPTA readily prevents induction of LTP but still allows for the induction of LTD (Bröcher et al., 1992; Kimura et al., 1990; Yoshimura et al., 1991). Second, the rise of intracellular $[Ca^{2+}]$ in postsynaptic spines increases with the frequency of the tetanus (Regehr and Tank, 1990) and the same is true for the probability of LTP induction. Third, in most cases induction of associative LTP requires, in addition to depolarization, the activation of NMDA receptor-gated conductances both in hippocampus (Collingridge et al., 1983) and in neocortex (Artola and Singer, 1987, 1990; but see following). This has led to the proposal that the second threshold, which discriminates between LTD and LTP, is associated with activation of NMDA receptor-gated conductances (Bear et al., 1987). Direct evidence for this proposal is now available. In visual cortex slices the same tetanic stimulus induces LTP when NMDA receptors are activatable and homosynaptic LTD when NMDA receptors are blocked (Artola et al., 1990). Activation of NMDA receptor-gated conductances can in turn be expected to cause particularly strong increases of $[Ca^{2+}]$ in the vicinity of the active synapses: First, it increases postsynaptic depolarization and thereby enhances activation of voltage-gated Ca^{2+} conductances, and second, it mediates a substantial influx of Ca^{2+} (MacDermott et al., 1986). Recent data from Ca^{2+} imaging support this notion. It has been shown for CA3 cells of the hippocampus that tetanus-induced increases of $[Ca^{2+}]$ reach much higher values in dendritic spines than in the dendritic shaft and that this large increase in the spine is mainly due to NMDA receptor-gated conductances (Müller and Connor, 1991). However, NMDA receptor activation is not an indispensable requirement for LTP induction. Under certain conditions, such as stimulation at very high frequencies (Grover and Teyler, 1990) or blockade of K^+ channels (Aniksztejn and Ben-Ari, 1991), associative LTP can be induced in hippocampal CA1 even in the presence of AP5. Likewise, NMDA receptor–independent LTP has been obtained in the visual cortex of young rats and kittens (Bear et al., 1992; Komatsu et al., 1988). This suggests that activation of NMDA receptor–gated conductances is not the only, but probably the most effective way to reach the very high $[Ca^{2+}]$ in the spine necessary to trigger LTP. Conversely, Ca^{2+} entry through NMDA receptor–gated channels need not always trigger LTP. There are many examples where synaptic transmission is not modified even if associated with a significant activation of NMDA receptors. The recent study of Dudek and Bear (1992) adds to this notion by indicating that activation of NMDA receptor-gated conductances can even contribute to LTD induction if this activation remains weak.

In conclusion, these results are all compatible with the interpretation that the critical variable for the differential induction of LTD and LTP is the amplitude of the surge of $[Ca^{2+}]$ in the postsynaptic compartment, LTD induction requiring less Ca^{2+} than LTP induction. Results from Ca^{2+} imaging support this interpretation by showing that stimulation conditions suitable for LTD induction cause less pronounced increases of Ca^{2+} than those which usually lead to LTP. If NMDA receptors are blocked, a condition that is compatible with LTD induction (Artola et al., 1990; Hirsch and Crepel, 1991; Stanton and Sejnowski, 1989), tetanic stimulation still leads to $[Ca^{2+}]$ increases in dendritic spines, but these are much smaller than if NDMA receptors are activated (Müller and Connor, 1991; Regehr et al., 1989).

Two possibilities may be considered to explain why Ca^{2+} apparently has opposite effects on synaptic transmission depending on the source of the Ca^{2+} surge and/or its amplitude. NMDA receptor-gated Ca^{2+} surges are with all likelihood maximal in the immediate vicinity of the postsynaptic receptors as this is the site where Ca^{2+} enters. Changes in $[Ca^{2+}]$ following activation of metabotropic glutamate receptors should be maximal close to the release sites from endoplasmic reticulum and those caused by voltage-dependent conductances should peak close to the membrane containing the respective channels. It is thus conceivable that Ca^{2+} provided by these different sources has differential actions on the various Ca^{2+}-activated second messenger cascades. Another possibility is that the differential effects of intracellular Ca^{2+} are solely concentration dependent. It has been proposed that intracellular Ca^{2+} can indeed have opposite effects depending on concentration because Ca^{2+}-regulated enzymes have different affinities for Ca^{2+} (Lisman, 1989). Based on this evidence, Lisman predicted that low levels of Ca^{2+} should lead to preferential activation of phosphatases while high levels should activate predominantly kinases. In the light of the recent evidence that the efficacy of glutamate receptor-gated ion channels can be changed by dephosphorylation and phosphorylation (Greengard et al., 1991; Wang et al., 1991), it is tempting to speculate that the Ca^{2+}-dependent depression and potentiation of excitatory transmission at glutamatergic synapses such as occurs with LTP and LTD is actually brought about by differential activation of Ca^{2+}-regulated enzymes with different Ca^{2+} affinity.

9 CHANGES OF INTRACELLULAR [Ca^{2+}] AS A COMMON TRIGGER FOR USE-DEPENDENT SYNAPTIC MODIFICATIONS

The data available on the induction of LTP and both homosynaptic and heterosynaptic LTD are all compatible with the hypothesis that the main determinant for the induction and the direction of a long-term synaptic modification is the amplitude of the [Ca^{2+}] increase in the postsynaptic compartment close to the modified synapse. The associative form of LTP appears to require very strong increases of [Ca^{2+}]. Under normal conditions of synaptic activation these are usually reached only when NMDA receptor-gated conductances contribute substantially to synaptic transmission. LTD, by contrast, appears to occur with [Ca^{2+}] surges of smaller amplitude such as can be reached by activation of voltage-gated Ca^{2+} conductances, activation of metabotropic glutamate receptors, and/or moderate activation of NMDA receptor–gated conductances. As the following examples illustrates, this hypothesis accounts well for the various conditions leading to LTP and homosynaptic and heterosynaptic LTD. In the neocortex and in the hippocampus, where excitatory synapses are endowed with NMDA receptors, the Ca^{2+} hypothesis predicts correctly that conditions which favor the activation of NMDA receptor–gated conductances, such as conjunction of presynaptic activity with strong postsynaptic depolarization, favor the occurrence of LTP. As NMDA receptor–gated conductances cannot be activated at inactive synapses because of the absence of the receptor-ligand, the Ca^{2+} hypothesis also accounts for the fact that there is no heterosynaptic LTP (but see Bradler and Barrionuevo, 1990). Furthermore, the Ca^{2+} hypothesis can explain why inputs become resistant to depression if they are themselves active and why this protective effect is abolished if NMDA receptors are blocked (see above and Artola et al., 1992). The assumption is that the active inputs, because they release transmitter, activate NMDA receptor–gated conductances and thereby raise [Ca^{2+}] in the spine above the range leading to LTD and into the range which induces LTP. Finally, since Purkinje cells are devoid of NMDA receptors, the Ca^{2+} hypothesis accounts for the nonccurrence of associative LTP in the synapses betweeen parallel fibers and Purkinje cells.

The Ca^{2+} hypothesis also accounts well for the conditions required to induce homosynaptic LTD in hippocampus and cortex. In both structures the synapses that can undergo LTD are endowed with NMDA receptors. This makes it more difficult to evoke the intermediate Ca^{2+} levels required for LTD induction. On the one hand, strong activation of NMDA receptor–gated conductances has to be avoided; on the other hand, enough Ca^{2+} has to be provided to reach the LTD threshold. In neocortex this can be achieved with precise control of the depolarization level of the postsynaptic neuron or with pharmacological blockade of NMDA receptors or, alternatively, by controlling the surge of intracellular [Ca^{2+}] with Ca^{2+} chelators. The fact that stimulation paradigms suitable for the induction of homosynaptic LTD have to be adjusted more precisely in the hippocampus than in the neocortex seems to indicate that in the former the LTD and LTP thresholds are either closer together or intracellular Ca^{2+} levels are more difficult to control.

The Ca^{2+} hypothesis also agrees well with the conditions which lead to the induction of heterosynaptic LTD, and this supports the proposal that the mechanisms responsible for homosynaptic and heterosynaptic LTD may actually be the same. The assumption is that inactive synapses depress whenever $[Ca^{2+}]$ in their postsynaptic compartment reaches the threshold for LTD, which is assumed to be the same for homosynaptic and heterosynaptic modifications. Because the synapses that are going to be modified are inactive, NMDA receptors cannot be activated and no precautions have to be taken to control Ca^{2+} influx through NMDA receptor-gated channels. Thus, in agreement with available data, all conditions that enhance postsynaptic depolarization and Ca^{2+}-entry also favor the occurrence of heterosynaptic depression.

Finally, it follows that inactive synapses should undergo depression even without stimulating other synaptic inputs to the neuron if the required $[Ca^{2+}]$ surge can be induced by other methods. Such has been shown to be the case with high-frequency antidromic stimulation and with increasing extracellular $[Ca^{2+}]$.

The hypothesis that the source and the amplitude of Ca^{2+} surges in the vicinity of synapses are key variables for the differential induction of LTD and LTP does not, of course, rule out additional factors determining the probability of occurrence of depression and potentiation. Thus, the lack of NMDA receptors may not be the only cause for the nonoccurrence of associative LTP in synapses between parallel fibers and Purkinje cells or between mossy fibers and CA3 pyramidal cells. In addition, it is conceivable that some of the Ca^{2+}-modulated second messenger systems are lacking. Lack of Ca^{2+}-dependent signal cascades could also explain why neither climbing fibers nor mossy fibers undergo LTD although activation leads to strong increases of postsynaptic Ca^{2+}. However, as it is still unknown which of the Ca^{2+}-dependent signaling cascades is responsible for the induction of LTP and LTD, the question of a synapse-specific differential expression of these mechanisms cannot yet be approached experimentally.

REFERENCES

Abraham, W. C., and Goddard, G. V. (1983) Asymmetric relationships between homosynaptic long-term potentiation and heterosynaptic long-term potentiation. *Nature* 305:717–718.

Abraham, W. C., and Wickens, J. R. (1991) Heterosynaptic long-term depression is facilitated by blockade of inhibition in area CA1 of the hippocampus. *Brain Res.* 546:336–340.

Alger, B. E., Megela, A. L., and Teyler, T. J. (1978) Transient heterosynaptic depression in the hippocampal slice. *Brain Res. Bull.* 3:181–184.

Andersen, P., Sundberg, S. H., Sveen, O., and Wigström, H. (1977) Specific long-lasting potentiation of synaptic transmission in hippocampal slices. *Nature* 266:736–737.

Andersen, P., Sundberg, S. H., Sveen, O. Swann, J. W., and Wigström, H. (1980) Possible mechanisms for long-lasting potentiation of synaptic transmission in hippocampal slices from guinea-pigs. *J. Physiol.* 302:463–482.

Aniksztejn, L., and Ben-Ari, Y. (1991) Novel form of long-term potentiation produced by a K$^+$-channel blocker in the hippocampus. *Nature* 349:67–69.

Artola, A., and Singer, W. (1987) Long-term potentiation and NMDA receptors in rat visual cortex. *Nature* 330:649–652.

Artola, A. and Singer, W. (1990) The involvement of *N*-methyl-D-aspartate receptors in induction and maintenance of long-term potentiation in rat visual cortex. *Eur. J. Neurosci.* 2:254–269.

Artola, A., Bröcher, S., and Singer, W. (1990) Different voltage-dependent thresholds for the induction of long-term depression and long-term potentiation in slices of the rat visual cortex. *Nature* 347:69–72.

Artola, A., Hensch, T., and Singer, W. (1992) A rise of [Ca^{2+}] in the postsynaptic cell is necessary and sufficient for the induction of long-term depression (LTD) in neocortex. *Soc. Neurosci.* 18:567.30.

Bear, M. F., Cooper, L. N., and Ebner, F. F. (1987) A physiological basis for a theory of synapse modification. *Science* 237:42–48.

Bear, M. F., Press, W. A., and Connors, B. W. (1992) Long-term potentiation in slices of kitten visual cortex and the effects of NMDA receptor blockade. *J. Neurophysiol.* 67:841–851.

Berridge, M. J., and Irvine, R. F. (1989) Inositol phosphates and cell signalling. *Nature* 341:197–205.

Bindman, L. J., Murphy, K. P. S. J., and Pockett, S. (1988) Postsynaptic control of the induction of long-term changes in efficacy of transmission at neocortical synapses in slices of rat brain. *J. Neurophysiol.* 60:1053–1965.

Bliss, T. V. P., and Lømo, T. (1973) Long-lasting potentiation of synaptic transmission in the dentate area of the anaesthetized rabbit following stimulation of the perforant path. *J. Physiol.* 232:331–356.

Bradler, J. E., and Barrionuevo, G. (1989) Long-term potentiation in hippocampal CA3 neurons: Tetanized input regulates heterosynaptic efficacy. *Synapse* 4:132–142.

Bradler, J. E., and Barrionuevo, G. (1990) Heterosynaptic correlates of long-term potentiation induction in hippocampal CA3 neurons. *Neuroscience* 35:265–271.

Bröcher, S., Artola, A., and Singer, W. (1992) Intracellular injection of Ca^{++} chelators blocks induction of long-term depression in rat visual cortex. *Proc. Natl. Acad. Sci. USA* 89:123–127.

Charpak, S., and Gähwiler, B. H. (1991) Glutamate mediates a slow synaptic response in hippocampal slice cultures. *Proc. Roy. Soc. Lond. (Biol.)* 243:221–226.

Charpak, S., Gähwiler, B. H., Do, K. Q., and Knöpfel, T. (1990) Potassium conductances in hippocampal neurons blocked by excitatory amino-acid transmitters. *Nature* 347:765–767.

Chattarji, S., Stanton, P. K., and Sejnowski, T. J. (1989) Commissural synapses, but not mossy fiber synapses, in hippocampal field CA3 exhibit associative long-term potentiation and depression. *Brain Res.* 495:145–150.

Collingridge, G. L., Kehl, S. J., and McLennan, H. (1983) Excitatory amino acids in synaptic transmission in the Schaffer collateral-commissural pathway of the rat hippocampus. *J. Physiol.* 334:33–46.

Collingridge, G. L., Herron, C. E., and Lester, R. A. J. (1988) Frequency-dependent *N*-methyl-D-aspartate receptor-mediated synaptic transmission in rat hippocampus. *J. Physiol.* 399:301–312.

Crepel, F., and Jaillard, D. (1991) Pairing of pre- and postsynaptic activities in cerebellar Purkinje cells induces long-term changes in synaptic efficacy in vitro. *J. Physiol.* 432:123−141.

Crepel, F., and Krupa, M. (1988) Activation of protein kinase C induces a long-term depression of glutamate sensitivity of cerebellar Purkinje cells. An in vitro study. *Brain Res.* 458:397−401.

Desmond, N. L., Colbert, C. M., Zhang, D. X., and Levy, W. B. (1991) NMDA receptor antagonists block the induction of long-term depression in the hippocampal dentate gyrus of the anesthetized rat. *Brain Res.* 552:93−98.

Dudek, S. M., and Bear, M. F. (1992) Homosynaptic long-term depression in area CA1 of hippocampus and effects of *N*-methyl-D-aspartate receptor blockade. *Proc. Natl. Acad. Sci. USA* 89:4363−4367.

Dunwiddie, T., and Lynch, G. (1978) Long-term potentiation and depression of synaptic responses in the rat hippocampus: localization and frequency dependency. *J. Physiol.* 276:353−367.

Ekerot, C.-F., and Kano, M. (1985) Long-term depression of parallel fibre synapses following stimulation of climbing fibres. *Brain Res.* 342:357−360.

Ekerot, C.-F., and Oscarsson, O. (1981) Prolonged depolarization elicited in Purkinje cell dendrites by climing fibre impulses in the cat. *J. Physiol.* 318:207−221.

Greengard, P., Jen, J., Nairn, A. C., and Stevens, C. F. (1991) Enhancement of the glutamate response by cAMP-dependent protein kinase in hippocampal neurons. *Science* 253:1135−1137.

Grover, L. M., and Teyler, T. J. (1990) Two components of long-term potentiation induced by different patterns of afferent activation. *Nature* 347:477−479.

Guthrie, P. B., Segal, M., and Kater, S. B. (1991) Independent regulation of calcium revealed by imaging dendritic spines. *Nature* 354:76−80.

Hirano, T. (1990a) Depression and potentiation of the synaptic transmission between a granule cell and a Purkinje cell in rat cerebellar culture. *Neurosci. Lett.* 119:141−144.

Hirano, T. (1990b) Effects of postsynaptic depolarization in the induction of synaptic depression between a granule cell and a Purkinje cell in rat cerebellar culture. *Neurosci. Lett.* 119:145−147.

Hirano, T. (1991) Differential pre- and postsynaptic mechanisms for synaptic potentiation and depression between a granule cell and a Purkinje cell in rat cerebellar culture. *Synapse* 7:321−323.

Hirsch, J. C., and Crepel, F. (1990) Use-dependent changes in synaptic efficacy in rat prefrontal neurons in vitro. *J. Physiol.* 427:31−49.

Hirsch, J. C., and Crepel, F. (1991) Blockade of NMDA receptors unmasks a long-term depression in synaptic efficacy in rat prefrontal neurons in vitro. *Exp. Brain Res.* 85:621−624.

Hirsch, J. C., and Crepel, F. (1992) Postsynaptic calcium is necessary for the induction of LTP and LTD of monosynaptic EPSPs in prefrontal neurons: An in vitro study in the rat. *Synapse* 10:173−175.

Ito, M., and Kano, M. (1982) Long-lasting depression of parallel fiber-Purkinje cell transmission induced by conjunctive stimulation of parallel fibers and climbing fibers in the cerebellar cortex. *Neurosci. Lett.* 33:253−258.

Ito, M., and Karachot, L. (1990) Receptor subtype involved in, and time course of, the long-term desensitization of glutamate receptors in cerebellar Purkinje cells. *Neurosci. Res.* 8:303−307.

Ito, M., Sakurai, M., and Tongroach, P. (1982) Climbing fibre induced depression of both mossy fibre responsiveness and glutamate sensitivity of cerebellar Purkinje cells. *J. Physiol.* 324:113−134.

Kano, M., and Kato, M. (1987) Quisqualate receptors are specifically involved in cerebellar synaptic plasticity. *Nature* 325:276–279.

Kimura, F., Tsumoto, T., Nishigori, A., and Yoshimura, Y. (1990) Long-term depression but not potentiation is induced in Ca^{2+}-chelated visual cortex neurons. *NeuroReport* 1:65–68.

Komatsu, Y., Fuji, K., Maede, J., Sakaguchi, H., and Toyama, K. (1988) Long-term potentiation of synaptic transmission in kitten visual cortex. *J. Neurophysiol.* 59:124–141.

Konnerth, A., Llano, I., and Armstrong, C. M. (1990) Synaptic currents in cerebellar Purkinje cells. *Proc. Natl. Acad. Sci. USA* 87:2662–2665.

Levy, W. B., and Steward, O. (1979) Synapses as associative memory elements in the hippocampal formation. *Brain Res.* 175:233–245.

Levy, W. B., and Steward, O. (1983) Temporal contiguity requirements for long-term associative potentiation/depression in the hippocampus. *Neuroscience* 8:791–797.

Linden, D. J., and Connor, J. A. (1991) Participation of postsynaptic PKC in cerebellar long-term depression in culture. *Science* 254:1656–1659.

Linden, D. J., and Connor, J. A. (1992) Long-term depression of glutamate currents in cultured cerebellar Purkinje neurons does not require nitric oxide signalling. *Eur. J. Neurosci.* 4:10–15.

Linden, D. J., Dickinson, M. H., Smeyne, M., and Connor, J. A., (1991) A long-term depression of AMPA currents in cultured cerebellar Purkinje neurons. *Neuron* 7:81–89.

Lisman, J. (1989) A mechanism for the Hebb and the anti-Hebb processes underlying learning and memory. *Proc. Natl. Acad. Sci. USA* 86:9574–9578.

Llano, I., Dreessen, J., Kano, M., and Konnerth, A. (1991) Intradendritic release of calcium induced by glutamate in cerebellar Purkinje cells. *Neuron* 5:577–583.

Llinas, R. R., and Sugimori, M. (1980) Electrophysiological properties of in vitro Purkinje cell dendrites in mammalian cerebellar slices. *J. Physiol.* 305:197–213.

Lynch, G. S., Gribkoff, V. K., and Deadwyler, S. A. (1976) Long-term potentiation is accompanied by a reduction in dendritic responsiveness to glutamic acid. *Nature* 263:151–153.

Lynch, G. S., Dunwiddie, T., and Gribkoff, V. (1977) Heterosynaptic depression: A postsynaptic correlate of long-term potentiation. *Nature* 266:737–739.

MacDermott, A. B., Mayer, M. L., Westbrook, G. L., Smith, S. J., and Barker, J. L., (1986) NMDA-receptor activation increases cytoplasmic calcium concentration in cultured spinal cord neurones. *Nature* 321:519–522.

Mayer, M. L., Westbrook, G. L., and Guthrie, P. B. (1984) Voltage-dependent block by Mg^{2+} of NMDA responses in spinal cord neurones. *Nature* 309:261–263.

Müller, W., and Connor, J. A. (1991) Dendritic spines as individual neuronal compartments for synaptic Ca^{2+} responses. *Nature* 354:73–76.

Nowak, L., Bregestovski, P., Ascher, P., Herbet, A., and Prochiantz, A. (1984) Magnesium gates glutamate-activated channels in mouse central neurones. *Nature* 307:462–465.

O'Dell, T. J., Hawkins, R. D., Kandel, E. R., and Arancio, O. (1991) Tests of the roles of two diffusible substances in long-term potentiation: Evidence for nitric oxide as a possible early retrograde messenger. *Proc. Natl. Acad. Sci. USA* 88:11285–11289.

Pockett, S., and Lippold, O. C. J. (1986) Long-term potentiation and depression in hippocampal slices. *Exp. Neurol.* 91:481–487.

Pockett, S., Brookes, N. H., and Bindman, L. J. (1990) Long-term depression at synapses in slices of rat hippocampus can be induced by bursts of postsynaptic activity. *Exp. Brain Res.* 80:196–200.

Regehr, W. G., Connor, J. A., and Tank, D. W. (1989) Optical imaging of calcium accumulation in hippocampal pyramidal cells during synaptic activation. *Nature* 341:533–536.

Regehr, W. G., and Tank, D. W. (1990) Postsynaptic NMDA receptor-mediated calcium accumulation in hippocampal CA1 pyramidal cell dendrites. *Nature* 345:807–810.

Ross, W. N., and Werman, E. (1987) Mapping calcium transients in the dendrites of Purkinje cells from the guinea-pig cerebellum in vitro. *J. Physiol.* 389:319–336.

Sakurai, M. (1987) Synaptic modification of parallel fibre-Purkinje cell transmission in vitro guinea-pig cerebellar slices. *J. Physiol.* 394:463–480.

Sakurai, M. (1990) Calcium is an intracellular mediator of the climbing fiber in induction of cerebellar long-term depression. *Proc. Natl. Acad. Sci. USA* 87:3383–3385.

Sastry, B. R., Chirwa, S. S., Goh, J. W., Maretic, H., and Pandanaboina, M. M. (1984) Verapamil counteracts depression but not long-lasting potentiation of the hippocampal population spike. *Life Sci.* 34:1075–1086.

Shibuki, K., and Okada, D. (1991) Endogenous nitric oxide release required for long-term synaptic depression in the cerebellum. *Nature* 349:326–328.

Sladeczek, R., Pin, J.-P., Recasens, M., Bockaert, J., and Weiss, S. (1985) Glutamate stimulates inositol phosphate formation in striatal neurones. *Nature* 317:717–719.

Stanton, P. K., and Sejnowski, T. J. (1989) Associative long-term depression in the hippocampus induced by hebbian covariance. *Nature* 339:215–218.

Stanton, P. K., Chattarji, S., and Sejnowski, T. J. (1991) 2-Amino-3-phosphonopropionic acid, an inhibitor of glutamate-stimulated phosphoinositide turnover, blocks induction of homosynaptic long-term depression, but not potentiation, in rat hippocampus. *Neurosci. Lett.* 127:61–66.

Wang, L.-Y., Salter, M. W., and MacDonald, J. F. (1991) Regulation of kainate receptors by cAMP-dependent protein kinase and phosphatases. *Science* 253:1132–1135.

White, G., Levy, W. B., and Steward, O. (1990) Spatial overlap between populations of synapses determines the extent of their associative interaction during the induction of long-term potentiation and depression. *J. Neurosci.* 64:1186–1198.

Wickens, J. R., and Abraham, W. C. (1991) The involvement of L-type calcium channels in heterosynaptic long-term depression in the hippocampus. *Neurosci. Lett.* 130:128–132.

Yoshimura, Y., Tsumoto, T., and Nishigori, A. (1991) Input-specific induction of long-term depression in Ca^{2+}-chelated visual cortex neurons. *NeuroReport* 2:393–396.

8 Theory of Synaptic Plasticity in Visual Cortex

Nathan Intrator, Mark F. Bear, Leon N. Cooper, and Michael A. Paradiso

1 INTRODUCTION

Because of its great complexity, visual cortex would not seem to be an auspicious region of the brain in which to carry out an investigation of synaptic plasticity or of the mechanisms and sites of memory storage. It is, in addition, almost certain that much of the architecture of visual cortex is preprogrammed genetically, leaving a relatively minor percentage to be shaped or modified by experience. However, the fact that visual cortex is accessible to single-cell electrophysiology, so that the output of individual cells can be measured, whereas the inputs can be controlled by varying the visual experience of the animal has made this a preferred area for experimentation and analysis. Thus over the past 30 years, a great deal of experimental and theoretical work has been done to investigate the responses of visual cortical cells, as well as the alterations in these responses under various visual rearing conditions.

It is widely believed that much of the learning and resulting organization of visual cortex as well as other parts of the central nervous system occurs due to modification of the efficacy or strength of at least some of the synaptic junctions between neurons, thus altering the relation between presynaptic and postsynaptic potentials. The vast amount of experimental work done in visual cortex—particularly area 17 of cat and monkey—strongly indicates that one is observing a process of synaptic modification dependent on the information locally and globally available to the cortical cells. Furthermore, it is known that small but coherent modifications of large numbers of synaptic junctions can result in distributed memories. Whether and how such synaptic modification occurs, what precise forms it takes, and what the physiological and/or anatomical bases of this modification are, are among the most interesting questions in this area. There is no need to assume that such mechanisms operate in exactly the same manner in all portions of the nervous system or in all animals. However, one would hope that certain fundamental similarities exist, so that a detailed analysis of the properties of these mechanisms in one preparation would lead to some conclusions that are generally applicable.

It is our hope that such a general form of modifiability manifests itself for at least some cells of visual cortex that are accessible to experiment. If so, one then may be able to distinguish between different cortical plasticity theories with theoretical tools and the aid of sophisticated experimental paradigms. Among the difficulties faced by theoreticians are (1) adequate representation of the visual environment; (2) knowledge of what the actual inputs to cortical cells are; (3) the appropriate rule for synaptic modification; and (4) an adequate representation of the complex architecture of visual cortex.

In this article, we give a short account of the BCM (Bienenstock, Cooper, and Munro) theory of visual cortical plasticity that has been developed over the past 10 years, address the difficulties mentioned above and compare the consequences of the theory with experiment. We discuss recent physiological experiments that seem to provide verification of some of the underlying assumptions of the theory, and finally, we initiate a comparison of the BCM theory with other theories that have been proposed. We assume that the reader has some familiarity with experiments demonstrating plasticity in visual cortex. A brief review may be found in Clothiaux et al. (1991).

2 BCM THEORY

In what follows we give a brief overview of the BCM theory of synaptic plasticity. For a more detailed account the reader is referred to the various references cited below.

2.1 Single Cell

A typical neuron in striate cortex receives thousands of afferents from other cells. Most of these afferents derive from the lateral geniculate nucleus (LGN) and from other cortical neurons. We have approached the analysis of this complex network in several stages. In the first stage we consider a single neuron with inputs from both eyes (i.e., LGN) but without intracortical interactions.

The output of this neuron (in the linear region) can be written

$$c = m^l \cdot d^l + m^r d^r,$$

where d^l (d^r) are the LGN inputs coming from the left (right) eye to the vector of synaptic junctions m^l (m^r). The neuron firing rate (in the linear region) is therefore the sum of the inputs from the left eye multiplied by the appropriate left-eye synaptic weights plus the inputs from the right eye multiplied by the appropriate right-eye synaptic weights. Thus the neuron integrates signals from the left and right eyes. (For simplicity, whenever possible we shall omit the left and right superscripts.) According to the theory presented by Bienenstock, Cooper, and Munro (BCM; 1982), the synaptic weight changes over time as a function of local and global variables: its change in time, $\dot{m}_j$, is given below:

$$\dot{m}_j = F(d_j, \ldots, m_j; d_k, \ldots, c; \bar{\bar{c}}; X, Y, Z).$$

Here variables such as $d_j, \ldots, m_j$ are designated local. These represent information (such as the incoming signal, d_j, and the strength of the synaptic junction,

m_j) available locally at the synaptic junction, m_j. Variables such as $d_k, \ldots, c$ are designated quasi-local. These represent information (such as c, the firing rate or depolarization of the postsynaptic cell, or d_k, the incoming signal to another synaptic junction) that may not be locally available to the junction m_j but is physically connected to the junction by the cell body itself, thus necessitating some form of internal communication between various parts of the cell and its synaptic junctions. Variables such as $\bar{c}$ (the time-averaged output of the cell) are averaged local or quasi-local variables. Global variables are designated $X, Y, Z, \ldots$. These latter represent information (e.g., presence or absence of neurotransmitters such as norepinephrine or the average activity of large numbers of cortical cells) that is present in a similar fashion for all or a large number of cortical neurons (distinguished from local or quasi-local variables presumably carrying detailed information that varies from synapse to synapse or cell to cell). Neglecting global variables, one arrives at the following form of synaptic modification equation:

$$\dot{m}_j = \phi(c, \Theta_m)d_j \tag{2.1}$$

so that the jth synaptic junction, m_j, changes its value in time as the product of the input activity (the local variable d_j) and a function ϕ of quasi-local and time-averaged quasi-local variables, c and Θ_m. Θ_m is a nonlinear function of some time averaged measure of cell activity that in the original BCM formulation was proposed as

$$\Theta_m = (\bar{c})^2. \tag{2.2}$$

In the BCM theory, this time average is replaced, for simplicity, by a spatial average over the environmental inputs ($\bar{c} \to m \cdot \bar{d}$). The shape of the function ϕ is given in figure 8.1 for two different values of the threshold Θ_m. The occurrence of negative and positive regions for ϕ results in the cell becoming selectively responsive to subsets of stimuli in the visual environment. This happens because the response of the cell is diminished to those patterns for which the output, c, is below threshold (ϕ negative), while the response is enhanced to those patterns for which the output, c, is above threshold (ϕ positive). The nonlinear variation of the threshold Θ_m with the average output of the cell contributes to the development of selectivity and the stability of the system (Bienenstock et al., 1982; Intrator and Cooper, 1992).

2.2   Cortical Network: Mean Field Theory

The actual cortical network is very complex. It includes different cell types, intracortical interactions, and recurrent collaterals. In what follows we present a method of analyzing this complex system. The first step is to divide the inputs to any cell into those from the LGN and those from all other sources. The activity of neuron i is affected by its input vector d from the LGN, and by the adjacent cortical neurons;

$$c_i = m_i \cdot d + \sum_j L_{ij}c_j, \tag{2.3}$$

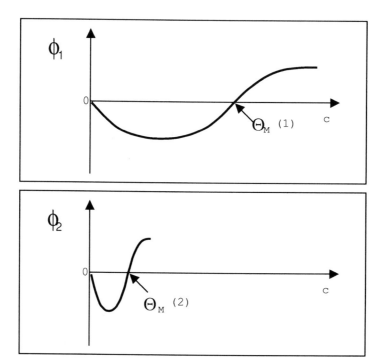

Figure 8.1 The ϕ function for two different Θ_m's.

where L_{ij} are the cortico-cortical synapses. Scofield and Cooper (1985; Cooper and Scofield, 1988) have analyzed a network extension of the single cell theory and a mean field approximation to the full network. Defining $\bar{c} = 1/N \sum_i c_i$, where N is the number of neurons in the network, the mean field approximation is obtained by replacing the inhibitory contribution of cell j, c_j by its average value (i.e., and average on all cells in the network) so that c_i becomes:

$$c_i = m_i \cdot d + \bar{c} \sum_j L_{ij}. \tag{2.4}$$

From a consistency condition it follows that $\bar{c} = \bar{m} \cdot d + \bar{c} L_0 = (1 - L_0)^{-1} \bar{m} \cdot d$, where $\bar{m} = 1/N \sum_i m_i$, and $L_0 = 1/N \sum_{ij} L_{ij}$, so that $c_i = (m_i + (1 - L_0)^{-1} \bar{m} \sum_j L_0) d$.

If we assume that the lateral connection strengths are a function only of the relative distance $i-j$, then L_{ij} becomes a circular matrix so that $\sum_i L_{ij} = \sum_j L_{ij} = L_0$, and

$$c_i = (m_i + L_0 (1 - L_0)^{-1} \bar{m}) d. \tag{2.5}$$

In the mean field approximation, one can therefore write $c_i(\alpha) = (m_i - \alpha) d$, with $\alpha = |L_0|(1 + |L_0|)^{-1} \bar{m}$.

When analyzing the position and stability of the fixed points using this approximation, it follows under some mild assumption on the evolution of the average synaptic weights, that there is a mapping

$$m_i' \leftrightarrow m_i(\alpha) - \alpha$$

Intrator et al.

such that for every neuron in such a network with synaptic weight vector m_i there is a corresponding neuron with weight vector m_i' that undergoes the same evolution (around the fixed points) subject to a translation α.

Although the averaged inhibition assumption used in the mean field theory is an approximation, the mean field network described above provides a powerful tool to analyze a certain type of network architecture in great detail, and to gain an intuitive understanding of a complex network in terms of the behavior of a single neuron.

2.3 Synapses with Varying Modifiability

In the equations above, all synapses are taken to be modifiable in the same way. However, the behavior of visual cortical cells in various rearing conditions suggests that some cells respond more rapidly to environmental changes than others. In monocular deprivation, for example, some cells remain responsive to the closed eye in spite of the very large shift of most cells to the open eye. Hubel and Wiesel (1959) and Singer (1977), found, using intracellular recording, that geniculo-cortical synapses on inhibitory interneurons are more resistant to monocular deprivation than are synapses on pyramidal cell dendrites. These results suggest that some LGN-cortical synapses modify rapidly, while others modify relatively slowly, with slow modification of some cortico-cortical synapses. Excitatory LGN-cortical synapses onto excitatory cells may be those that modify primarily. Since these synapses are formed exclusively on dendritic spines, this raises the possibility that the mechanisms underlying synaptic modification exist primarily in axo-spinous synapses. To embody these facts we introduce two types of LGN-cortical synapses: those (m_i) that modify according to the modification rule discussed in BCM and those (z_k) that remain relatively constant. In a cortical network with modifiable and nonmodifiable LGN-cortical synapses, and nonmodifiable cortico-cortical synapses L_{ij}, the synaptic evolution equations become

$$\dot{m}_i = \phi(c_i, \Theta_m^i)d,$$

$$\dot{z}_k = 0,$$

$$\dot{L}_{ij} = 0. \tag{2.6}$$

As will be discussed below, such a network is capable of explaining the variety of experiments considered.

3 THE BCM THEORY AND THE NEUROBIOLOGY OF SYNAPTIC MODIFICATION

The BCM theory and its recent extensions originated as an attempt to account for the varied consequences of different visual environments on the developing visual cortex. In cats, the circuitry of the visual cortex can be modified by simple manipulations of visual experience during a "critical period" in the first few months of postnatal development. For example, one such manipulation, monocular deprivation, leads to a disconnection of the inputs from the deprived eye that renders the animal behaviorally blind through that eye. The goal of the BCM theory is to develop a model of synaptic modification that accounts for those striking changes in visual cortex that result from alterations in the patterns and amount of activity arising at the two retinae. While the theory aims to provide a physiologically plausible account of synaptic plasticity, it does not address the mechanism by which plasticity diminishes at the end of the critical period. A number of possible mechanisms have been proposed to account for the short duration of the plastic period, but at present it is not clear that the length of the critical period is determined by the same mechanism as that underlying synaptic change.

The validity of the BCM theory, as with any theory, can be tested in two ways. The first is to derive predictions or consequences of the theory in various situations that can be compared with experimental results. There is a considerable experimental literature on visual cortical plasticity reaching back 30 years which facilitates such comparisons with the BCM theory. The second approach is to attempt to verify the underlying assumptions of the theory, particularly those assumptions that distinguish it from others. In the case of the BCM theory, the most important and unique assumptions concern the form of the synaptic modification function ϕ and the movement of the modification threshold. Over the last 5 years we have made significant progress using both of these approaches, and this work is summarized briefly below.

3.1 Comparison of Theory and Experiment

In work recently published by Eugene Clothiaux and colleagues (Clothiaux et al., 1991) the consequences of the BCM theory were compared in detail with the results of experiments on what were called "classical" rearing conditions. These conditions include normal binocular vision, monocular deprivation, reverse suture, strabismus, binocular deprivation, as well as the restoration of normal binocular vision after various forms of deprivation. Comparisons with the pharmacological manipulations that affect visual cortical plasticity (e.g., Bear et al., 1990; Greuel et al., 1987; Reiter and Stryker, 1988) were not considered and remain an area that is ripe for further work. The modifications considered by Clothiaux et al. were those that occur in kitten visual cortex during the second postnatal month after brief (approx. 2 weeks) changes in visual experience. Particular attention was given to the manner in which the theory predicts that changes in visual experience should affect the binocularity of cortical neurons and the selectivity of these neurons for the stimulus pattern (e.g., its orientation). These properties of binocularity and selectivity distinguish cortical neurons from those in the retina and thalamus. A review of the experimental literature as it relates to the modification of these properties may be found in Clothiaux et al. (1991).

All theories of visual cortical plasticity have to make some assumptions as to how the initial visual scenes are converted into LGN firing rates and how this information reaches visual cortex. We wish to model the input to visual cortex that arises from the regions of the two retinae that view the same point in visual space. For simplicity, Clothiaux et al. assumed that LGN activity is a direct reflection of retinal ganglion cell activity. Two types of LGN-cortical input were modeled: (1) activity elicited when visual contours are presented to the retinae, which we call "pattern" input; and (2) activity that arises in the absence of visual contours, which we call "noise." From our point of view the important distinction between pattern and noise input is the degree of correlation that the two types of input produce in the LGN. For a specific input pattern the activity of one LGN neuron is assumed to have a predictable relationship (i.e., correlation) to the activity of other LGN neurons whereas for noise the activity of one LGN neuron is independent of the activity of the other LGN neurons. (Addition of local correlations such as those suggested by the work of Mastronarde (1989) does not alter the results.) Differences between distinct patterns (for example, between various stimulus orientations) are reflected by the differences in their distribution of activity across the LGN. Using this type of pattern input distorted by noise, and noise alone, Clothiaux et al. were able to reproduce both the outcome and kinetics of synaptic change in visual cortex resulting from normal visual experience and a wide variety of visual deprivation conditions.

As one example of the quantitative nature of these results, consider the simulation of the effects of monocular deprivation (figure 7 in Clothiaux et al., 1991). Beginning from a state in which the simulated neuron is binocularly responsive and selective, substituting pattern input through one eye with noise leads to a rapid synaptic disconnection of the "deprived" eye. Mathematical analysis provides a complete account of the factors on which this result depends if it is governed by the principles of the BCM theory. For example, for this result to be obtained using the BCM theory it is necessary that the neuron be selective (i.e., that it respond vigorously only to a fraction of the patterns that are presented to the "open eye") before the ocular dominance changes, and that the deprived eye inputs carry noise (i.e., that they be active). The prediction that the ocular dominance shift depends on neuronal selectivity was tested by Paradiso and colleagues (Ramoa et al., 1988). They found that cortical infusion of the GABA receptor antagonist bicuculline, which greatly reduces orientation selectivity in visual cortex, eliminates the ocular dominance shift that normally results from monocular deprivation. The second prediction—that the disconnection of the deprived eye depends on noise—has never been tested explicitly, but there are some indications that it is also correct. For example, clinical observations in humans led Jampolsky (1978) to conclude that the effects of monocular diffusion (resulting from lid suture) are more severe than the effects of monocular occlusion (resulting from an opaque eye-patch or contact lens).

To determine the time equivalence of each iteration for the parameters used, the behavior of the model under monocular deprivation can be compared to the results of the corresponding experiment. Equivalence was established between the number of computer iterations and the duration of deprivation required for complete disconnection of the deprived eye

(Clothiaux et al. 1991). Thus, using a fixed set of parameters, one has a direct correspondence between the temporal dynamics of synaptic change in the theory and experiments. This can be used to analyze and compare kinetics and outcome of theory and experiment for other manipulations. For example, in "reverse suture," the deprived eye is opened and the open eye is closed after a period of initial monocular deprivation. Experimentally, it is observed that the newly closed eye shows a greatly reduced response in about 24 hr, but that the recovery of the response to the newly open eye generally does not begin for another 1–2 days (Mioche and Singer, 1989). The same difference in the time required to obtain the initial effect and the reversal is seen with the model. The correspondence of theory and experiment is thus very close. The theoretical explanation for this result is that recovery requires that the modification threshold slide nearly to zero and, using the same parameters that were fixed for monocular deprivation, this requires approximately 24 hr. Similar comparisons for the other experimental manipulations are discussed in detail in Clothiaux et al. (1991). We conclude that when the predictions of the theory have been tested, they are in good agreement with what is seen experimentally.

3.2 Neurobiological Foundations for the Assumptions of the BCM Theory

Recent advances in our understanding of excitatory amino acid (EAA) receptors have suggested a possible physiological basis of the BCM form of synaptic modification. In 1987, Bear and colleagues proposed that the modification threshold Θ_m of the BCM theory related to the membrane potential at which the N-methyl-D-aspartate (NMDA) receptor–dependent Ca^{2+} flux reached the threshold for inducing synaptic long-term potentiation (LTP). In support of the hypothesis that NMDA receptor mechanisms play a role in synaptic plasticity, Bear and co-workers have found that the pharmacological blockade of NMDA receptors with the competitive antagonist AP5 disrupts the physiological (Bear et al., 1990; Kleinschmidt et al., 1987) and anatomical (Bear and Colman, 1990) consequences of monocular deprivation in striate cortex. Although the interpretation of these experiments is compromised by the finding that AP5 reduces visually evoked responses (Fox et al., 1989), the data indicate that activity evoked in visual cortex in the absence of NMDA receptor activation is not sufficient to produce loss of closed-eye responsiveness in MD.

In the past several years our work has focused on the synaptic plasticity that can be evoked in brain slices to better investigate the assumptions of the BCM theory and to address possible underlying mechanisms (Bear et al., 1992; Connors and Bear, 1988; Dudek and Bear, 1992; Kirkwood et al., 1993; Press and Bear, 1990). Hippocampus, particularly CAl and dentate gyrus, is an advantageous preparation because robust and long-lasting experience-dependent synaptic modifications can be evoked in this structure. Serena Dudek in Bear's lab (1992) recently tested a theoretical prediction that patterns of excitatory input activity that consistently fail to activate target

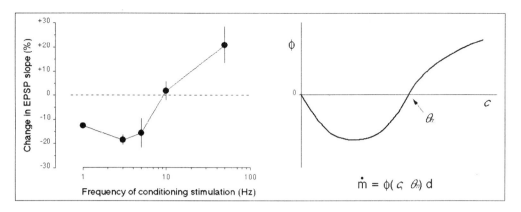

Figure 8.2 Comparison of experimental observations with BCM ϕ function for synaptic modification. (Data replotted from Dudek and Bear 1992.)

neurons sufficiently to induce synaptic potentiation will instead cause a specific synaptic depression. To realize this situation experimentally, the Schaffer collateral projection to CA1 in rat hippocampal slices was stimulated electrically at frequencies ranging from 0.5 to 50 Hz. Nine hundred pulses at 1–3 Hz consistently yielded a depression of the CA1 population EPSP that persisted without signs of recovery for more than 1 hr following cessation of the conditioning stimulation. This long-term depression was specific to the conditioned input and could be prevented by application of NMDA receptor antagonists. This result was surprising in that NMDA receptors are known to participate in the induction of long-term potentiation, an increase in synaptic effectiveness. Indeed, at higher stimulation frequencies the depression was replaced by a potentiation. If the effects of varying stimulation frequency in the experiments of Dudek and Bear are explained by different values of post-synaptic response (perhaps the integrated postsynaptic depolarization or Ca^{2+} level) during the conditioning stimulation, then it can be seen from figure 8.2 that their data are in striking agreement with assumptions of the BCM theory.

Of course, as striking as this similarity is, Dudek's work was performed in hippocampus and the BCM theory was developed for visual cortex. And, although these two forms of synaptic plasticity (depression and potentiation) have been reported in the sensory neocortex (cf. Artola et al., 1990), evidence to date has indicated that they occur with far lower probability, usually require pharmacological treatments for their induction, and are elicited by stimulation patterns that differ dramatically from those that are effective in hippocampus (see discussion in Bear et al., 1992). Together, these data have been taken as support for the view that hippocampus and sensory neocortex may be quite distinct with respect to their capability for synaptic change. However, a direct comparison of plasticity of synaptic responses evoked in adult rat hippocampal field CA1 with those evoked in adult rat and immature cat visual cortical layer III has now been carried out by Alfredo Kirkwood and colleagues in Bear's lab (1993). In the neocortical preparations they have stimulated the direct input to layer III from layer IV rather than using the traditional approach of stimulating the white matter, and find, contrary to the prevailing view, that very similar forms of plasticity, LTP and LTD, are evoked with precisely the same types of stimulation in the three types of cortex without the use of pharmacological treatments. Further, in all three preparations, both LTP and LTD depend on activation of NMDA receptors. These data suggest, first, that hippocampus should not be considered as a privileged site for plasticity in the adult brain and, second, that a common principle may govern experience-dependent synaptic plasticity, both in CA1 and throughout the superficial layers of the neocortex. We believe that this work represents an important advance towards a general theory of experience-dependent synaptic plasticity in the mammalian brain.

It is our opinion that in its entirety this work gives strong justification for a form of modification similar to that assumed by the BCM theory. However, the question of the sliding modification threshold is still open. Although more work remains to be done on this question, we note that two recent studies have shown that the sign and magnitude of a synaptic modification in both hippocampus (Huang et al., 1992) and the Mauthner cell of goldfish (Yang and Faber, 1991) have been shown to depend on the recent history of synaptic activation.

4   REFORMULATION AND EXTENSION OF THE BCM THEORY

In order to compare the BCM theory with other theories of synaptic plasticity as well as to exhibit its information processing and statistical properties, the following formulation proves convenient.

4.1   Objective Function Formulation

In a recent statistical formulation of the BCM theory (Intrator and Cooper, 1992), the threshold Θ_m was defined (In the notation of Intrator and Cooper, d is replaced by x) as

$$\Theta_m = E[(d \cdot m)^2],$$

and an energy function that corresponds to a risk function in statistical decision theory was presented:

$$R_m = -\mu\{\tfrac{1}{3}E[(d \cdot m)^3] - \tfrac{1}{4}E^2[(d \cdot m)^2]\}. \tag{4.1}$$

It was shown that the differential equations describing synaptic weight modification are a stochastic approximation of the negative gradient of the risk, hence tending to minimize this risk (see Intrator and Cooper, 1992, for review). This formulation permits us to demonstrate the connection between the unsupervised BCM learning procedure and various statistical methods, in particular, that of exploratory projection pursuit (Friedman, 1987). It also provides a general method for stability analysis of the fixed points of the theory and enables us to analyze the behavior and the evolution of the network under various visual rearing conditions. In the next few sections we shall use this formulation to extend the theory to nonlinear neurons, and consequently to a network of feedforward inhibitory neurons.

4.2 Nonlinear Neurons

From statistical considerations that are motivated by the projection pursuit ideas, it is more effective to consider a nonlinear neuron that is less sensitive to possible outliers in the data. This is done by defining the neuron's activity as $c = \sigma(d \cdot m)$, where σ usually represents a smooth sigmoidal function. It is also desirable to have the ability to shift the projected distribution (of the input data) so that one of its peaks is at zero, by introducing a threshold β so that the projection is defined to be $c = \sigma(d \cdot m + \beta)$. From the biological viewpoint, β can be considered as spontaneous activity. The modification equations for finding the optimal threshold β are easily obtained by observing that this threshold effectively adds one dimension to the input vector and the vector of synaptic weights so that $d = (d_1, \ldots, d_n, 1)$, $m = (m_1, \ldots, m_n, \beta)$, and therefore, β can be found by using the same synaptic modification equations. For the rest of the paper we shall assume that this threshold is added to the projection, without specifically writing it.

For the nonlinear neuron, Θ_m is defined to be $\Theta_m = E[\sigma^2(d \cdot m)]$. The gradient of the risk becomes:

$$-\nabla_m R_m = \mu E[\phi(\sigma(d \cdot m), \Theta_m)\sigma'd], \qquad (4.2)$$

where σ' represents the derivative of σ at the point $(d \cdot m)$. Note that the multiplication by σ' reduces sensitivity to outliers of the differential equation since for outliers σ' is close to zero. The gradient decent procedure is valid, provided that the risk is bounded from below (cf. Intrator and Cooper, 1992).

4.3 Networks with Feedforward Inhibition: Application to Classification

Intrator and Cooper (1992) have extended the single cell theory to a feedforward inhibition network which does not require the mean field approximation; nor does it require that the cortico-cortical synapses L_{ij} be constant. Thus it is possible to study networks with varying amounts of excitation and inhibition.

The activity of neuron k in the network is $c_k = d \cdot m_k$, where m_k is the synaptic weight vector of neuron k. The *inhibited* activity and threshold of the k'th neuron are given by

$$\tilde{c}_k = c_k - \eta \sum_{j \neq k} c_j, \qquad \tilde{\Theta}_m^k = E[\tilde{c}_k^2]. \qquad (4.3)$$

The relation between the feed forward inhibition network and the mean field network is discussed in Intrator and Cooper (1992).

For the feedforward network the risk for node k is given by:

$$R_k = -\mu\{\tfrac{1}{3}E[\tilde{c}_k^3] - \tfrac{1}{4}E^2[\tilde{c}_k^2]\}, \qquad (4.4)$$

and the total risk is given by

$$R = \sum_{k=1}^{N} R_k .$$ (4.5)

It follows that the gradient of R becomes:

$$\frac{\partial R}{\partial m_k} = \frac{\partial R_k}{\partial m_k} - \eta \sum_{j \neq k} \frac{\partial R_j}{\partial m_j}$$

$$= \mu \left[E[\phi(\tilde{c}_k, \tilde{\Theta}_m^k) d] - \eta \sum_{j \neq k} E[\phi(\tilde{c}_j, \tilde{\Theta}_j) d] \right].$$ (4.6)

The equation performs a constraint minimization in which the derivative with regard to one neuron can become orthogonal (when $\eta \to 1$) to the sum over the derivatives of all other synaptic weights. Nevertheless, the coupling between the neurons is very simple to calculate and does not require any matrix inversion. Equation (4.6) therefore, allows a simple computational algorithm that performs exploratory projection pursuit of several projections in parallel.

When the nonlinearity of the neuron is included, the inhibited activity is defined (as in the single neuron case) as $\tilde{c}_k = \sigma(c_k - \eta \sum_{l \neq k} c_l)$. $\tilde{\Theta}_m^k$, and R_k are defined as before. However, in this case

$$\frac{\partial \tilde{c}_k}{\partial m_j} = -\eta \sigma'(\tilde{c}_k) d, \qquad \frac{\partial \tilde{c}_k}{\partial m_k} = \sigma'(\tilde{c}_k) d.$$ (4.7)

Therefore the total gradient becomes:

$$\dot{m}_k = \frac{\partial R}{\partial m_k} = \mu \left\{ E[\phi(\tilde{c}_k, \tilde{\Theta}_m^k) \sigma'(\tilde{c}_k) d] - \eta \sum_{j \neq k} E[\phi(\tilde{c}_j, \tilde{\Theta}_m^j) \sigma'(\tilde{c}_j) d] \right\}.$$ (4.8)

This biologically motivated system of equations has many desirable statistical properties and has been applied to various nontrivial feature extraction tasks such as phoneme recognition (Intrator, 1992) and three-dimensional object recognition (Intrator and Gold, 1993).

5   COMPARISON OF BCM WITH OTHER VISUAL CORTICAL PLASTICITY THEORIES

In order to compare ideas concerning visual cortical plasticity, it is important to analyze separately the different components that make up a theory, and to compare theories feature by feature. We consider a theory as being composed of the following three components:

• Synaptic modification equations

• Model of the input environment

• Network architecture

In some cases, there are interactions between these components that are not explicitly defined. For example, several theories are said to have the property of being able to develop orientation selectivity prenatally, that is, using random noise as an input environment (Linsker, 1986; Miller et al., 1989). However, under closer examination, it turns out that they have architectual constraints that actually yield very different input environments. Inputs to the network become strongly locally correlated after the first layer due only to network architecture (the arborization function). The arborization function determines the density of synapses as a function of planar distance from their target cell. This correlated input can then drive the higher level of cells to develop orientation-selective cells. When the arborization function is uniform, all the weights of all layers will become positively saturated; thus no selectivity will develop.

5.1   Comparison Based on Synaptic Modification Equations

To examine the effect of the synaptic modification equations in isolation, we shall fix the network inputs to be the same, and fix the architecture as well. The simplest architecture that would already yield a significant difference between several models is of a single cortical neuron receiving input from a single source (single eye).

In the correlation of activity models (Kammen and Yuille, 1988; Linsker, 1986; Miller et al., 1989; Sejnowski, 1977; Yuille et al., 1989) the input is defined in terms of the correlation of activity in the presynaptic afferents, whereas in the BCM model the input is defined in terms of the presynaptic activity. For reasons that will become clear, it is difficult to transform the correlation of activity models to a presynaptic activity models; however, we can rewrite the BCM model as a correlation of activity model.

To simplify notation and without loss of generality we shall assume that the input activity in each ganglion cell has zero mean. First we show how the transformation from input activity to correlation activity is done by expanding on footnote 15 of Miller et al. (1989). This will be done in the simple case of a single cortical neuron with no interaction between LGN inputs coming from the two eyes. Miller's rule has the following form:

$$\frac{dS(\alpha, t)}{dt} = \lambda A(-\alpha)[c(t) - c_1]a_\sigma(\alpha, t) - \gamma S(\alpha, t) - \varepsilon' A(-\alpha), \tag{5.1}$$

where α is the afferent location, A is the arbor function representing the number (or in the limit, the density of) afferents coming from location α, $a_\sigma(\alpha, t)$ is the afferent activity at location α, the subscript σ represents an addition of threshold and saturation effects, and c_1 is a constant. $c(t)$ is the neuronal activity, which in this simple case of no lateral interactions is given by $c(t) = \sum_\beta S(\beta, t)a_\sigma(\beta, t) + c_2$ where c_2 is some constant. $\gamma S(\alpha, t) + \varepsilon' A(-\alpha)$ are decay functions of the synaptic weights. Substituting $c(t)$ into (5.1), denoting $c_3 = c_2 - c_1$, and taking the average over the input space (at a given afferent location) we obtain

$$\frac{dS(\alpha, t)}{dt} = \lambda A(-\alpha) \left\{ \sum_\beta S(\beta, t) E(a_\sigma(\beta, t) a_\sigma(\alpha, t)) + c_3 E(a_\sigma(\alpha, t)) \right\}$$

$$- \gamma S(\alpha, t) - \varepsilon' A(-\alpha). \tag{5.2}$$

Using $C(\alpha, \beta)$ to represent the correlation of activity $C(\alpha, \beta) \stackrel{\text{def}}{=} E(a_\sigma(\alpha, t) a_\sigma(\beta, t))$ we get

$$\frac{dS(\alpha, t)}{dt} = \lambda A(-\alpha) \left\{ \sum_\beta S(\beta, t) C(\alpha, \beta) - c_1 E[a_\sigma(\alpha, t)] \right\} - \gamma S(\alpha, t) - \varepsilon' A(-\alpha),$$

$$\tag{5.3}$$

which is a simple case of equation (1) in Miller et al. (1989).

Analogous reformulation is done below for the BCM modification equation (for the purpose of the comparison d is replaced by $a(\alpha, t)$ below)

$$\frac{dm(\alpha, t)}{dt} = \lambda \phi(c(t), \Theta_m) a(\alpha, t), \tag{5.4}$$

for the synaptic weight m (in Miller's notation this is S); for simplicity we omit decay terms and assume a uniform arbor function.

Using a simple form of the modification function, $\phi(c, \Theta_m) \stackrel{\text{def}}{=} c(c - \Theta_m)$ (Bienenstock et al., 1982), substituting $c(t) = \sum_\beta m(\beta) a(\beta, t)$, and taking the average over the input space at a given afferent location we obtain

$$\frac{dm(\alpha, t)}{dt} = \lambda E \left\{ a(\alpha) \sum_{\beta\gamma} m(\beta) a(\beta) m(\gamma) a(\gamma) \right\} - E \left\{ a(\alpha) \sum_\beta m(\beta) a(\beta) \right\} \Theta_m. \tag{5.5}$$

Wherever it is clear, we omit the dependency of $a(\alpha)$ on t (assuming it is a stationary process). Using the same correlation function as defined above, and defining the third-order correlation $\tilde{C}(\alpha, \beta, \gamma)$ of the input activity to be $\tilde{C}(\alpha, \beta, \gamma) = E[a(\alpha) a(\beta) a(\gamma)]$, yields

$$\frac{dm(\alpha, t)}{dt} = \lambda \left\{ \sum_{\beta, \gamma} \tilde{C}(\alpha, \beta, \gamma) m(\beta) m(\gamma) - \Theta_m \sum_\beta m(\beta) C(\alpha, \beta) \right\}. \tag{5.6}$$

Using a definition for the threshold $\Theta_m \stackrel{\text{def}}{=} E[\sum_\alpha a(\alpha) m(\alpha)]^2$ (Intrator, 1990; Intrator and Cooper, 1992) and using the second-order correlation function C, Θ_m becomes $\Theta_m = \sum_{\gamma, \delta} C(\gamma, \delta) m(\gamma) m(\delta)$. Therefore, equation (5.6) becomes

$$\frac{dm(\alpha, t)}{dt} = \lambda \left\{ \sum_{\beta, \gamma} \tilde{C}(\alpha, \beta, \gamma) m(\beta) m(\gamma) - \sum_{\beta\gamma\delta} C(\alpha, \beta) C(\gamma, \delta) m(\beta) m(\gamma) m(\delta) \right\}.$$

$$\tag{5.7}$$

A few important observations follow. The correlation based models use only the first- and second-order statistical information of the data (in other words, the mean and covariance matrix of input activity), whereas the BCM theory utilizes in addition the third-order statistics of the input activity. Therefore, without going into the details of the limiting behavior, this already suggests that correlation-based models are less sensitive to the input environment. Analysis shows that in many cases the correlation of activity models find the principal components of the input environment (Granger et al., 1989;

Kohonen, 1984; Miller et al., 1989; Oja, 1982; Sanger, 1989; Yuille et al., 1989). In the following section we discuss some properties of principal components in information processing.

Comparison Based on the Information Extraction Properties   It now becomes relevant to ask what type of structure can be extracted from first and second moments only, and what constitutes an *interesting structure*. The first question is quite old and its answer is well known. First and second moments contain information about the principal components of the input distribution, which are those directions that can minimize L^2 error between the original data and the reconstructed data based only on the first few leading components. Another way to view principal components is to observe that they maximize the variance of the projected distribution, namely the variance of the new random variable that is the projection of the inputs onto the principal components.

Principal Components and Maximum Information Preservation   Networks that extract principal components from data are numerous (e.g., Granger et al., 1989; Kammen and Yuille, 1988; Linsker, 1986; Miller et al., 1989; Oja, 1982; Sanger, 1989; Sejnowski, 1977; Yuille et al., 1989). Linsker presented the principles guiding synaptic modification in his layered network and showed that the development rule causes a cell to develop so as to maximize the variance of its output activity, subject to the constraint on the total connection strength and on each synaptic value (Linsker, 1988). Linsker then describes the connection of this rule to principal component analysis and to the principle of *maximum information preservation* taken from information theory. This principle is optimal when the goal is to accurately reconstruct the input, but is not optimal when the goal is classification. This is shown in the following simple example (figure 8.3; see also Duda and Hart, 1973, p. 212). Two clusters, each belonging to a different class, are presented. The goal is to find

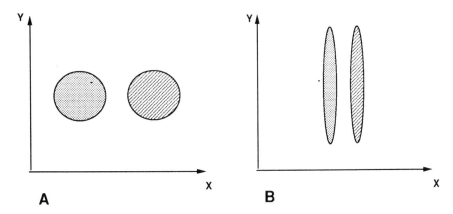

Figure 8.3   Principal components find useful structure in data (A) and fail when the variance of each cluster is different in each direction (B).

a single-dimensional projection that will capture the structure information in the data. In figure 8.3B different clusters have different variance in either direction, whereas in figure 8.3A the variance in both directions is equal. Clearly, the structure in the data is conveyed in the x projection; however, in the first example the variance is maximized in the y projection. This projection also minimizes the mean squared error (MSE) and is therefore superior for maximum information preservation. In the second example, because the variance of each cluster is equal in both directions, the projection that captures the most structure in the data and preserves maximum information is the x projection.

Another way to view what principal components do to the data is to observe that they define a new system of coordinates in which the covariance matrix is diagonal; namely, they eliminate the second-order correlation in the data i.e., correlation between the projections of the input data onto any two principal components. It is important to note here that this procedure does not eliminate higher order correlation in the data.

Finding Other Interesting Low-Dimensional Structure in Data   This problem has recently been discussed in the context of a statistical method called projection pursuit (PP) (see Huber, 1985, for review). This method seeks structure that is exhibited by (linear) projections of the data and is therefore relevant to neural network theory, since the activity of a neuron is believed to be a function of the projection of the inputs on the vector of synaptic weights. Diaconis and Freedman (1984), have shown that for most high-dimensional clouds, most low-dimensional projections are approximately normal. This finding suggests that important information in the data is conveyed in those directions whose single-dimensional projected distribution is far from Gaussian. For example, some known measures of deviation from normality are skewness and kurtosis, which are functions of the first four moments of the distribution. These moments contain information about statistical correlations up to fourth order. Intrator (1990) has shown that a BCM neuron (given by equation 4.8) can find structure in the input distribution that exhibits deviation from normality in the form of multimodality in the projected distributions. This type of deviation, which is measured by the first three moments of the distribution, is particularly useful for finding clusters in high-dimensional data (since clusters can not be found directly in the data due to its sparsity) and is thus useful for classification or recognition tasks. Below, we give another interpretation of this projection index in light of the previous discussion.

If we assume that the retina is performing decorrelation of the inputs (Atick and Redlich, 1992) then the covariance matrix $C(\alpha, \beta)$ is diagonal (assuming that the inputs have zero mean) and so for eigen values $e(\alpha)$, equation (5.7) becomes:

$$\frac{dm(\alpha, t)}{dt} = \lambda \left\{ \sum_{\beta, \gamma} \tilde{C}(\alpha, \beta, \gamma) m(\beta) m(\gamma) - e(\alpha) m(\alpha) \sum_{\gamma} e(\gamma) m^2(\gamma) \right\}. \tag{5.8}$$

Table 8.1 Assumptions about Input Environment: Two Models

	Clothiaux et al. (1991)	Miller et al. (1989)
Normal rearing	Patterned input (correlated activity within the eye with addition of noise)	Locally correlated input from both eyes
	Correlation between eyes	No correlation between eyes
Monocular deprivation	Patterned input from the open eye	Same correlation structure as normal rearing
	Uncorrelated noise from the deprived eye	Reduced activity to the deprived eye
Strabismus	Patterned input from each eye	Locally correlated input from both eyes
	No correlation between eyes	Anticorrelations between eyes

This suggests that the BCM synaptic modification equation is performing third-order decorrelation of the inputs subject to some penalty related to the size of the weights. When the second-order statistics of the input data is not decorrelated, then the modification equation can be thought of trying to find some balance between third-order correlation and second-order correlation in the data.

5.2 Comparison Based on Assumptions About the Input Environment

In table 8.1 we summarize the different assumptions about the environment used by our group and by Miller and colleagues to model classical visual deprivation experiments. What is apparent from this comparison is the different emphasis given to between-eye and within-eye correlations in activity. To quote Mastronarde (1984):

Some of the strongest evidence on the importance of correlated firing in development comes from cases where local correlations in activity are induced by sensory stimulation; e.g., formation of binocular cells in visual cortex requires binocularly corresponding visual input to the two eyes (Hubel and Wiesel, 1965). There has been growing interest in a more restricted question: what is the role in development of the correlated activity that occurs in the spontaneous discharge?

In work we have chosen to focus on the influence of activity induced by sensory stimulation on the development of visual cortex.

5.3 Comparison Based on Network Architecture

Although it is possible that network architecture plays an important role in comparison of varuous ideas on visual cortical plasticity, in this chapter we have not done any analysis of different architecture. This will be dealt with in subsequent work.

6   CONCLUDING REMARKS

We have given a short account of the BCM theory of synaptic plasticity, including comparison with experiments in visual cortex and possible cellular and molecular basis for the fundamental modification equations. In addition, we have shown that correlation-based models and BCM theory differ in the type of structure for which they search. Correlation models include first- and second-order statistics of input correlations, while BCM modification also includes third-order statistics.

Evidence exists for a principal component type preprocessing that may be taking place in the retina; we suggest that BCM modification further preprocesses the visual inputs by reducing (extracting) third-order statistical correlations. Extracting third-order statistics from the visual environment is a natural extension and complements the extraction of second-order statistics that may be done in the retina.

Statistical theory tells us that finite-order statistics of the data is not sufficient to uniquely characterize the data distribution. However, the addition of the third-order moment adds important feature such as skewness to the description of the distribution (see Kendall and Stuart, 1977, for review), and in this case, it adds information about multimodality (Intrator, 1992). The method of principal components is sufficient for finding clusters in data when the variance of each cluster is relatively constant in all directions, since then directions that maximize the variance also maximize the information conveyed for the purpose of classification. When this is not the case, the example (figure 8.3) shows that the direction that maximizes the variance of the projection does not necessarily carry information useful for separation of the two clusters although it does find the direction that will minimize the mean squared error between the reconstructed signal and the input; this is dictated by the principle of maximum information preservation.

It is possible that the principle of maximum information preservation is useful in retinal processing, in which an order of magnitude reduction in the number of cells occurs. We suggest that this principle is not general enough to account for processing done in early visual cortex and that such statistical properties provide a convenient framework for comparison of various plasticity theories.

ACKNOWLEDGMENT

Research was supported by the Office of Naval Research, the Army Research Office, and the National Science Foundation.

REFERENCES

Artola, A., Bröcher, S., and Singer, W. (1990) Different voltage dependent thresholds for the induction of long-term depression and long-term potenation in slices of rat visual cortex. *Nature* 347:69–72.

Atick, J. J., and Redlich, N. (1992) What does the retina know about natural scenes. *Neural Computation* 4:196–210.

Bear, M. F., and Colman, H. (1990) Binocular competition in the control of geniculate cell size depends upon visual corical NMDA receptor activation. *Proc. Natl. Acad. Sci. USA* 87:9246–9249.

Bear, M. F., Cooper, L. N., and Eben, F. F. (1987) A Physiological basis for a theory of synapse modification. *Science* 237:42–48.

Bear, M. F., Gu, Q., Kleinschmidt, A., and Singer, W. (1990) Disruption of experience-dependent synaptic modification in the striate cortex by infusion of an NMDA receptor antagonist. *J. Neurosci.* 10:909–925.

Bear, M. F., Press, W. A., and Connors, B. W. (1992) Long-term potentiation of slices of kitten visual cortex and the effects of NMDA receptor blockade. *J. Neurophysiol.* 67:841–851.

Bienenstock, E. L., Cooper, L. N., and Munro, P. W. (1982) Theory for the development of neuron selectivity: Orientation specificity and binocular interaction in visual cortex. *J. Neurosci.* 2:32–48.

Clothiaux, E. E., Bear, M. F., and Cooper, L. N. (1991) Synaptic plasticity in visual cortex: Comparison of theory with experiment. *J. Neurophysiol.* 66:1785–1804.

Connors, B. W., and Bear, M. F. (1988) Pharmacological modulation of long term potentiation in slice of visual cortex. *Soc. Neurosci. Abstr.* 14:298.8.

Cooper, L. N., and Scofield, C. L. (1988) Mean-field theory of a neural network. *Proc. Natl. Acad. Sci. USA* 85:1973–1977.

Diaconis, P., and Freedman, D. (1984) Asymptotics of graphical projection pursuit. *Ann. Stat.* 12:793–815.

Duda, R. O., and Hart, P. E. (1973) *Pattern Classification and Scene Analysis.* John Wiley, New York.

Dudek, S. M., and Bear, M. F. (1992) Homosynaptic long-term depression in area CA1 of hippocampus and the effects on NMDA receptor blockade. *Proc. Natl. Acad. Sci. USA* 89:4363–4367.

Fox, K., Sato, H., and Daw, N. (1989) The location and function of NMDA receptors in cat and kitten visual cortex. *J. Neurosci.* 9:2443–2454.

Friedman, J. H. (1987) Exploratory projection pursuit. *J. Am. Stat. Assoc.* 82:249–266.

Granger, R., Ambrose-Ingerson, J., and Lynch, G. (1989) Derivation of encoding characteristics of layer II cerebral cortex. *J. Cog. Neurosci.* 1:61–87.

Greuel, J. M., Luhmann, H. J., and Singer, W. (1987) Evidence for a threshold in experience-dependent long-term changes of kitten visual cortex. *Dev. Brain Res.* 34:141–149.

Huang, Y. Y., Colino, A., Selig, D. K., and Malenka, R. C. (1992) The influence of prior synaptic activity on the induction of long-term potentiation. *Science* 255:730–733.

Hubel, D. H., and Wiesel, T. N. (1959) Integrative action in the cat's lateral geniculate body. *J. Physiol.* 148:574–591.

Hubel, D. H., and Wiesel, T. N. (1965) Bimocular interaction in striate contex of kittens reared with artificial squint. *J. Neurophysiol.* 28:1041–1059.

Huber, P. J. (1985) Projection pursuit (with discussion). *Ann. Stat.* 13:435–475.

Intrator, N. (1990). A neural network for feature extraction. In D. S. Touretzky and R. P. Lippmann (eds.), *Advances in Neural Information Processing Systems*, Vol. 2. Morgan Kaufmann, San Mateo, CA, pp. 719–726.

Intrator, N. (1992) Feature extraction using an unsupervised neural network. *Neural Computation* 4:98–107.

Intrator, N., and Cooper, L. N. (1992) Objective function formulation of the BCM theory of visual cortical plasticity: Statistical connections, stability conditions. *Neural Networks* 5:3–17.

Intrator, N., and Gold, J. I. (1993) Three-dimensional object recognition of gray level images: The usefulness of distinguishing features. *Neural Computation* 5:61–74.

Jampolsky, A. (1978) Unequal visual inputs and strabismus management: A comparison of human and animal strabismus. In *Symposium on Strabismus (Transactions of New Orleans Academy of Ophthalmology)*. Mosby, St. Louis, p. 358.

Kammen, D., and Yuille, A. (1988) Spontaneous symmetry-breaking energy functions and the emergence of orientation selective cortical cells. *Biol. Cybern.* 59:23–31.

Kendall, M., and Stuart, A. (1977) *The Advanced Theory of Statistics*, Vol. 1. Macmillan, New York.

Kirkwood, A., Gold, S. M. D. J. T., Aizenman, C., and Bear, M. F. (1993) Common forms of synaptic plasticity in hippocampus and neocortex in vitro. *Science*, 260:1518–1521.

Kleinschmidt, A., Bear, M. F., and Singer, W. (1987) Blockage of NMDA receptors disrupts experience-dependent plasticity of kitten striate cortex. *Science* 238:355–358.

Kohonen, T. (1984) *Self-Organization and Associative Memory*. Springer-Verlag, Berlin.

Linsker, R. (1986) From basic network principles to neural architecture (series). *Proc. Natl. Acad. Sci. USA* 83:7508–7512, 8390–8394, 8779–8783.

Linsker, R. (1988) Self-organization in a perceptual network. *IEEE Comput.* 88:105–117.

Mastronarde, D. N. (1989) Correlated firing of cat retinal ganglion cells. *Trends Neurosci.* 12:75–80.

Miller, K. D., Keller, J., and Stryker, M. P. (1989) Ocular dominance column development: Analysis and simulation. *Science* 240:605–615.

Mioche, L. and Singer, W. (1989) Chronic recordings from single sites of kitten striate cortex during experience-dependent modifications of receptive-field properties. *J. Neurophysiol.* 62:85–197.

Oja, E. (1982) A simplified neuron model as a principal component analyzer. *Math. Biol.* 15:267–273.

Press, W. A., and Bear, M. F. (1990) Effects of disinhibition on LTP induction in slices of visual cortex. *Soc. Neurosci. Abstr.* 16:348.9.

Ramoa, A. S., Paradiso, M. A., and Freeman, R. D. (1988) Blockade of intracortical inhibition in kitten striate cortex: Effects on receptive field properties and associated loss of ocular dominance plasticity. *Exp. Brain Res.* 73:285–296.

Reiter, H. O., and Stryker, M. P. (1988) Neural plasticity without action potentials: Less active inputs become dominant when kitten visual cortical cells are pharmacologically inhibited. *Proc. Natl. Acad. Sci. USA* 85:3623–3627.

Sanger, T. D. (1989) Optimal unsupervised learning in a single-layer linear feedforward neural network. *Neural Networks* 2:459–473.

Scofield, C. L., and Cooper, L. N. (1985) Development and properties of neural networks. *Contemp. Phys.* 26:125–145.

Sejnowski, T. J. (1977) Storing covariance with nonlinearly interacting neurons. *J. Math. Bio.* 4:303–321.

Intrator et al.

Singer, W. (1977) Effects of monocular deprivation on excitatory and inhibitory pathways in cat striate cortex. *Exp. Brain Res.* 134:508−518.

Yang, X., and Faber, D. S. (1991) Initial synaptic efficacy influences induction and expression of long-term changes in transmission. *Proc. Natl. Acad. Sci. USA* 88:4299−4303.

Yuille, A., Kammen, D., and Cohen, D. (1989) Quadrature and the development of orientation selective cortical cells by hebb rules. *Biol. Cybern.* 61:183−194.

9

A Theoretical and Experimental Strategy for Realizing a Biologically Based Model of the Hippocampus

Theodore W. Berger, German Barrionuevo, Gilbert Chauvet, Donald N. Krieger, and Robert J. Sclabassi

1 INTRODUCTION

Research on the neurobiological substrates of learning and memory has progressed substantially during the past two decades, with a convergence of evidence identifying several brain systems critical for memory function (Berger and Bassett, 1992; Thompson et al., 1983) and several putative cellular and biochemical mechanisms of learning-induced synaptic plasticity (Brown et al., 1990; Byrne, 1987; Clements et al., 1991; Ito, 1989; Jaffe and Johnston, 1990; Linden and Routtenberg, 1989; Madison et al., 1991; Sejnowski, 1991; Staubli et al., 1992). It is becoming widely recognized, however, that further progress in understanding the relationship between neuronal processes and mnemonic processes will require the use of mathematical models and computer simulations of the dynamic properties expressed by networks of neurons (Anderson and Rosenfeld, 1988; Byrne and Berry, 1989; Carpenter et al., 1987; Hanson and Burr, 1990; Levy et al., 1985, 1989; Sejnowski et al., 1988; Zipser, 1992; Zornetzer et al., 1990). In response to this development, an increasing number of investigators are exploring the use of more theoretical approaches to determine how interactions among neural elements of a brain system can result in "emergent" properties that are not necessarily predictable from the activities of its single neurons, and that more formally parallel the cognitive characteristics of mnemonic operations (Ambros-Ingerson et al., 1990; Bienenstock et al., 1982; Cooper and Schofield, 1988; Finkel and Edelman, 1985; Gingrich and Byrne, 1987; Gluck and Thompson, 1987; Grossberg and Schmajuk, 1989; Holmes and Levy, 1990; Klopf, 1988; Lee et al., 1988; Lockery et al., 1989; McNaughton and Morris, 1987; Mpitsos et al., 1988; Qian and Sejnowski, 1990; Schmajuk and DiCarlo, 1991; Traub et al., 1991; Treves and Rolls, 1992; Zador et al., 1990; Zipser and Andersen, 1988). One of the most important issues regarding this goal is how to ensure a sufficient degree of identity between mathematical models of neural networks and functional properties of the real brain so that the focus of neural network research remains biologically meaningful, and thus, likely to identify the basis for the unique information processing and storage capabilities of the brain. In addition, without sufficient biological constraints, it is not always obvious how characteristics of the model can be verified experimentally.

2 STRATEGIES FOR MODELING NEURAL NETWORKS

We have been attempting to develop a solution to this general problem in our studies of network properties of the mammalian hippocampal formation (Berger et al., 1987, 1991, 1992; Sclabassi et al., 1988b, 1992). The hippocampal formation is composed of five subsystems: the entorhinal, dentate, hippocampal (CA3 and CA1 regions), and subicular cortices (figure 9.1). A single population of projection neurons provides the only output from each subsystem (except in the case of the entorhinal cortex), and is the source of monosynaptic, excitatory input to the projection neurons of other subsystems. The five cortical regions are interconnected in the form of a closed feedback loop, such that activity within any one subsystem modulates activity of the other subsystems. Interneurons within each subsystem also modulate output of the projection neurons through local feedforward and feedback pathways. Our strategy in developing a biologically based model of this neural network has involved the complementary use of two different approaches: (1) application of nonlinear systems anaylsis, through which the functional dynamics resulting from interaction among the various neuronal populations can be characterized experimentally, and (2) application of an n-level field theory, through which is realized a continuous representation of the physiological and anatomical mechanisms underlying those dynamics. The rationale for each approach and their interrelationship is as follows.

2.1 Modeling Network Properties as Input/Output Functions

The approach that is the most well-developed is based on the principles of nonlinear theory (Berger et al., 1987a, 1989; Sclabassi et al., 1988a, 1989b). In this approach, functional properties of a network of neurons are quantitatively characterized as input/output functions, that is, the transformation of an input signal into an output signal. The input/output characterizations are formally expressed as the kernels of a functional power series and are arrived at experimentally by recording neuronal output to randomized input signals (Krausz, 1975; Marmarelis and Marmarelis, 1978; Marmarelis and Naka, 1972; Sclabassi et al., 1977). Thus, the dynamic properties of neural networks can be observed directly and, due to the general nature of the analytic approach, at all levels of network organization: population activity, single cell activity, and the activity of sub/cellular processes.

To use the dentate gyrus as an example, its transformational properties are assessed experimentally by stimulating perforant path fibers of the entorhinal cortex with a train of electrical impulses having an exponential distribution of interimpulse intervals that approximates a Poisson process. The responses of granule cells, the output neurons of the dentate, are measured using extracellular recording of population field potentials or intracellular recording from single granule cells. Cross-correlation procedures are used to estimate the linear and higher-order nonlinear components of the relationship between

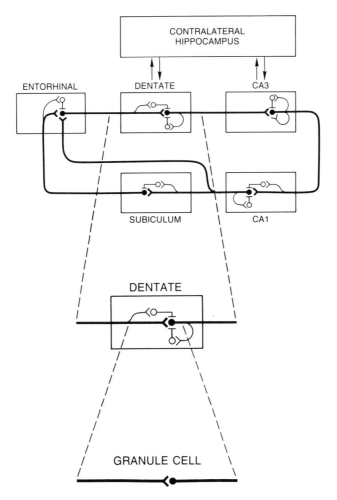

Figure 9.1 Schematic representation of the five subsystems of the hippocampal formation: entorhinal cortex, dentate gyrus, hippocampal CA3 region, hippocampal CA1 region, subiculum. The schematized filled neurons represent the population of projection neurons for each subsystem, e.g., granule cells of the dentate gyrus. The filled pathway connecting the entorhinal cortex and the dentate gyrus represents the fibers of the perforant path. The schematized open neurons represent a subset of the interneuron populations known to exist within each subsystem. The system is represented in only two spatial dimensions, though the fundamental organizational characteristics shown here are repeated throughout the longitudinal axis of the hippocampus. In the lower panels, the dentate gyrus is used as an example to illustrate conceptually the reduction of one subsystem into progressively simplified preparations.

A Biologically Based Model of the Hippocampus

temporal poperties of the input (sequence of interimpulse interval) and the magnitude or probability of granule cell output.

2.2 Theoretical and Experimental Decomposition

When kernels are computed for the dentate gyrus of an intact system, they must reflect (1) the intrinsic membrane properties of granule cells, (2) feedback and feedforward modulation by local interneurons, and (3) modulation of granule cell and/or interneuron activity by connectivity with other subsystems of the hippocampal formation (see figure 9.1). The contribution of these various sources can be distinguished by characterizing the input/output properties of the dentate both when it is interconnected with the remaining subsystems of the hippocampal formation (closed-loop condition) and after experimental procedures have isolated it from the other network elements (open-loop condition).

Likewise, the functional properties of an individual, isolated granule cell must reflect (see figure 9.2): (1) the amount of neurotransmitter released per impulse by perforant path afferents, (2) the receptor and channel kinetics of the ligand-dependent conductances initiated by the released neurotransmitter (NMDA and AMPA receptor–mediated components of glutamatergic input), (3) passive membrane properties of granule cells which deterrnine the amplitude, time-course, and spatial distribution of the resulting membrane potentials (MEMBRANE), and (4) voltage-dependent conductances (vdc and THRESHOLD) that will vary with level of depolarization. The contribution of these different sources can be determined by characterizing input/output

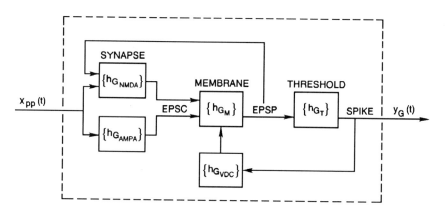

Figure 9.2 Schematic representation of a single granule cell of the dentate gyrus, defined as a multiloop feedback system. $x_{pp}(t)$ represents the input from the perforant path; EPSC represents the postsynaptic currents produced by the nonlinear dynamics of synaptic processes and are represented separately for each of two glutamate receptor subtypes, $\{h_{Gampa}\}$, $\{h_{Gnmda}\}$; EPSP represents the postsynaptic potentials resulting from the translation of PSCs due to passive membrane properties, $\{h_{Gm}\}$; nonlinearities due to threshold events, $\{h_{Gt}\}$, result in spike output, $y_G(t)$; and feedback modulation due to postspike voltage-dependent conductances $\{h_{Gvdc}\}$.

Berger et al.

properties of a individual granule cell after pharmacological elimination of voltage-dependent conductances, and a progressive truncation of the sequence of events underlying the transition from synaptic currents to action potential generation.

Although a large and complex neural system, the structural organization of the hippocampal system is amenable to such an evaluation of open-loop properties. Each of the dentate gyrus, hippocampus (CA3 and CAI), subiculum and entorhinal cortices has one, or at the most two, populations of output neurons that are homogeneous with respect to structural and functional characteristics (Lorente de Nó, 1934). Thus, activity of the projection cells provides a measure of the integrated activity of all cell populations within a subsystem and defines the primary input to the next subsystem. Each population of principal neurons is segregated from other intrinsic cell types through a high degree of lamination, so their activity can be sampled independently of the activity of other cell populations (Andersen et al., 1971a). Connectivity between the subsystems is topographic (Swanson et al., 1978), which allows them to be isolated from each other experimentally. Because of this combination of characteristics, the activity of the principal neurons that connect the subsystems together (granule and pyramidal neurons) can be studied both when the principal neurons participate in the network and when the dynamic input of other subsystems is removed. The activity of the principal neurons also can be characterized at several different levels of analysis. Their uniform structure and orientation provides the opportunity for measuring activity at the population level in vivo (Andersen et al., 1971a); the susceptability of the hippocampus to in vitro slice preparation allows a cellular analysis of biophysical variables (Spruston and Johnston, 1992).

Through a progressive experimental decomposition of the hippocampus, the resulting kernel functions can provide biologically based measurements of the nonlinear dynamics of the subcellular components of the projection neurons of each hippocampal subsystem, the extent to which the dynamics intrinsic to the principal neurons are modulated by local interneurons, and the extent to which the dynamics of each subsystem are modulated by connectivity with other subsystems.

2.3   Nonparametric and Parametric Models

A model of the hippocampus that is a composite of the input/output functions of its subsystems would constitute a "nonparametric" or "external" model (Casti, 1988), because there are few underlying assumptions which constrain fitting of the data, and the biological processes responsible for the input/output relationship are not represented explicitly. There are advantages and disadvantages to nonparametric models. The disadvantages we hope to overcome through parallel development of a parametric model (see next section). The advantages, particularly as they relate to modeling neural systems, are the following. First, functional characteristics of the system that result from interactions among its elements are measured directly, so that all mathematical representations of network properties are based on biologically determined constraints of the system. Likewise, predictions based on the computer simulations can be verified experimentally. Second, direct experimental monitoring of each element within the network is not required for accurate specification of the input/output characteristics of that element. For example, through characterizations of input/output properties of dentate granule cells, both in the presence and absence of the $GABA_A$ receptor antagonist, bicuculline, the input/output properties of the inhibitory basket cell population can be computed. This determination by decomposition, through the use of known interconnectivity among network elements, not only is possible computationally but is complementary to many modern neurobiological techniques, such as neurotoxins, pharmacological antagonists, and antibodies. Third, it follows that mathematical representations of the network can be expanded to accommodate the contribution of any new element. When investigated in the closed-loop condition, the input/output functions represent the combined activities of all subpopulations of neurons, both known and unknown, both observable and unobservable. In contrast to a parametric model, no assumptions are made as to the numbers or types of other elements (interneuron or subcellular entity) that may be contributing to projection neuron activity. As a result, as new molecular entities and new local circuit neurons become identified and can be manipulated specifically, their respective contribution to the system dynamics can be added. Thus, a nonparametric model can develop with increasing complexity as our experiments progress and as qualitatively different dimensions of neuronal structure and function are discovered. Finally, because of their theoretical definition as impulse responses, the kernels allow prediction of the response to any arbitrary input signal. As such, the kernels allow hypothesis testing to be readily extended to the behaving animal—arbitrary input signals can be defined on the basis of principal neuron responses recorded during conditioning or other behavioral conditions.

The alternative to an input/output model, a "parametric" or "internal" model, is one in which the underlying biological processes are represented explicitly. The major advantages are succinctness of the mathematical expressions and interpretability, in the sense that manipulations of one biological process may have functional consequences represented within several orders of nonlinearity. Formulating a series of hypotheses that can be mapped into tractable experiments is more readily accomplished in the context of a parametric model. In parallel to the nonparametric model, we also are developing a parametric model of the hippocampus, that is, a model in which each neurobiological process considered is represented explicitly through a different parameter, and the spatial relations between neurons are included as a set of geometrical constraints. We are developing such a model using formalisms of a two-level field theory described by Chauvet (Chauvet, 1993a, b). Included in the model at this stage is a population of perforant path fibers and terminals and a population of granule cell bodies and dendrites; no other populations of neurons or subsystems are considered (Chauvet and Berger, submitted). In other words, the model assumes the equivalent of an open-loop condition for granule cells—the very conditions we recently have created as a step in achieving a nonparametric model. Just as a nonparametric modeling approach has weaknesses, the potential weakness of a parametric model is the validity of the underlying assumptions. Our strategy is to use both types of models in a complementary, manner. Specifically, the behavior of the parametric model will be compared with the behavior of the nonparametric, input/output model. Because the input/output model is determined experimentally, it can be used as a source of biological constraints on the parametric model.

3   NONLINEAR MODEL OF THE HIPPOCAMPUS

3.1   General Experimental and Analytical Procedures

Preparations   All experiments were conducted using the hippocampus of male New Zealand white rabbits. For experiments conducted in vivo, bipolar stimulating electrodes were implanted chronically in the perforant path and a recording electrode was implanted ipsilaterally in the dendritic or cell body layer of the dentate gyrus. Anesthetized preparations were maintained continuously on gaseous anesthesia. Chronically implanted preparations were allowed 1–2 weeks to recover from surgery, and all data were collected while animals were awake and mildly restrained in a Plexiglas body holder. For experiments conducted in vitro, transverse slices (300–600 μm thickness) of the hippocampus were prepared and maintained according to standard procedures. Under visual control, bipolar stimulating electrodes were positioned near the fissure of the dentate gyrus, where perforant path fibers enter the molecular layer of the dentate; a recording electrode was positioned in the granule cell body layer.

Random Impulse Train Stimulation   Perforant path fibers were stimulated with a random-interval train of electrical impulses: a series of 4064 impulses with interimpulse intervals drawn from a Poisson distribution. For most experiments conducted to date, the mean interevent interval (Δ) of the random train has been 500 ms and the range of intervals is 1–5000 ms. Throughout delivery of the random train, evoked activity is recorded from granule cells of the dentate gyrus. Recordings of extracellular population spike and EPSP responses were used to monitor activity of populations of granule cells; intracellular recordings were used to monitor the activity of single neurons.

Analytical procedures   Nonlinear input/output properties of the dentate are defined as the kernels of a functional power series:

$$y(t) = G_i[h_i, x(t)] \tag{1}$$

where $y(t)$ is the output of dentate granule cells, (G_i) is a set of mutually orthogonal functionals, and (h_i) is a set of symmetric kernels which characterize the relationship between the input and output. The functionals are defined as:

$$G_0(t) = 0 \tag{2}$$

$$G_1(t) = \int h_1(\tau)x(t - \tau)\,d\tau \tag{3}$$

$$G_2(t) = 2 \int\int h_2(\tau, \tau + \Delta)x(t - \tau)x(t - \Delta - \tau)\,d\Delta\,d\tau \tag{4}$$

$$G_3(t) = 6 \int\int\int h_3(\tau, \tau + \Delta_1, \tau + \Delta_1 + \Delta_2)x(t - \tau)x(t - \tau - \Delta_1)$$
$$\times x(t - \tau - \Delta_1 - \Delta_2)\,d\Delta_1\,d\Delta_2\,d\tau \tag{5}$$

When considering neurobiological systems which transmit information via all-or-none action potentials, it is most appropriate to model the input as a series of point process events (Krausz, 1975), in which case the input, $x(t)$, is a zero mean Poisson process. For each impulse in the train, τ is the observation period following each impulse at time t, and Δ is the time interval since a preceding impulse. The first four kernels of the series were obtained using cross-correlation techniques (Lee and Schetzen, 1965), and were normalized relative to the first order kernel.

Interpretation of Kernel Functions   It may be helpful to clarify interpretation of kernels in the context of real data. In initial experiments, we characterized nonlinear response properties of granule cells as reflected in population field potentials recorded in vivo from both anesthetized and chronically implanted, unanesthetized animals (Berger et al., 1988a, b). The *first order kernel*, $h_1(\tau)$, is the average of all evoked granule cell responses, occurring with a latency of τ, during random train stimulation (see figure 9.3, top). The first order kernel represents the best linear model of the system, that is, it would be the best predictor of granule cell output if output depended only on stimulus intensity and there were no time-dependent processes that modulated granule cell excitability. When a relatively low stimulus intensity is used for random-impulse train stimulation (one that evokes a population spike amplitude approximately 10% of maximum when the perforant path is stimulated at 0.5 Hz), first order kernels showed that the average population spike amplitude was 2.2 ± 0.3 mV ($\pm$SEM), a value that depends on stimulus intensity (Balzer et al., submitted). The first order kernel accounts for 35–45% of the variance in granule cell output for the conditions of an in vivo preparation and low stimulus intensity.

The *second order kernel*, $h_2(\tau, \Delta)$, represents the modulatory effect of a preceding stimulus occurring Δ ms earlier on granule cell response (with a latency of τ) evoked by the most current stimulation impulse, that is, systematic facilitation or suppression of granule cell output not predicted by the first order kernel. In general terms, the second order kernel can be interpreted as a generalized recovery function, namely, the probability (in addition to that provided by the first order kernel) that a granule cell will reach threshold, as a function of time since a previous perforant path volley. Second order kernels

First Order Kernel

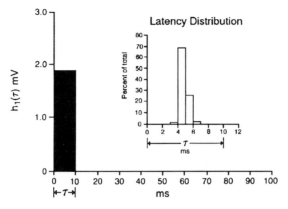

Second Order Kernel

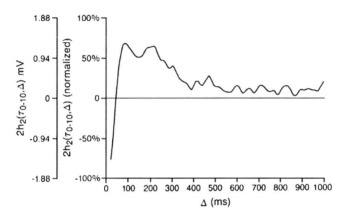

Third Order Kernel

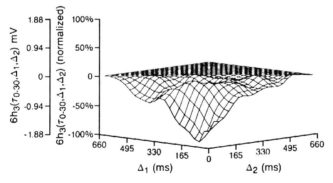

Figure 9.3 First (top), second (middle) and third order kernels (bottom) for dentate granule cells recorded from a representative in vivo preparation. Inset in the top panel shows the latency distribution of population spike responses evoked by the entire 4064-impulse random train. Both second and third order kernel values are expressed in absolute millivolts (mV; outside axis) and as a percentage of the first order kernel magnitude (normalized; inside axis).

A Biologically Based Model of the Hippocampus

indicated that granule cell output exhibited prominent nonlinearities in response to several ranges of interstimulus intervals: population spike amplitude was almost completely suppressed when preceding impulses occurred within 10–30 ms (figure 9.3, middle), and there was a marked facilitation of spike amplitude when preceding impulses occurred within 50–500 ms; a smaller magnitude facilitation occurred in response to intervals between 500–1000 ms. Intervals greater than 1000 ms induced no consistent change in spike amplitude. The second order kernel accounts for an additional 20–30% of the variance in granule cell output for the conditions of an in vivo preparation and low stimulus intensity. It is important to realize that the second order kernel is not equivalent to a paired impulse function (see Berger et al., 1988b).

The *third order kernel*, $h_3(\tau, \Delta_1, \Delta_2)$, represents the modulatory effect of any two preceding stimuli occurring Δ_1 ms and Δ_2 ms earlier on granule cell response evoked by the most current stimulation impulse, that is, systematic facilitation or suppression of granule cell output not predicted by the first and second order kernels. The third order kernel can be interpreted as a family of conditional recovery functions, that is, the probability (in addition to that provided by the lower order kernels) that a granule cell will reach threshold as a function of time (Δ_2) since a previous perforant path input, given the occurrence of a perforant path input $\Delta_1 + \Delta_2$ ms earlier. Prominent third order nonlinearities were expressed when the intervals separating any pair of preceding intervals was less than or equal to 200–300 ms. In response to these stimulus patterns, granule cell output was reduced by an average maximum of 60% of the first order kernel, with the magnitude of suppression inversely related to interval length (figure 9.3, bottom). To clarify further by example, third order nonlinearites observed in vivo reflect primarily increased $GABA_A$ receptor–mediated feedback inhibition due to facilitation-induced recruitment of granule cells. The third order kernel accounts for an additional 10–15% of variance in granule cell output for the conditions of an in vivo preparation and low stimulus intensity.

There also is a *zero order kernel*, h_0, which traditionally is defined as the best estimate of that part of the system output that is not dependent on the input, for example, the resting membrane potential upon which synaptic input is superimposed. For reasons that are detailed elsewhere (Sclabassi et al., 1988a), in our analyses to date, $h_0 \rightarrow 0$. Because it does not contribute significantly to the results, h_0 will be ignored in the review here.

3.2   Analysis of the In Vivo Hippocampal Dentate Gyrus: Interactions Between Subsystems

Contribution of the Commissural System to Nonlinear Response Properties of Dentate Granule Cells   Commissural projections to and from the contralateral hippocampus provide a major source of feedback to the dentate gyrus. The commissural system of the dentate gyrus arises from polymorphic neurons of the hilar region (Berger et al., 1981), which receive direct excitatory input from the perforant path, as well as indirect input from granule cell collaterals (Claiborne et al., 1986; Scharfman and Schwartzkroin, 1988). Polymorphic cells provide monosynaptic, excitatory input to granule cells and inhibitory interneurons of the contralateral dentate (Buszàki and Eidelberg, 1981; Douglas et al., 1983). Thus, the commissural pathway generates a feedback excitation, with an embedded feedforward inhibition.

The contribution of commissural connections to nonlinearities of granule cells was determined by conducting random impulse train stimulation of the perforant path in vivo before and after removal of the rostral tip of the contralateral hippocampus where commissural fibers converge (Berger et al., 1990). Results showed that acute removal (1–24 hr) of the commissural feedback loop increased the magnitudes of first order kernels, second order kernel facilitation, and third order kernel suppression; second order kernel suppression was unchanged (figure 9.4). Second and third order nonlinearities continued to be expressed in response to the same interstimulus intervals characteristic of the intact system, however. In intact preparations, electrical stimulation of commissural afferents (constant frequency of 2 Hz) simultaneously with random impulse train stimulation of the perforant path ($\lambda = 2$ Hz) resulted in a virtual complement of the effects of surgical removal of commissural feedback, that is, decreases in the magnitude of first, second, and third order kernel values with no shift in the intervals associated with nonlinearities.

These findings indicate that commissural feedback is not sufficiently time-locked to each perforant volley to provide the basis for interval-specific non-linearities. Instead, the commissural system appears to contribute to the gain of nonlinearities resulting from other pathways and cellular mechanisms. These results also may be interpreted with respect to the known physiology of commissural afferents. The feedforward inhibition driven by commissural fibers has been shown to predominate over the monosynaptic, excitatory input to granule cells (Deadwyler et al., 1974; Douglas et al., 1983). The substantial increase in facilitation following transection of commissural connections is consistent with the loss of the stronger feedforward inhibition, whereas the stability of the suppression of spike amplitude in response to shorter interstimulus intervals is consistent with the comparatively weaker excitatory feedback.

Differences Between Nonlinearities of Granule Cells Expressed in Response to Medial and Lateral Perforant Path Input   We recently have begun an analysis of the lateral perforant path as well. The two pathways can be distinguished electrophysiologically using established criteria (McNaughton and Barnes, 1977). Our initial results have revealed that, in marked contrast to the medial perforant path, second order kernels for the lateral perforant path display inhibition for almost all inter-impulse intervals within the range of 10–1000 ms. In some preparations, a slight facilitation (10–20%) of population spike amplitude is seen in response to intervals of 50–100 ms.

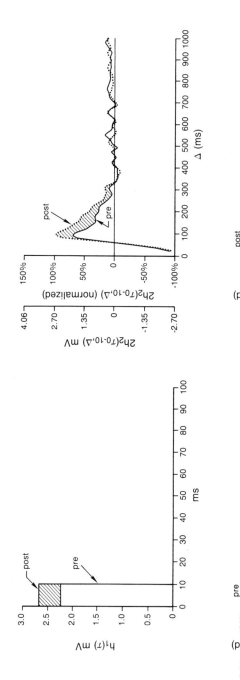

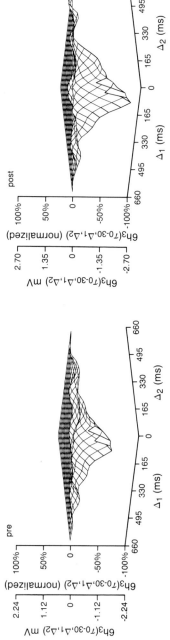

Figure 9.4 Acute effects of unilateral hippocampectomy on first and second order kernels (top) and on third order kernels (bottom) for the granule cell population spike of the contralateral dentate. The data were collected 48 hr after surgery.

In further contrast to the medial perforant path, third order kernels indicate almost exclusively facilitative interactions.

The medial and lateral perforant paths transmit information from associational neocortical and olfactory brain regions, respectively (Wilson and Steward, 1978), and terminate onto spatially restricted, nonoverlapping regions of granule cell dendrites (Steward, 1976). The contrasting nonlinear response properties of the two components of the perforant path indicate that functional characteristics of the dentate gyrus (and thus, the entire hippocampus) may be determined in part by the modality of stimuli being processed. Neural representations associated with nonolfactory stimuli would be subject to the transformations characteristic of the medial perforant path, whereas those associated with olfactory stimuli would be subject to the transformations characteristic of the lateral path. Associations of nonolfactory and olfactory cues (e.g., Eichenbaum et al., 1989; Staubli et al., 1984) would involve a cross-modulation of the activities propagated along the medial and lateral perforant paths, respectively.

Feedforward Projections of Perforant Path Afferents to Hippocampal Pyramidal Neurons   Functional characterizations of the hippocampus have been based primarily on its intrinsic trisynaptic circuitry, formed by successive excitatory projections from the entorhinal cortex to the dentate gyrus, from dentate granule cells to CA3 pyramidal cells, and finally from CA3 pyramidal cells to CA1 pyramidal cells. Despite anatomical endence for additional monosynaptic projections from entorhinal to CA3 and CA1 (Steward, 1976), few in vivo electrophysiological studies of the direct pathway have been conducted to test the validity of the cascade model of the hippocampus. We stimulated axons of entorhinal cortical neurons in vivo and recorded evoked single and population spike responses in the dentate, CA3, and CA1 of hippocampus, to determine if pyramidal cells are driven primarily via monosynaptic or trisynaptic pathways. Our results showed that neurons within the three subfields of the hippocampus discharge simultaneously in response to input from a given subpopulation of entorhinal cortical neurons, and that the initial monosynaptic excitation of pyramidal cells then is followed by weaker excitatory volleys transmitted through the trisynaptic pathway (see Berger and Yeckel, 1991; Yeckel and Berger, 1990). In addition, we found that responses of CA3 pyramidal cells often precede those of dentate granule cells, and that excitation of CA3 and CA1 pyramidal cells can occur in the absence of dentate granule cell excitation.

These results argue that instead of the traditionally assumed cascade relationship between the three subsystems of the hippocampus, excitatory input from the entorhinal cortex initiates a two-stage feedforward excitation of pyramidal cells, with the dentate gyrus providing feedforward excitation of CA3, and with both the dentate and CA3 providing feedforward excitation of CA1 (figure 9.5).

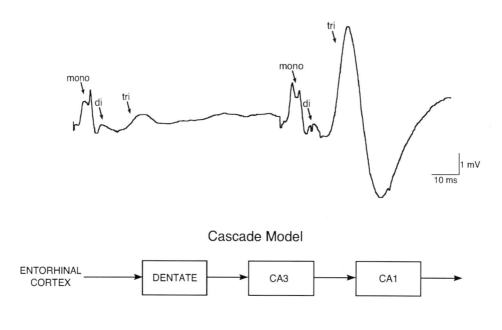

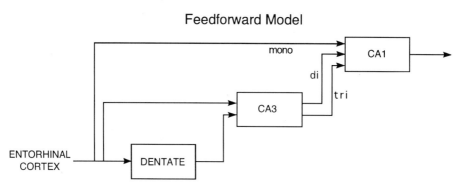

Figure 9.5 (Top) Demonstration of feedforward excitation of CA1 pyramidal cells by paired-impulse stimulation of input from the entorhinal cortex. Arrows identify the monosynaptically evoked population spikes (mono), followed by a disynaptically evoked single action potential (di; second impulse), and the trisynaptic (tri) population EPSP (calibration; 10 ms and 1 mV). (Middle) Schematic representation of the traditional model of sequential propagation of activity through the trisynaptic pathway. (Bottom): Schematic representation of the proposed model of two-phase feedforward excitation of CA1 pyramidal cells.

3.3 Analysis of the In Vitro Hippocampal Dentate Gyrus: Interactions Within Subsystems

As discussed above, an essential component of our approach is to experimentally characterize input/output properties of progressively simplified components of the hippocampal system so that dynamic properties intrinsic to individual hippocampal neurons can be distinguished from dynamic properties that arise from synaptic interconnections among the neurons. One means for substantially reducing the influence of other subsystems is to utilize the hippo-

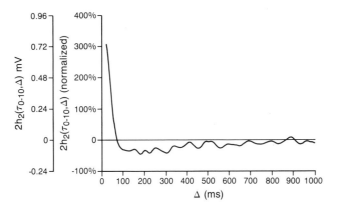

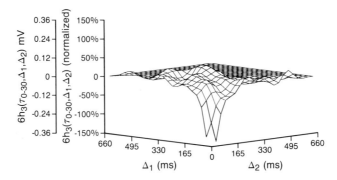

Figure 9.6 Second and third order kernels for dentate granule cells recorded from a 600 μm thick in vitro hippocampal slice preparation.

campal slice preparation, which typically consists of tissue sections (600 μm in thickness) cut perpendicular to the longitudinal axis of the hippocampus and maintained in vitro. When sectioned in this manner, slices contain granule cells and their projections to CA3, and CA3 pyramidal cell projections to CA1. In addition, the distal ends of perforant path axons and their synaptic input to the dentate gyrus remain intact and functionally viable. In contrast, all connections with the contralateral hippocampus and the ipsilateral entorhinal cortex are removed, thus eliminating feedback to the dentate from the other subsystems of the hippocampal formation. Input/output properties of granule cells were studied in the context of this slice preparation using simultaneous intracellular and field potential recordings (Harty et al., 1992a, submitted).

The average first bin value of first order kernels was significantly smaller (0.3 ± 0.03 mV; N = 12) than first order kernels obtained from in vivo preparations, consistent with the reduced nature of the in vitro slice preparation. Second order nonlinearities (figure 9.6, top) were qualitatively different than those exhibited by in vivo preparations. Instead of suppression of granule cell output in response to short interimpulse intervals, a robust facilitation was observed. The facilitation was greater in magnitude (with respect to normal-

A Biologically Based Model of the Hippocampus

ized kernel values, 241 ± 27%) and occurred maximally in response to shorter intervals (10–20 ms) compared to data from in vivo preparations. In further contrast, facilitation in slices occurred only in response to intervals less than 100–150 ms, a much narrower range than was observed in vivo. Finally, data from slices consistently exihibited suppression to intervals of 150–800 ms; interstimulus intervals within the same range produced facilitation or no effect for in vivo preparations. Third order kernels from slices revealed suppression of a larger magnitude (normalized values, average maximum of 90%), in response to a narrower range of intervals (< 90 ms) than was observed for the in vivo dentate gyrus. Third order nonlinearities for in vitro slices also included a facilitation in response to input patterns of $\Delta_1 = 100$–200 ms and $\Delta_2 = 300$–400 ms, which was not observed in vivo.

Of particular interest was the finding of a strong and consistent parallel between intracellular and field potential measures (examples shown in figure 9.8), indicating that the population field potentials provide an accurate measure of the behavior of the individual elements. The difference in relative magnitudes of facilitation and suppression in higher order kernels (see figure 9.8) is due only to a scaling factor: extracellular measures can reflect facilitation at a population level, namely, recruitment, whereas intracellular measures cannot; because this facilitation is included in the first order kernel, total suppression is more difficult to achieve at the population level.

Contribution of GABAergic Interneurons Differences between the second and third order properties of the in vivo and in vitro dentate gyrus could not be accounted for on the basis of differences in the number of granule cells tested in each preparation. Increasing stimulation intensity so as to recruit responses from more granule cells in vitro did not markedly alter higher order kernels: facilitation and suppression were observed to the same ranges of intervals, and kernel values changed only slightly.

GABAergic interneurons of the dentate gyrus provide powerful feedforward and feedback inhibition of granule cells (McCarren and Alger, 1985; Ribak et al, 1990; Ribak and Seress, 1983). One of the inhibitory postsynaptic potentials initiated by these interneurons is mediated by $GABA_A$ receptors, and has both a short latency to onset and a rapid time to peak (within 20 ms); decay is exponential (figure 9.7, left). Thus, the inhibitory effect of this interneuron population within second order kernels should be revealed by interstimulus intervals corresponding to such a time course. The suppression of the population spike when $\Delta = 10$–30 ms for in vivo preparations is consistent with this hypothesis. The lack of similar suppression in second order kernels of in vitro slices suggests that connections between granule cells and GABAergic interneurons are reduced within a 600-μm slice. Processes of GABAergic interneurons are known to travel preferentially in parallel with the longitudinal axis of the hippocampus (Struble et al., 1978), and thus, perpendicular to the plane of section. If the cell bodies of the interneurons that are the origin of GABAergic input lie outside the boundaries of the slice, then

GABA_A Inhibition

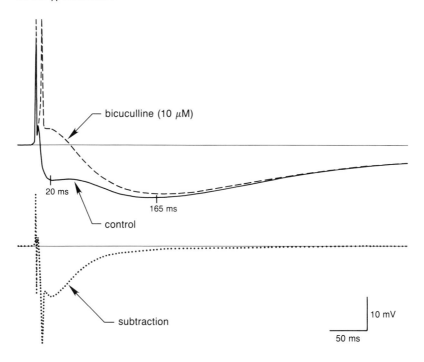

bicuculline (10 μM)

20 ms

165 ms

control

subtraction

10 mV

50 ms

GABA_B Inhibition

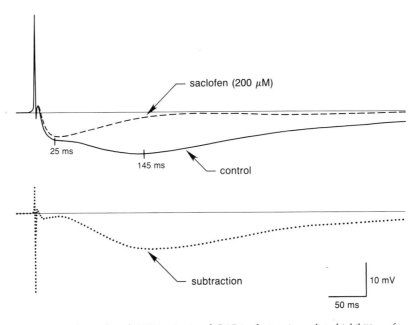

saclofen (200 μM)

25 ms

145 ms

control

subtraction

10 mV

50 ms

Figure 9.7 Examples of GABA_A (top) and GABA_B (bottom)–mediated inhibition of granule cells in vitro evoked by perforant path input. Cells have been depolarized to −50 mV to enhance the magnitude of hyperpolarizing potentials.

A Biologically Based Model of the Hippocampus

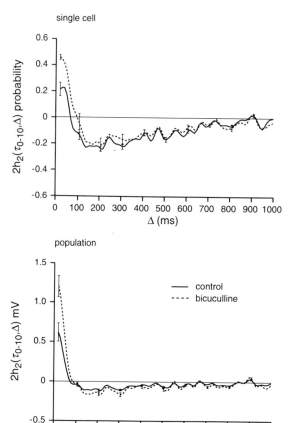

single cell

population

control
bicuculline

Figure 9.8 Effects of the GABA$_A$ receptor antagonist, bicuculline (left panels), and the GABA$_B$ receptor antagonist, saclofen (right panels), on second order nonlinearities of granule cells of the in vitro dentate gyrus. Kernels obtained in the absence and presence of antagonist are represented by a solid line and a dotted line, respectively. Data are shown for simultaneous intracellular (top panels) and extracellular (bottom panels) recordings.

pharmacological blockade of GABA$_A$ receptors should not result in a major alteration of granule cell nonlinearities.

Application of the GABA$_A$ receptor antagonist bicuculline (10–20 μM) resulted in a small, though significant, increase in second order kernel facilitation (figure 9.8, left). The presence of a residual GABAergic influence was supported by the results of experiments in which the postsynaptic effect of GABA was enhanced by adding the GABA$_A$ allosteric agonist alphaxalone (Barker et al., 1987) to the slice media In the presence of alphaxalone (1–3 μM), the second order facilitation induced by short interstimulus intervals was replaced with a suppression equivalent (relative to the first order kernel) to that observed in vivo (figure 9.9).

GABA$_B$ Receptor–mediated Inhibition of Dentate Granule Cells

GABA also induces a bicuculline-insensitive slow IPSP, which is a potassium-

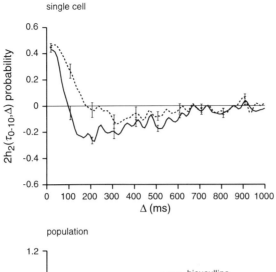

single cell

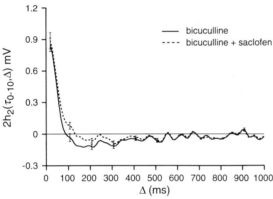

population

- bicuculline
- - - bicuculline + saclofen

Figure 9.8 (cont.)

dependent hyperpolarization resulting from activation of GABA$_B$ receptors (Alger and Nicoll, 1982; Newberry and Nicoll, 1985). The latency-to-peak of the GABA$_B$-mediated IPSP is approximately 100–200 ms (see figure 9.7, right), corresponding to the peak of the second order kernel suppression observed in vitro which also is bicuculline-insensitive (see figure 9.8, left). Confirming the hypothesis that these second order nonlinearities reflected the contribution of GABA$_B$ receptor activation, we found that suppression was greatly reduced by the GABA$_B$ receptor antagonist, saclofen (see figure 9.8, right).

Dentate Granule Cells in "Thin" Slices and "Mini" Slices: Possible Open-loop Condition The results of experiments using 600-μm slices suggested that there may be relatively few GABAergic interneurons which both receive granule cell and/or perforant path input and terminate onto granule cells within a 600-μm distance. Thus, the magnitude of feedforward and feedback inhibition should be inversely related to slice thickness. To test this hypothesis, we examined input/output properties of dentate granule cells

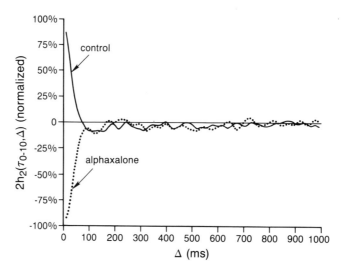

Figure 9.9 Effects of the GABA_A receptor allosteric agonist, alphaxalone, on second order kernel properties of the in vitro dentate gyrus. Kernels obtained in the absence and presence of alphaxalone are represented by a solid line and a dotted line, respectively. Note the selective enhancement of second order kernel suppression to interstimulus intervals < 100 ms.

using 300-μm "thin" slices. First order kernels were smaller in magnitude than those for 600-μm slices (data not shown), consistent with a further reduction in the size of the granule cell population. Although second order nonlinearities of granule cells recorded from "thin" slices were virtually identical to those obtained using thicker slices (in terms of the direction of nonlinearities and the intervals associated with nonlinearities), second order kernels for "thin" slices were not altered by bicuculline. This finding suggests that the anatomical connections required for significant GABAergic inhibition are established over a distance greater than 300 μm, and that feedforward/feedback modulation of dentate granule cell activity by GABAergic interneurons is effectively eliminated in "thin" slices.

Polymorphic and GABAergic cell populations are only two of several classes of interneurons known to exist within the dentate gyrus (Amaral, 1978; Gulyas et al., 1991; Sloviter and Nilaver, 1987). Some interneurons lying beneath the granule cell layer in the hilus of the dentate, such as those containing somatostatin and the hilar mossy cells, are thought to have projections that ramify more locally than those of GABAergic interneurons and, thus, might significantly modulate granule cell activity even within a 300 μm slice.

To test this possibility, we created "mini" slices that were 600 μm in thickness but that consisted of approximately one-half of the dentate gyrus separated surgically from the remaining slice. This isolated dentate slice preparation was reduced further by a second knife cut just below the granule cell layer, made to eliminate the possibility of feedback from any population of interneurons in the hilus. Because GABA-containing cells and processes are partially embedded in the granule cell layer and are not susceptible to surgical manipulation, however, any connections with GABAergic interneurons would remain intact within such a "mini" slice.

Input/output properties of granule cells within "mini" slices were not distinguishable from those of whole slices, indicating that surgical separation of the dentate from the remaining hippocampus did not result in tissue damage, and that feedback provided from hilar interneurons within the limits of a slice is not substantial (third order nonlinearities have not yet been examined). Also attesting to the physiological viability of the "mini" slice preparation was the finding that, in contrast to the effects of the hilar knife cut, application of bicuculline increased second order facilitation to the same extent as in "whole" slices; thus, inhibition by GABAergic interneurons within the layer subjacent to granule cells remains intact.

Although other interneuron systems remain to be examined, it would appear likely that thin slice preparations, and particularly "thin-mini" slices, will provide the basis for an open-loop characterization of dentate granule cells, and because of the common structural features shared by the three subfields of the hippocampus, open-loop properties of CA3 and CA1 pyramidal cell regions as well. The results from one "thin-mini" slice would represent the functional dynamics of, roughly, 1–2% of the total population of granule cells or pyramidal cells. The possibility of heterogeneities as a function of spatial location is a proposed area of investigation. When completed, data from these analyses will provide the foundation for modeling the three major intrinsic cell populations of the hippocampus for the three-dimensional structure of the hippocampal system.

3.4 Nonlinearities in Granule Cell Synaptic Responses

Characteristics of the Closed-loop System We also have analyzed nonlinearities of granule cell synaptic responses to perforant path input, recorded either intracellularly in vitro or as a population EPSP in vivo, to determine if the nonlinearities in population spike amplitude can be accounted for on the basis of synaptic processes. Stimulation intensities were equivalent to those used for analysis of the population spike, namely, low-intensity suprathreshold. Second order nonlinearities for the population EPSP were significantly different than those observed for the population spike (figure 9.10). Second order nonlinearities for the EPSP were exclusively facilitative, and occurred in response to a smaller range of intervals than seen for the population spike, with maximum facilitation of the EPSP occurring in response to a smaller value of Δ. In further contrast to the population spike, no significant third order nonlinearities were found for the population EPSP.

These findings strongly suggest that some second order nonlinearities (when $\Delta = 10$–40 ms and when $\Delta > 300$ ms) and virtually all third order nonlinearities are due to processes initiated by action potential generation, such as feedback from other neuron populations activated by granule cell output and intrinsic voltage-dependent conductances.

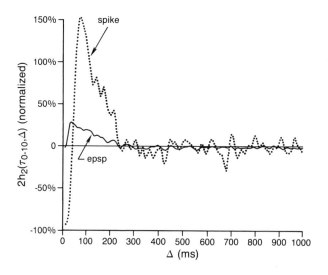

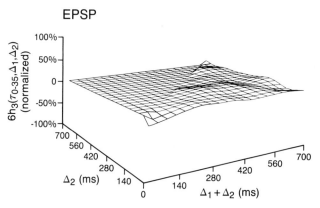

Figure 9.10 Second and third order nonlinearities of the population synaptic response (EPSP) of dentate granule cells in response to perforant path input. In the upper panel, an example second order kernel for the population spike is shown for comparison.

Pharmacological Dissociation In Vivo Between AMPA and NMDA Receptor–mediated Components of Glutamatergic Perforant Path Input Glutamatergic synaptic transmission in the perforant path is mediated by α-amino-3-hydroxy-5-methy-4-isoxazoleproprianate (AMPA) and N-methyl-D-aspartate (NMDA) receptor subtypes (Collingridge and Lester, 1989). AMPA and NMDA receptors are characterized by very different kinetic properties, which should be reflected in different nonlinear response profiles. We have developed procedures that will allow study in vivo of the relative contribution of the two classes of glutamatergic receptor subtypes that mediate perforant path input to granule cells. Specifically, we have examined population EPSPs recorded from the dentate molecular layer while administering the AMPA receptor antagonist, CNQX (6-cyano-7-nitroquinaxaline-2,3-dione), and/or the NMDA receptor antagonist, D-APV, by microinfusion through a multibarrelled pipette positioned 100–500 μm from the recording site (Blanpied and Berger, 1992).

CNQX (25–50 μM) reduced the evoked EPSP by 70–95% without affecting the afferent fiber volley; subsequent addition of D-APV (50–100 μM) substantially reduced the residual response (figure 9.11). For greater resolution of the component sensitive to D-APV, digitized responses evoked during the application of CNQX and D-APV were subtracted from those evoked in the presence of CNQX alone. Residuals revealed that D-APV eliminated a negative-going potential with a peak latency 25–200% longer than control (10.0 ms vs. 5.1 ms control), consistent with analyses from whole-cell recordings, and a peak amplitude of up to 20% of the control.

Consistent with the voltage-dependent block of the NMDA channel by Mg^{2+}, amplitude of the NMDA component was found to be strongly frequency dependent, that is, it was greatly enhanced (200% of the amplitude to a single impulse) by the depolarization that accompanies the temporal summation of high-frequency stimuli (e.g., 2–5 impulses delivered with a 2-ms interstimulus interval). These results indicate that the NMDA-mediated component of perforant path input to dentate granule cells may be studied effectively in vivo in the presence of CNQX, and predict that nonlinearities specific to NMDA receptor activation will be associated with high-frequency components of the random train.

Bidirectional, Activity-dependent Modification of NMDA Receptor–mediated Synaptic Transmission   One of our goals in developing a mathematical model of the hippocampus is to study the functional consequences of activity-dependent changes in the interactions among interconnected neurons. One important component of this effort is to identify the range of conditions (e.g., activity patterns, levels of excitability) that constitute prerequisites for synaptic plasticity; the limits of these conditions then will be incorporated within the model. Although it has been estabrished that AMPA receptor–mediated synaptic transmission can undergo both long-term potentiation (LTP) and long-term depression (LTD), the extent to which NMDA receptor–dependent synaptic events are susceptible to activity-dependent modification is less certain. There have been conflicting reports as to whether NMDA receptor–mediated activity expresses LTP, and it was not known if NMDA receptors express LTD. These issues are important ones to resolve because activity-dependent modification of AMPA receptor function is dependent on concurrent activation of the NMDA receptor subclass. Thus, any enhancement or decrement in NMDA receptor function has the potential for a cascading effect through the regulation of AMPA receptor function.

Experiments were conducted during intracellular recordings from granule cells of the hippocampal dentate gyrus in vitro (Xie et al., 1992). In the presence of the AMPA receptor antagonist CNQX (10 μM), robust LTP of NMDA receptor–mediated synaptic potentials was induced by brief high- (50 Hz) and lower- (10 Hz) frequency tetanic stimuli of glutamatergic afferents (60 $\pm$ 6% and 43 $\pm$ 12%) (tracings 4 and 5 in figure 9.12). In contrast, hyperpolarization of the granule cell membrane potential to -100 mV during 10-Hz tetanic stimuli resulted in LTD of NMDA receptor–mediated synaptic

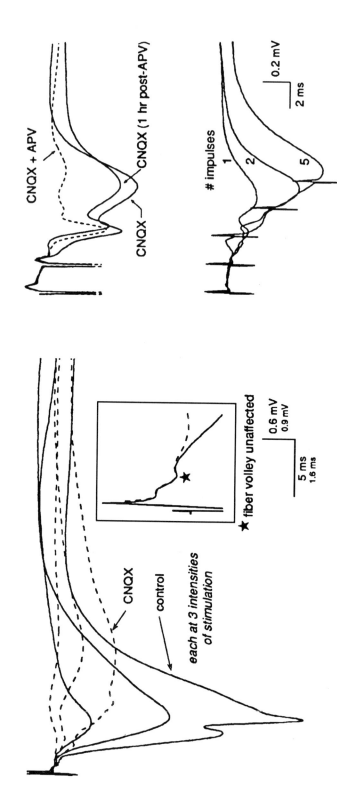

Figure 9.11 (Left) Blockade of AMPA mediated component of granule cell population EPSP in vivo. (Right, top) Blockade of CNQX resistant component with D-APV. (Right, bottom) Enhancement of NMDA component with high-frequency stimulation.

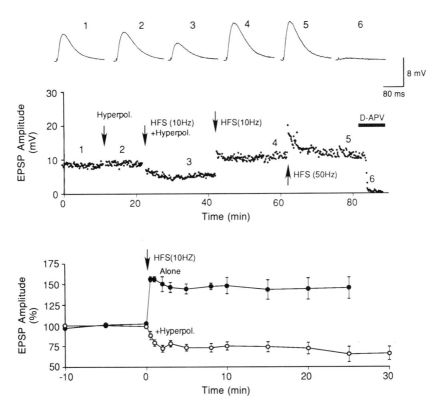

Figure 9.12 The induction of long-term potentiation (LTP) or long-term depression (LTD) of NMDA receptor–mediated synaptic responses depends on the level of postsynaptic membrane polarization. (Top) In this cell EPSPs were taken at −80 mV during a 10-min baseline period (1). No change in the size of this response was observed after intracellular injection of hyperpolarizing current pulses (−0.23 nA, 2 sec in duration, repeated four times at intervals of 5 sec) (2). The passage of current produced a 20-mV hyperpolarization of the soma. Intracellular current injection then was repeated in conjunction with 10-Hz tetanic stimuli of perforant path afferents. Simultaneous synaptic activation and intracellular hyperpolarization caused LTD of NMDA receptor-mediated EPSPs (3). A second 10-Hz tetanus in the absence of current injection induced LTP of the previously depressed response (4). No further enhancement was observed after additional tetanic stimuli delivered at 50-Hz. (Bottom) Group data showing posttetanic changes in EPSP amplitudes induced in cells receiving either 10-Hz tetanus alone (filled circles, n = 3) or in conjunction with hyperpolarizing current injection (open circles, n = 8). Tetanic stimulation was delivered at time zero and at the same intensity as test stimulus.

potentials (−34 ± 8%) (tracing 3 in figure 9.12). Increases in $[Ca^{2+}]_i$ appear to play a critical role in the induction of both LTP and LTD, because when $[Ca^{2+}]_i$ was buffered by intracellular injections of the calcium chelator BAPTA prior to tetanization, the induction of both LTP and LTD was prevented. These findings provide the first evidence for the induction of both LTP and LTD of NMDA receptor–mediated synaptic transmission and demonstrate that the level of postsynaptic depolarization can determine which of the two forms of synaptic plasticity is expressed in response to an identical afferent signal. These constraints on the induction of synaptic plasticity will be important to integrate into a model of the hippocampus, both in terms of "learning rules" for the nonparametric model and in terms of molecular dynamics for the parametric model (see below).

3.5 Effect of LTP on Nonlinear Response Properties of Dentate Granule Cells

We have begun an investigation of the consequences of synaptic plasticity on input/output properties of the hippocampus, by initially using the induction of LTP in perforant path afferents in vivo because of the robustness of the phenomenon and the degree of experimental control (Balzer et al., 1989). Using chronically implanted preparations, a Poisson-distributed impulse train was used to characterize dentate granule cell response to medial perforant path input. LTP then was induced through the delivery of brief (20 ms) bursts of 400 Hz (total of 80 impulses/day) given over the course of 3–5 days. The same intensity random impulse train then was used to characterize input/output properties of granule cells for a second time. Results showed that the magnitude of first order kernels was increased substantially post LTP induction, confirming the potentiating effects of high-frequency tetanus. Higher orders kernels also were altered markedly, however, with the common effect across kernel order and interstimulus interval being a reduction in the magnitude of nonlinearities. This consequence of LTP persisted even when the intensity used for random-impulse train stimulation was reduced so that approximately the same number of granule cells (equivalent population spike amplitudes) were activated per impulse in response to low-requency (0.2 Hz) stimulation. In contrast, the identical experimental procedures induced no change in the nonlinear response properties of the population EPSP (Balzer et al., 1991). We interpret these results as indicating that after the induction of LTP the amount of current injection that can be initiated by a potentiated synapse is near maximum, so that alternative synaptic inputs to the same neuron activated by feedback pathways exert relatively little influence on postsynaptic cell excitability; thus, output of the postsynaptic cell comes to depend almost exclusively on stimulus intensity and to a much lesser extent on interstimulus interval. The effects of several other experimental manipulations that also induce synaptic plasticity also have been examined (Robinson et al., 1991, 1993).

3.6 Computer Simulations of the Input/Output Model

Transputer-based Network   Using procedures like those outlined above, input/output models can be obtained for different subsystems, or components of subsystems, of the hippocampal formation. The behavior of the subsystem (and ultimately, combinations of subsystems) is simulated using convolutions of the kernels with a specified input. We have begun implementing a computational model of the global, functional network properties of the hippocampus on a set of parallel processors called transputers (Krieger et al., 1988; Solomon et al., 1989). Each transputer element includes a 10 MIPS processor with 4

KBytes of on-chip high-speed cache, private random access memory, and four 2-way 10 Mbit–sec links for establishing communication with other transputer elements. Convolution integrals utilizing experimentally determined kernels (through the third order) for each subsystem in the network are represented on the transputers. Thus, the simulations are implemented on a hardware network of parallel processors, which compute a predicition of the input/ output behavior of the subsystem, cell population, or subcellular process (depending on the level of the representation), based on a history of stimuli and representation of the measured kernels obtained by nth-order convolutions. The rationale for utilizing a transputer-based system includes the following: (1) given their parallel configuration, computations for each subsystem can be conducted simultaneously, as in the operation of the real, biological system; (2) data from the processor of each transputer is transmitted directly to the processors of other transputers, so the computation speed is very high; (3) the linkage between any two transputers can be reconfigured easily (electronic switching), so that the consequences of different configurations of network elements can be investigated, and the model can evolve in parallel with experimental investigations (e.g., so as to include feedforward input from entorhinal cortex to the CA3 and CA1 pyramidal cell fields).

Prediction of Response to Arbitrary Inputs   In our first attempts to simulate the functional properties of the dentate gyrus, the experimentally determined kernels were convolved with the input to predict granule cell output (Sclabassi et al., 1992; Solomon et al., 1989). Simulation studies have been performed using the first and second order terms of the series, and the first, second, and third order terms, for data obtained from the intact, in vivo hippocampal formation and for the in vitro hippocampal slice preparation. For the intact hippocampus, the granule cells are conceptualized as a feedforward element, as is the contralateral hippocampus. All other elements are lumped into the system feedback element. The slice preparation represents the open-loop system, where the contralateral hippocampus has been removed, the trisynaptic pathway is open, and the local inhibitory feedback has been removed. The models were used to predict the results of arbitrarily chosen paired and triplet inputs, that is, stimuli not given using a random train format.

For the results shown figure 9.13, the nonlinear properties of the dentate gyrus in vivo first were characterized using the first, second, and third order kernels obtained from random train stimulation. The same preparation then was stimulated using a set of paired impulses, with the separation between the impulses in a pair (Δ) systematically varied from 10 to 500 ms. The average value of the predicted response to the first impulse was subtracted from the amplitude of the population spike produced by the second impulse to give an estimate of the nonlinear residual. The same experiment then was performed computationally, using the kernels as a model. The top panel of figure 9.13 summarizes the results when only the first and second order kernels were used as the model. The bottom panel summarizes the results when the first, second,

1st and 2nd Order Kernels

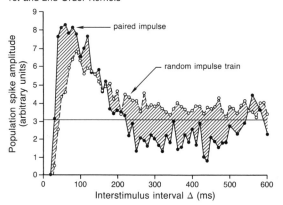

1st, 2nd, and 3rd Order Kernels

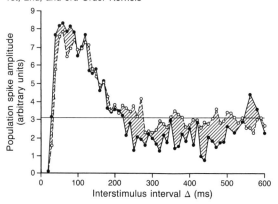

Figure 9.13 Transputer-based simulation of closed-loop input/output properties of the dentate gyrus. Experimentally determined kernel characterizations (open circles) are used to predict population spike amplitudes (closed circles) evoked by paired impulse inputs (interimpulse intervals ranging from 10 to 1200 ms). (Top) Predictions based on first and second order kernels only. (Bottom) Predictions based on first, second, and third order kernels.

and third order kernels were used to predict responses; obviously, inclusion of the third order kernel improves accuracy of the prediction.

Multidimensional Laplace Transforms and Fourier Transforms Our approach in modeling the hippocampus as a set of input/output functions is based on the concept that a neuronal network consists of multiple homogeneous populations of neurons, each of which may be treated as a unit with its own dynamics, and that these neuronal populations interact with each other through network connectivity to produce global network properties. The strategy we have been pursuing is to take advantage of the topology of the hippocampal system to decompose it into a number of irreducible subsystems, which can be characterized independently of each other, either experimentally or computationally, and then recombined to produce a global solution. The subsystem models are developed in terms of nth order convolution operators.

Berger et al.

The nth order kernel may be interpreted as an nth order impulse response and may be transformed using multidimensional Laplace transforms. This has the advantage of yielding algebraic relationships between the inputs and outputs of system elements that may be manipulated more easily than the convolution operators in the time domain. In addition, the characterization and utilization of these higher order transform pairs allows both the time and frequency domain properties of the subsystems and the recombined systems to be studied.

We have defined the higher-order Laplace transforms for assumed relationships between various subsystems and components of the hippocampus (Sclabassi et al., 1990, 1992). Among the cases that have been solved to date are the cascade, negative feedback, and combined negative feedback and positive feedforward configurations. Software for computing one- and two-dimensional Fourier transforms has been written and evaluated both with defined test data as well as experimental data (Kosanović, 1992).

Computation of Kernels for "Unobservable Elements": Estimation of kernels for GABAergic Inhibitory Interneurons In the context of the above studies, we have computed the kernels for $GABA_A$ receptor–mediated inhibitional, although the GABAergic interneurons were not recorded from directly. We used the following strategy: the kernels for the in vitro dentate were-determined experimentally in presence of alphaxalone, that is, when $GABA_A$ receptor–mediated inhibition is enhanced; for this condition, the relationship between granule cells, the feedthrough element, and basket cells, the feedback element, may be represented as follows:

$$E_1(S) = \frac{A_1(S)}{1 - A_1(S)B_1(S)}$$

$$E_2(S_1, S_2) = \frac{A_1(S_1)A_1(S_2)A_1(S_1 + S_2)B_2(S_1, S_2) + A_2(S_1, S_2)}{[1 - A_1(S_1)B_1(S_1)][1 - A_1(S_2)B_1(S_2)][1 - A_1(S_1 + S_2)B_1(S_1 + S_2)]}$$

$$
\begin{aligned}
E_3(S_1, S_2, S_3) = &\{A_1(S_1, S_2, S_3)[\tfrac{2}{3}B_2(S_1, S_2 + S_3)E_1(S_1) \cdot E_2(S_2, S_3) \\
&+ \tfrac{2}{3}B_2(S_2, S_1 + S_3)E_1(S_2) \cdot E_2(S_1, S_3) \\
&+ \tfrac{2}{3}B_2(S_3, S_1 + S_2)E_1(S_3) \cdot E_2(S_1, S_2) \\
&+ B_3(S_1, S_2, S_3)E_1(S_1)E_1(S_2)E_1(S_3)] \\
&+ \tfrac{2}{3}\{A_2(S_1, S_2 + S_3)[1 + B_1S_2(S_1)E_1S_2(S_1)] \\
&\cdot [B_1(S_2 + S_3)E_2(S_2, S_3) + B_2(S_2, S_3)E_1(S_2)E_1(S_3)] \\
&+ A_2(S_2, S_1 + S_3)[1 + B_1(S_2)E_1(S_2)] \\
&\cdot [B_1(S_1 + S_3)E_2(S_1, S_3) + B_2(S_1, S_3)E_1(S_1)E_1(S_3)] \\
&+ A_2(S_3, S_1 + S_2)[1 + B_1(S_3)E_2(S_3)] \\
&\cdot [B_1(S_1 + S_2)E_2(S_1, S_2) + B_2(S_1, S_2)E_1(S_1)E_1(S_2)]\} \\
&+ A_3(S_1, S_2, S_3)[1 + B_1(S_1)E_1(S_1)][1 + B_1(S_2)E_1(S_2)]
\end{aligned}
$$

$$\cdot [1 + B_1(S_3)E_1(S_3)]\}/$$
$$\cdot [1 - A_1(S_1 + S_2 + S_3)B_1(S_1 + S_2 + S_3)]$$

Input/output properties then were measured again in the presence of bicuculline, that is, when all $GABA_A$ receptor–mediated inhibition was eliminated. The higher order Laplace transforms shown above were used to solve for B (Sclabassi et al., 1991):

$$B_3(S_1, S_2, S_3) = \{E_3(S_1, S_2, S_3)[1 - A_1(S_1 + S_2 + S_3)B_1(S_1 + S_2 + S_3)]$$
$$- A_3(S_1, S_2, S_3)[1 + B_1(S_1)E_1(S_1)][1 + B_1(S_2)E_1(S_2)]$$
$$\cdot [1 + B_1(S_3)E_1(S_3)]$$
$$- \tfrac{2}{3}\{A_2(S_1, S_2 + S_3)[1 + B_1(S_1)E_1(S_1)]$$
$$\cdot [B_1(S_2 + S_3)E_2(S_2, S_3) + B_2(S_2, S_3)E_1(S_2)E_1(S_3)]$$
$$+ A_2(S_2, S_1 + S_3)[1 + B_1(S_2)E_1(S_2)]$$
$$\cdot [B_1(S_1 + S_3)E_2(S_1, S_3) + B_2(S_1, S_3)E_1(S_1)E_1(S_3)]$$
$$+ A_2(S_3, S_1 + S_2)[1 + B_1(S_3)E_1(S_3)]$$
$$\cdot [B_1(S_1 + S_2)E_2(S_1, S_2) + B_2(S_1, S_2)E_1(S_1)E_1(S_2)]\}$$
$$- \tfrac{2}{3}A_1(S_1 + S_2 + S_3)[B_2(S_1, S_2 + S_3)E_1(S_1)E_2(S_2, S_3)$$
$$+ B_2(S_2, S_1 + S_3)E_1(S_2)E_2(S_1, S_3)$$
$$+ B_2(S_3, S_1 + S_2)E_1(S_3)E_2(S_1, S_2)\}/$$
$$\cdot [E_1(S_1)E_1(S_2)E_1(S_3)A_1(S_1 + S_2 + S_3)]$$

When converted back into the time domain, this computational procedure allows for an explicit expression of the contribution of the GABAergic interneuron population, as it acts through $GABA_A$ receptors.

4 A TWO-LEVEL FIELD THEORY–BASED MODEL OF THE HIPPOCAMPUS

The ultimate objective of the studies reviewed above is to develop experimentally based input/output characterizations of "elemental functional units" of the hippocampus which then can be used as building blocks in an attempt to construct a model of the dynamics of the global system. Having achieved what we believe can be described as an "elemental functional unit," that is, a small population of perforant path fibers and their granule cell targets with only minimal feedback from any other cell population, we have begun to develop the corresponding parametric model. Again, the strategy is to use the experimentally based nonparametric model to constrain assumptions that must be made in developing the parametric model.

The model we are developing is based on an n-level field theory, that is, a continuous representation in which the state variables of the system are defined in real space, r, and time, T. The dynamics of two monosynaptically

Berger et al.

connected populations of neurons can be formulated at the level of neurons, i.e., the neural network, and at the level of synapses, i.e., the level of one neuron, by the general field equation:

$$H\psi(r_0, T_0) = \Gamma(r_0, T_0) \tag{5}$$

where $\psi(r_0, T_0)$ is the field variable at (r_0, T_0), and $\Gamma(r_0, T_0)$ is the source. H is a space-time differential operator, e.g.,

$$H \equiv \frac{\partial}{\partial T} - D\nabla^2 + H_1 \tag{6}$$

with the diffusion operator, ∇^2, and the interaction operator, H_I, which transports the field ψ from one point to another. Field variables are: (1) soma membrane potential, ψ, or the integration of all synaptic inputs, voltage-dependent and ion-dependent conductances that determine cell output, and (2) synaptic efficacy, μ. In previous work by Chauvet (1992a,b), field equations including nonlocal operators for soma membrane potential and synaptic efficacy have been determined using an extension of Hodgkin-Huxley equations. These two field variables have been shown to evolve according to the equations:

$$\frac{\partial \psi(r_0, T_0)}{\partial t} = \nabla_r(D^r \nabla_r \psi(r_0, T_0)) +$$

$$+ \int_{D_R(r_0)} \rho_1(r)\psi(r, T) \int_{D_s(r, r_0)} B(r_0, T_0, r, T)\pi_0(s, r; r_0)\mu(s, t)\, ds\, dr$$

$$+ \Gamma_\psi[\psi(r_0, T_0^-), \psi_{refr}]$$

$$\frac{\partial \mu(s, t)}{\partial t} = \nabla_s[D^s \nabla_s \mu(s, t)]$$

$$+ \int_{D_R(r_0)} \rho_1(r') \int_{D_s(r', r_0)} \mu_0(s', t')\pi_0(s', r'; r_0)A(s, s')\, ds'\, dr' + \Gamma_\mu(s, t)$$

$$s \equiv s(r, r_0)$$

$$D_R(r_0) = \bigcup_{r'} D_s(r', r_0)$$

where $T = T_0 - d/v_\psi$, $d = \|r - r_0\|$, v_ψ is the transport velocity of the ψ-interaction, namely, the neural activity, and $t' = t - \|s - s'\|/v_\mu$, with v_μ being the velocity of the μ-interaction. Thus, the above equations are the two 2-1evel field equations for the synaptic and neuronal activity of a population of neurons and their respective populations of synapses at two corresponding points $(s(r, r_0), t)$ and (r, T) in space-time of a neural network. The neural tissue is characterized by two geometrical functions: the density of presynaptic neurons, ρ_1, and the density-connectivity π of synapses. $D_s(r, r_0)$ is the space of synapses in neurons localized in r_0, which correspond to neurons in r. Space $D_R(r_0)$ is the neural integration space that is the union of subspaces $D_s(r, r_0)$.

The first term on the right of the ψ field equation represents the local diffusion of activity from r to points $r + dr$ (e.g., ephaptic coupling), which can be substantial in the case of the hippocampus where the cell body densities are very high. The second term is the nonlocal interaction operator, which represents the influence of synaptic input from all other neurons on a given cell at r. The third term represents the local effect of the source, that is, the local transformations that drive the soma membrane potential (or more precisely, the membrane potential at the site of action potential generation) to threshold.

The first term on the right of the nonlocal equation for the synaptic efficacy represents the local space diffusion from s to points $s + ds$. The second term is the nonlocal interaction operator which represents the influence of all distant synapses on the given synapse at s. The third term represents the local effect of the source, that is, the local transformation that allows the value of μ to be modified (e.g., a change in the conformation of receptors).

Synaptic plasticity is introduced into the above model by assuming, similar to Hebb's postulate (Hebb, 1949), that synaptic efficacy μ is in direct relation with the product of presynaptic and postsynaptic activities:

$$\mu_0 = h \langle X(r, T) \rangle \langle X(r_0, T_0) \rangle$$

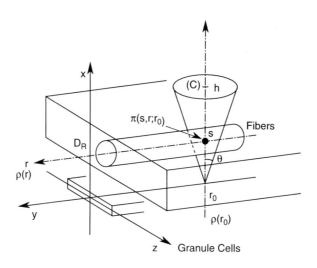

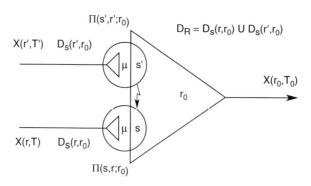

Figure 9.14 Geometrical model used to incorporate morphological and anatomical constraints characteristic of granule cells and perforant path fibers.

where activity $X(r, T)$ is the stimulating frequency in the perforant path fibers, and $X(r_0, T_0)$ is the output activity of the granule cells, and in a more biologically meaningful manner through mechanistic definitions of presynaptic and postsynaptic efficacy.

A geometrical model has been constructed to represent the morphological and anatomical features of the system (figure 9.14): the set of perforant path fibers is approximated by a cylinder, but, because of the laminar distribution of entorhinal afferents within the granule cell dendritic region: (1) the set of activated fibers within the dentate gyrus has been represented as a layer having a "width" $D_R(I)$ that is a function of I; (2) the dendritic tree for one granule cell is represented as a cone. The cone is defined by its angle 2θ and its height h; (3) the intersection of the layer and the cone is a truncated cone (C). In mathematical terms, the cell bodies of perforant paths fibers with density $\rho_1 r$ are located at r; they act on granule cells with density ρ_0, r_0 located at r_0. The density of synapses between neurons at r_0, in the continuous space of neurons, and neurons at $r \neq r_0$, is described by the density-connectivity function $\pi(s, r, r_0)$, that is, the probability of having a connection via a synaptic contact at s in the space of synapses.

We have used the first generation of this model to predict the population behavior of the extracellular field potentials (population spike and population EPSP) generated by the combined activity of a set of granule cells activated by a volley of excitatory input from a set of perforant path axons (figure 9.15; Chauvet and Berger, 1990, submitted; Costalat et al., 1991). Perhaps the most important point is that what is included in this parametric model is what we hypothesize to be remaining *functionally* in the thin-mini dentate hippocampal slice. A comparison of the behaviors of the input/output model and the field theory–based model will provide a test of that hypothesis.

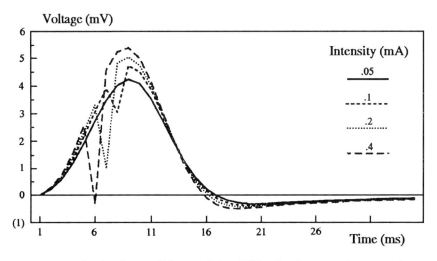

Figure 9.15 Simulated extracellular population EPSP and spike potentials generated using the field theory–based model. Simulated responses are shown as a function of stimulation intensity.

A Biologically Based Model of the Hippocampus

5 CONCLUSIONS

A combined theoretical-experimental strategy can be formulated for developing biologically constrained mathematical models of neural systems typical of the mammalian brain, that is, those with large numbers of heterogeneous populations of neurons and with a complex interconnecting circuitry. As outlined here, that strategy consists of a dual theoretical approach in which nonlinear systems analytic techniques are used to generate input/output functions describing the functional dynamics of major subsystems of the neural network under study. The global system then is modeled as the composite of the input/output functions for all subsystems. This nonparametric model captures the functional properties that emerge from the interaction of all system elements: those known and unknown, those observable and unobservable. As such, the input/output model may provide essential constraints in the formulation of a parametric model, in which the mechanisms underlying the functional properties are represented explicitly. For developing a parametric model, an n-level field theory approach was described which has the advantages of a continuous representation in space and time, and includes formalisms for relating the different hierarchical levels of the nervous system. Through such an approach, the effect of molecular events on network dynamics can be described.

ACKNOWLEDGMENTS

This research was supported by the Office of Naval Research (N00014-90-J-4000) the Air Force Office of Scientific Research (89-0197), NIH (NS 52488), and NIMH (MH00343).

REFERENCES

Alger, B. E., and Nicoll, R. A. (1982) *Journal of Physiology* 328:125–141.

Amaral, D. G. (1978) *Journal of Comparative Neurology* 182:851–914.

Amaral, D. G., and Witter, M. P. (1989) *Neuroscience* 31:571–591.

Amaral D. G., Dolorfo C., and Alvarez-Royo P. (1991) *Hippocampus* 1:415–436.

Ambros-Ingerson, J., Granger, R., and Lynch, G. (1990) *Science* 247:1344–1348.

Andersen, P., Bliss, T. V. P., and Skrede, K. K. (1971a) *Experimental Brain Research* 13:208–221.

Andersen, P., Bliss, T. V. P., and Skrede, K. K. (1971b) *Experimental Brain Research* 13:222–238.

Anderson, J. A., and Rosenfeld, E. (1988) *Neurocomputing.* Cambridge, Mass.: MIT Press.

Bakst, I., Avendano, C., Morrison, J. H., and Amaral, D. G. (1986) *Journal of Neuroscience* 6:1452–1462.

Balzer, J. R., Sclabassi, R. J., and Berger, T. W. (1989) *Society for Neuroscience Abstracts* 15:403.

Balzer, J. R., Sclabassi, R. J., and Berger, T. W. (1991) *Society for Neuroscience Abstracts* 17:386.

Balzer, J. R., Sclabassi, R. J., and Berger, T. W., submitted.

Barker, J. L., Harrison, N. L., Lange, G. D., and Owen, D. G. (1987) *Journal of Physiology* 386:485−501.

Berger, T. W., and Bassett, J. L. (1992) In *Learning and Memory: The Biological Substrates*, I. Gormezano and E. A. Wasserman (eds.). Hillsdale, N. J.: Erlbaum, pp. 275−320.

Berger, T. W., and Sclabassi, R. J. (1988) In *Long-term Potentiation: From Biophysics to Behavior*, P. W. Landfield and S. A. Deadwyler (eds.). New York: Liss, pp. 467−497.

Berger, T. W., and Yeckel, M. F. (1991) In *Long-Term Potentiation: A Debate of Current Issues*, M. Baudry and J. Davis (eds.). Cambridge, Mass.: MIT Press, pp. 327−356.

Berger, T. W., Semple-Rowland, S., and Bassett, J. L. (1981) *Brain Research* 215:329−336.

Berger, T. W., Berry, S. D. and Thompson, R. F. (1986) In *The Hippocampus*, R. L. Isaacson and K. H. Pribram (eds.). New York: Plenum, pp. 203−239.

Berger, T. W., Robinson, G. B., Port, R. L., and Sclabassi, R. J. (1987) *Advanced Methods of Physiological System Modeling, Vol. I*, V. Z. Marmarelis (ed.). Los Angeles: Biomedical Simulations Resource, pp. 73−103.

Berger, T. W., Eriksson, J. L., Ciarolla, D. A., and Sclabassi, R. J. (1988a) *Journal of Neurophysiology* 60:1077−1094.

Berger, T. W., Eriksson, J. L., Ciarolla, D. A., and Sclabassi, R. J. (1988b) *Journal of Neurophysiology* 60:1095−1109.

Berger, T. W., Harty, T. P., Barrionuevo, G, and Sclabassi, R. J. (1989) In *Advanced Methods of Physiological System Modeling, Vol. II*, V. Z. Marmarelis (ed.). New York: Plenum, pp. 113−128.

Berger, T. W., Weikart, C. L., and Sclabassi, R. J. (1990) *Society for Neuroscience Abstracts* 16:739.

Berger, T. W., Barrionuevo, G., Levitan, S. P., Krieger, D. N., and Sclabassi, R. J. (1991) In *Neurocomputation and Learning: Foundations of Adaptive Networks*, J. W. Moore and M. Gabriel (eds.). Cambridge, Mass.: MIT Press, pp. 283−352.

Berger, T. W., Harty, T. P., Xie, X., Barrionuevo, G., and Sclabassi, R. J. (1992) *Proceedings of the IEEE 34th Midwest Symposium on Circuits and Systems*, pp. 91−97.

Blanpied, T. A., and Berger, T. W. (1991) *Society for Neuroscience Abstracts* 17:1035.

Blanpied, T. A., and Berger, T. W. (1992) *Hippocampus*, 2:373−388

Brown, T. H., Kairiss, E. W., and Keenan, C. L. (1990) *Annual Review of Neuroscience* 13:475−511.

Buonomano, D. V., and Byrne, J. H. (1990) *Science* 249:420−423.

Buzsáki, G. (1986) *Brain Research* 398:242−252.

Buzsáki, G., and Eidelberg, E. (1981) *Brain Research* 230:346−350.

Byrne, J. H. (1987) *Physiological Reviews* 67:329−439.

Byrne, J. H., and W. O. Berry (eds.) (1989) *Neural Models of Plasticity: Experimental and Theoretical Approaches*. New York: Academic Press.

Carpenter, G. A., Cohen M. A., Grossberg, S., Kohonen, T., Oja, E., Palm, G., Hopfield, J. J., and Tank, D. W. (1987) *Science* 235:1226−1229.

Chauvet, G. (1993a) *Journal of Mathematical Biology* 31:475−486

Chauvet, G. (1993b) *Journal of Mathematical Biology* in press.

Chauvet, G., and Berger, T. W. (1990) *Society for Neuroscience Abstracts* 16:739.

Chauvet, G., and Berger, T. W., submitted.

Claiborne, B. J., Amaral, D. G., and Cowan, W. M. (1986) *Journal of Comparative Neurology* 246:435–458.

Clements, M. P., Bliss, T. V. P., and Lynch, M. A. (1991) *Neuroscience* 45:379–389.

Collingridge, G. L., and Lester, R. (1989) *Pharmacological Review* 40:143–210.

Cooper, L. N., and Scofield, C. L. (1988) *Proceedings of the National Academy of Sciences* 85:1973–1977.

Costalat, R., Genet, S., Thiels, E., Berger, T. W., and Chauvet, G. (1991) *Society for Neuroscience Abstracts* 17:1037.

Deadwyler, S. A., West, J. R., Cotman, C. W., and Lynch, G. S. (1974) *Journal of Neurophysiology* 37:167–184.

Douglas R. M., McNaughton, B. L., and Goddard, G. V. (1983) *Journal of Comparative Neurology* 219:285–294.

Eichenbaum, H., Wiener, S. I., Shapiro, M. L., and Cohen, N. J. (1989) *Journal of Neuroscience* 9:2764–2775.

Finkel, L. H., and Edelman, G. M. (1985) *Proceedings of the National Academy of Sciences, USA* 82:1291–1295.

Gingrich, K. J., and Byrne, J. H. (1987) *Journal of Neurophysiology* 57:1705–1715.

Gluck, M. A., and Thompson, R. F. (1987) *Psychological Review* 94:176–191.

Grossberg, S., and Schmajuk, N. A. (1989) *Neural Networks* 2:79–102.

Gulyas, A. I., Toth, K., Danos, P., and Freund, T. F. (1991) *Journal of Comparative Neurology* 312:371–378.

Hanson, S. J., and Burr, D. J. (1990) *Behavioral and Brain Sciences* 13:471–518.

Harrison, N. L., Vicini, S., and Barker, J. L. (1987) *Journal of Neuroscience* 7:604–609.

Harty, T. P., Barrionuevo, G., Sclabassi, R. J., and Berger, T. W. (1991) *Society for Neuroscience Abstracts* 17:1037.

Harty, T. P., Berger, T. W., Sclabassi, R. J., and Barrionuevo, G. (1993a) submitted for publication.

Harty, T. P., Berger, T. W., Sclabassi, R. J., and Barrionuevo, G. (1993b) submitted for publication.

Hebb, D. O. (1949) *The Organization of Behavior: A Neuropsychological Theory.* New York: Wiley.

Hestrin, S., Nicoll, R. A., Perkel, D. J., and Sah, P. (1990) *Journal of Physiology* 422:203–225.

Holmes, W. R., and Levy, W. B. (1990) *Journal of Neurophysiology* 63:1148–1168.

Hopfield, J. J. (1982) *Proceedings of the National Academy of Science* 79:2554–2558.

Ishizuka, N., Weber, J., and Amaral, D. G. (1990) *Journal of Comparative Neurology* 295:580–623.

Ito, M. (1989) *Annual Review of Neuroscience* 12:85–102.

Jaffe, D., and Johnston, D. (1990) *Journal of Neurophysiology* 64:948–960.

Klopf, A. H. (1988) *Psychobiology* 16:85–125.

Kosanović, B. (1992) M.S.E.E. Thesis, University of Pittsburgh.

Krausz, H. (1975) *Biological Cybernetics* 19:217–230.

Krieger, D., Solomon, J., Levitan, S., Berger, T., Barrionuevo, G., Larimore, W., and Sclabassi, R. (1988) *Proceedings of the 19th Annual Pittsburgh Conference on Modeling and Simulation* 19:2397–2401.

Krieger, D., Berger, T. W., Levitan, S., and Sclabassi, R. J. (1990) *Advances in Computers and Mathematics in Medicine* 20:231–246.

Krieger, D. N., Berger, T. W., and Sclabassi, R. J. (1992) *IEEE Transactions on Biomedical Engineering* 39:420–424.

Lee, C., Rohrer, W. H., and Sparks, D. L. (1988) *Nature* 332:357–360.

Lee, Y. W., and Schetzen, M. (1965) *International Journal of Control* 2:237–254.

Levy, W. B., Anderson, J. A., and Lehmkuhle, S. (1985) *Synaptic Modification, Neuron Selectivity, and Nervous System Organization.* Hillsdale, N.J.: Erlbaum.

Levy, W. B., Colbert, C. M., and Desmond, N. L. (1989) In *Neuroscience and Connectionistic Theory*, M. Gluck and D. Rumelhart (eds.). Hillsdale, N.J.: Erlbaum, pp. 187–235.

Linden, D. J., and Routtenberg, A. (1989) *Brain Research Reviews* 14:279–296.

Lockery, S. R., Wittenberg, G., Kristan, W. B., and Cottrell, G. W. (1989) *Nature* 340:468–471.

Lorente de Nó, R. (1934) *Journal of Psychological Neurology* 46:113–177.

Madison, D. V., Malenka, R. C., and Nicoll, R. A. (1991) *Annual Review of Neuroscience* 14:379–397.

Marmarelis, P. Z., and Marmarelis, V. Z. *Analysis of Physiological Systems: The White Noise Approach.* New York: Plenum, 1978.

Marmarelis, P. Z., and Naka, K.-I. (1972) *Science* 175:1276–1278.

Marmarelis, V. Z. (1987) In *Advanced Methods of Physiological System Modeling.* Los Angeles: Biomedical Simulations Resource, pp. 73–103.

McCarren, M., and Alger, B. E. (1985) *Journal of Neurophysiology* 53:557–71.

McNaughton, B. L., and Barnes, C. A. (1977) *Journal of Comparative Neurology* 175:439–454.

McNaughton, B. L., and Morris, R. G. M. (1987) *Trends in Neurosciences* 10:408–415.

Michelson, H. B., and Wong, R. K. S. (1991) *Science* 253:1420–1423.

Mpitsos, G. J., Burton, R. M., and Creech, H. C. (1988) *Brain Research Bulletin* 21:539–546.

Newberry, N. R., and Nicoll, R. A. (1985) *Journal of Physiology* 360:161–185.

Nicoll, R. A., Kauer, J. A., and Malenka, R. C. (1988) *Neuron* 1:97–103.

Qian, N., and Sejnowski, T. J. (1990) *Proceedings of the National Academy of Sciences* 87:8145–8149.

Ribak, C. E., and Seress, L. (1983) *Journal of Neurocytology* 12:577–597.

Ribak, C. E., Nitsch, R., and Seress, L. (1990) *Journal of Comparative Neurology* 300:449–461.

Robinson, G. B., Sclabassi, R. J., and Berger, T. W. (1991) *Brain Research* 562:17–25.

Robinson, G. B., Fluharty, S. J., Zigmond, M. J., Sclabassi, R. J., and Berger, T. W. (1993) *Brain Research*, 614:21–28.

Rugh, W. J. (1981) *Nonlinear Systems Theory: The Volterra/Wiener Approach.* Baltimore: John Hopkins University Press.

Scharfman, H. C., and Schwartzkroin, P. A. (1988) *Journal of Neuroscience* 8:3812–3821.

Schmajuk, N. A., and DiCarlo, J. J. (1991) *Behavioral Neuroscience* 105:82–110.

Sclabassi, R. J., Hinman, C. L., Kroin, J. S., and Risch, H. (1977) *Proceedings of the Joint Automatic Control Conference*, IEEE, New York, 12:787–795.

Sclabassi, R. J., Eriksson, J. L., Port, R. L., Robinson, G. B., and Berger, T. W. (1988a) *Journal of Neurophysiology*, 60 : 1066–1076.

Sclabassi, R. J., Krieger, D. N., and Berger, T. W. (1988b) *Annals of Biomedical Engineering* 16 : 17–34.

Sclabassi, R. J., Krieger, D. N., Biedka, T., and Berger, T. W. (1989a) *Society for Neuroscience Abstracts* 15 : 403.

Sclabassi, R. J., Krieger, D. N., Solomon, J., Samosky, J., Levitan, S., and Berger, T. W. (1989b) In *Advanced Methods of Physiological System Modeling, Vol. II*, V. Z. Marmarelis (ed.). New York: Plenum, pp. 129–146.

Sclabassi, R. J., Biedka, T., Solomon, J., Krieger, D., Barrionuevo, G., and Berger, T. W. (1990) *Society for Neuroscience Abstracts* 16 : 738.

Sclabassi, R. J., Paul, J., Kosanović, B., Krieger, D., Barrionuevo, G., and Berger, T. W. (1991) *Society for Neuroscience Abstracts* 17 : 1037.

Sclabassi, R. J., Krieger, D. N., Solomon, J., Kosanović, B., and Berger, T. W. (1992) *Proceedings of the IEEE 34th Midwest Symposium on Circuits and Systems*, pp. 114–117.

Sejnowski, T. J. (1991) *Current Biology* 1 : 38–40.

Sejnowski, T. J., Koch, C., and Churchland, P. S. (1988) *Science* 24 : 1299–1306.

Sloviter, R. S. (1991) *Hippocampus* 1 : 31–40.

Sloviter, R. S., and Nilaver, G. (1987) *Journal of Comparative Neurology* 256 : 42–60.

Solomon, J. M., Krieger, D. N., Berger, T. W., and Sclabassi, R. J. (1989) *Society for Neuroscience Abstracts* 15 : 402.

Sørensen, K. E., and Shipley, M. T. (1979) *Journal of Comparative Neurology* 188 : 313–334.

Spruston, N., and Johnson, D. (1992) *Journal of Neurophysiology* 67 : 508–529.

Staubli, U., Ivy, G., and Lynch, G. (1984) *Proceedings of the National Academy of Sciences* 81 : 5885–5887.

Staubli, U., Ambros-Ingerson, J., and Lynch, G. (1992) *Hippocampus* 2 : 49–58.

Steward, O. (1976) *Journal of Comparative Neurology* 167 : 285–314.

Struble, R. G., Desmond, N. L., and Levy, W. B. (1978) *Brain Research* 152 : 580–585.

Swanson, L. W., and Cowan, W. M. (1977) *Journal of Comparative Neurology* 172 : 49–84.

Swanson, L. W., Wyss, J. M., and Cowan, W. M. (1978) *Journal of Comparative Neurology* 181 : 681–716.

Thiels, E., Weisz, D. J., and Berger, T. W. (1992) *Neuroscience* 46 : 501–509.

Thompson, R. F., Berger, T. W., and Madden, J., IV. (1983) *Annual Review of Neuroscience* 6 : 447–491.

Traub, R. D., Miles, R., and Wong, R. K. S. (1989) *Science* 243 : 1319–1325.

Traub, R. D., Wong, R. K. S., Miles, R., and Michelson, H. (1991) *Journal of Neurophysiology* 66 : 635–650.

Treves, A., and Rolls, E. T. (1992) *Hippocampus* 2 : 189–200.

Volterra, V. (1959) *Theory of Functionals and of Integral and Integro-differential Equations*. New York: Dover Publications.

Wiener, N. (1958) *Nonlinear Problems in Random Theory*. New York: Wiley.

Wilson, M., and Bower, J. M. (1992) *Journal of Neurophysiology* 67 : 981–995.

Wilson, R. C., and Steward, O. (1978) *Experimental Brain Research* 33:523–534.

Xie, X., Berger, T. W. and Barrionuevo, G. (1992) *Journal of Neurophysiology* 67:1009–1013.

Yeckel, M. F., and Berger, T. W. (1990) *Proceedings of the National Academy of Sciences* 87:5832–5836.

Yeckel, M. F., and Berger, T. W. (1991) *Society for Neuroscience Abstracts* 17:385.

Zador, A., Koch, C., and Brown, T. H. (1990) *Proceedings of the National Academy of Sciences* 87:6718–6722.

Zipser, D. (1992) *Neuroscience* 47:853–862.

Zipser, D., and Andersen, R. A. (1988) *Nature* 331:679–684.

Zornetzer, S., Davis, J., and Lau, C. (eds.) (1990) *An Introduction to Neural and Electronic Networks*. San Diego: Academic Press.

10 Synaptic Plasticity, Learning, and Memory

Steven P. R. Rose

1 MEMORY AND THE HEBB SYNAPSE

The suggestion that learning and memory might be functions of synaptic plasticity is now both commonplace and almost universally attributed to Donald Hebb, who in his book *The Organization of Behavior* in 1949 offered the following hypothetical explanation for how learning might occur:

Let us assume then that the persistence or repetition of a reverberatory activity (or "trace") tends to induce lasting cellular changes that add to its stability. The assumption can be precisely stated as follows: *When an axon of cell A is near enough to excite a cell B and repeatedly or persistently takes part in firing it, some growth process or metabolic change takes place in one or both cells such that A's efficiency, as one of the cells firing B, is increased*

The most obvious and I believe much the most probable suggestion concerning the way in which one cell could become more capable of firing another is that synaptic knobs develop and increase the area of contact between the afferent axon and efferent [cell body]. There is certainly no direct evidence that this is so.... There are several considerations, however, that make the growth of synaptic knobs a plausible perception.

The attractiveness of Hebb's ideas to classical learning psychologists lay in the fact that this formulation appeared to elegantly translate the known rules of association learning into a cellular script, as the two inputs, strong and weak, into the postsynaptic neuron could be regarded as representing respectively the unconditioned and the conditioning stimulus, and the changed response of the postsynaptic neuron was represented by the CR.

As all historians of science know, no idea is entirely novel, and in this case Hebb's ideas can be traced back to the neuroanatomist Ramón y Cajal, and beyond him to the Italian psychiatrist Eugenio Tanzi, who as long ago as the 1880s—even before it was clear that neurons were distinct cells separated by synaptic junctions, but were still regarded as comprising a syncytium, or polynucleated network within the brain—suggested:

Perhaps every representation immediately determines a functional hypertrophy of the protoplasmic processes and axons concerned: molecular vibrations become more intense and diffuse themselves, momentarily altering the form of the dendrites; and thus, if the conditions are favourable, new expansions and collaterals originate and become permanent.... (Tanzi, English translation 1909)

But despite Tanzi's prescience, neural network modelers now speak routinely of "Hebb synapses," by which they mean postsynaptic neurons receiving two synapses, one of which is capable of causing the postsynaptic cell to fire, while the other is initially too weak so to do. If, however, weak inputs occur in close temporal contiguity with those from the strong synapse, they will be strengthened so as to in due course be capable in their own right of causing the postsynaptic cell to fire. Hebbian mechanisms are thus heterosynaptic, and learning—that is, the change in responsiveness of the postsynaptic neuron to a previously insufficient synapse—is a postsynaptic mechanism. Later generations of modelers have produced a number of variants on these rules, so as to consider the possibility of anti-Hebbian neurons whose responsiveness is weakened rather than strengthened by training, or homosynaptic rather than heterosynaptic mechanisms (Singer, 1987, 1990). One of the greatest challenges to Hebbian orthodoxy came in the late 1970s and early 1980s with the claim by Kandel and his colleagues that the mechanisms of habituation, sensitisation and even associative learning could be mimicked by a dissected *Aplysia* neuron and its single input in what was essentially a presynaptic mechanism (Goelet et al., 1986). Kandel went on to speak of learning as a single synapse phenomenon and of a "cellular alphabet" of memory formation. Although there has more recently been a retreat from this extreme reductionism (Dudai, 1989), there is no doubt that it has profoundly influenced thinking about synaptic plasticity and memory over the past decade. Echoes of the presynaptic/postsynaptic controversy find their way also into the literature of LTP (see chapters 4, 5).

Accepting Hebbianism as a theory was unproblematic; demonstrating in practice that memory formation involves modulation of synaptic plasticity, and even more, unraveling the molecular mechanisms of that plasticity, has been much harder (Thompson, 1992). In this chapter I will review some of the evidence from my own laboratory that training animals on simple tasks does indeed result in changes in synaptic biochemistry, morphology, and electrophysiology that are compatible with the idea that memory fomlation involves modulation of synaptic connectivity. However, I will also argue that to demonstrate this is not thereby to accept that the Hebbian proposition is all that needs to be said about the neurobiology of memory, just as not all learning is reducible to simple associationsim.

If synaptic mechanisms are in some way to form the neural representations of memory, they must match in important respects the characteristic features of memory at the behavioral level. One such is its time dimension. Although a single trial is often enough to establish a memory, it has been known for many years, initially from observations on human memory, later from animal experiments, that memory formation occupies a number of distinct phases, stretching over at least an hour. The early phases of memory are very labile and can be disrupted in humans and nonhuman animals by electroshock, hypothermia, or concussion, or simply, in humans, through failure of internal reinforcement or rehearsal (as in remembering number strings, for instance) Once having survived this short-term phase, however, memories appear to be very stable, often in humans lasting a lifetime. This is interpreted as demonstrating that there are both short- and long-term forms of memory, possibly with other intermediate stages (Gibbs and Ng, 1977). Although the progression between the forms is subjectively perceived as a seamless transition, McGaugh (1964) argued convincingly that the two are in fact processed independently, short-term memory declining as long-term memory becomes established. Certain pharmacological interventions, such as administration of protein synthesis inhibitors, will prevent the establishment of long-term memory while leaving short-term memory unimpaired (Davis and Squire, 1984) so that memory decays over an hour or so; other agents result in more rapid declines and are presumed to be affecting earlier memory phases.

It follows that there must be synaptic mechanisms—probably independent —which correspond to both short- and long-term forms of memory. In a simple version of the Hebbian model, one would expect to find that the same synapse, transiently strengthened during the short-term memory phase, has this strengthening confirmed and stamped in by more substantive molecular processes during long-term memory. But the fact that short- and long-term memory are separable also means that the cellular "mobilizing processes," such as the synthesis of membrane constituents to be inserted at the synapse, must be occurring contemporaneously with the distinctive synaptic events that represent short-term memory. Some of these mobilizing processes may be what is sometimes dismissively called "biochemical housekeeping," but if we are to properly understand the cellular and molecular mechanics of memory, it will be necessary to try to identify them and to distinguish them from other concomitants of memory formation—that is, to identify the necessary, sufficient, and specific cellular correspondents of memory (Rose, 1981, 1992).

Surprisingly, many, if not most studies on synaptic plasticity occurring during or as a result of learning have focused on the early events rather than on mechanisms that might confer longer-term changes in synaptic connectivity, and have tended to disregard the implications of the psychological evidence for the separability of the phases. One example of the way in which this thinking has trapped theoreticians is the speculation that synaptic transients involving phosphorylation of membrane proteins could produce, in the protein kinases of the membrane, a sort of autocatalytic response which resulted in their lasting covalent modification (Crick, 1984). In this way synapses could "learn" without any need for reference back to the neuron's protein synthetic machinery or the synthesis of new membrane constituents. The argument behind such a purely synaptic model is that it provides a mechanism for specificity, marking and modifying a single synapse rather than all the many that a particular neuron makes—and such specificity is certainly a requirement of Hebbian mechanisms. The early calpain hypothesis of Lynch and Baudry (1984) suggests one way of achieving synaptic specificity and is biochemically more plausible than the autocatalytic model (although its authors would no longer maintain it in the form originally presented). However, it still assumes that synaptic biochemistry can be stably modified more or less autonomously from the rest of the neuron and, as will be seen below, the evidence points strongly to the occurence of learning-induced gene expression as a necessary step in long-term memory formation.

One way of looking at the synaptic modulations involved in memory formation is as a special case of the neuronal and synaptic plasticity that occurs during development, when, as is well known, there is an initial efflorescence and overproduction of synaptic connections, followed by a period of pruning and what Changeux and Danchin (1976) and Edelman (1984, 1989) have described as synaptic specification and stabilization and Singer (1987) as experience- or activity-dependent plasticity. Viewing memory processes in this light allows analogies to be drawn from the cellular events occurring in development, analogies which certainly can be compatible with Hebbian mechanisms, as Singer (1990) has shown.

If we accept for the moment that learning involves some variant of a Hebbian mechanism and try to define this mechanism in cellular and molecular terms, the initial processes must be, as specified earlier, the contiguous release of neurotransmitter from two synapses from different neurons, one strong and one weak, onto a postsynaptic cell. The contiguity results in the weak synapse being strengthened. To achieve this requires that a signal pass from the post-synaptic cell *back to* the weak presynaptic cell, thereby triggering some process, at the presynaptic and/or postsynaptic side, which strengthens subsequent signals or their reception. This hypothetical signal has been termed a *retrograde messenger*, and as will become clear below, some considerable effort is now being devoted to identifying such a messenger from a range of more or less plausible candidates.

Thus the initial events in learning are synaptic. For transient synaptic changes to be stabilized, however, the signals need to go beyond the synapse to the neuronal nucleus, where they result in the synthesis of new proteins destined to be transported back to the synapse so as permanently to modify its structure. If experiment is to match theory, we therefore need to track a biochemical cascade of processes that travel from postsynaptic to presynaptic side of the cleft, from synapse to nucleus and back to synapse again, within the time scale imposed by the behavioral evidence concerning the consolidation of long-term memory.

2 GOD'S ORGANISMS

Hebb formulated his hypothesis in 1949. Yet it took another quarter century before it could begin to yield experimental results. The delay was partly about technique, the need for methods of sufficient biochemical and morphological sophistication to reliably detect small changes in synaptic molecules or structures. But partly it was about the need to develop appropriate experimental learning systems in which to search for synaptic change. For a variety of reasons (see Dudai, 1989; Rose, 1992 for a more detailed discussion), the learning models beloved of classical psychology—adult rats and pigeons in Skinner boxes trained to press levers or peck at illuminated panels for reward, or to run mazes to avoid punishment—proved inappropriate. Learning such tasks was superimposed on a lifetime of other learning experience, and hunting for small synaptic changes in unknown regions of the brain proved somewhat harder than looking for needles in haystacks. What was needed was novel learning systems in which large changes might be presumed to be occurring in small brain regions, ideally in which the circuitry was already known. The hunt for such novel systems (on the basis of the old biologists' dictum that for every research problem, God has created precisely the appropriate organism in which to study it) led Bliss, Lømo and their successors to LTP, Singer to experience-dependent plasticity in the visual system, Thompson to the rabbit nictitating membrane, Kandel and Alkon to their favored molluscs, and Horn, Bateson, and myself to the day-old chick.

As a model for the study of learning the chick has a number of advantages; it is a precocial animal and therefore has an urgent neccessity within hours of hatching to learn a number of survival skills, including recognizing and following its mother (imprinting; Horn, 1985, 1991) and distinguishing edible food. It has a large and accessible brain and a minimal blood-brain barrier. Its unossified skull means that drugs, isotopes, and other agents can be injected directly and precisely to specific brain locations without cannulation, anesthesia, or other major disruptive intervention. Chicks can be readily hatched in the laboratory, and large numbers of experimental subjects are therefore potentially available (Andrew, 1991). There are concomitant disadvantages: working with a young animal means that learning-associated changes are superimposed on rapid developmental events; and by comparison with laboratory mammals, avian neural circuitry is not well mapped. My laboratory's task of choice has been one-trial passive avoidance learning, originally introduced by Cherkin (1969). This task takes advantage of the fact that day-old chicks rapidly peck at small bright objects in their field of view; if the object, such as a small chrome or colored bead, is dipped in a bitter-tasting liquid (generally methylanthranilate, MeA) the chick will peck once, show a strong disgust response, and avoid similar but dry beads subsequently. Upwards of 80% of chicks learn the task in a single trial and recall it for at least 48 hr. By contrast with most learning tasks, which require extended training over many trials or sessions, the one-trial learning event is thus very sharply timed, making it possible to distinguish between neurobiological processes associated with the context of learning itself, such as visual or motor activity, and those involved in the consolidation of memory. To study the effects of learning this task, biochemical, morphological, or physiological measures can be compared in chicks trained on the MeA-coated bead with those which have instead been offered a water-coated bead (W) to peck at training, and which consequently peck rather than avoid a dry bead on test. Other controls can include untrained birds, or birds which have pecked the MeA bead but have been rendered amnesic by mild electroshock or pharmacological intervention. In passive avoidance, amnesia is reflected in the MeA-trained birds *pecking* at the dry bead on test; the fact that they have to perform a specific act which demands motivation, visual and motor coordination is important because it implies that any pharmacological treatment resulting in apparent amnesia is not exerting its effect simply by nonspecific behavioral mechanisms. By timing drug injections in relation to training, the sequence of synaptic events associated with memory formation can be identified, and by varying the time between training and interventive procedure and test, one can infer which stage of the memory consolidation any intervention affects (Gibbs and Ng, 1977).

None of the controls individually prove unambiguously that a particular neurobiological event is an aspect of the memory formation process; taken together they enable one to establish a plausible sequence (see Rose, 1981 for a discussion of the question of controls in memory research). Because this chapter is primarily concerned with synaptic mechanisms rather than the behavioral issues, this question will not be further pursued here, and the following sections will review the evidence for the several stages involved in the synaptic modification, selection, and stabilization involved in memory formation. Although the results are derived from the study of the chick passive-avoidance model, it will be clear that there are strong analogies with the early events of LTP, widely regarded as a physiological analog—if not directly a mechanism—of memory, and clearly our own research strategy has in part been to draw on the LTP literature so as to test out its biochemical claims in the context of real vertebrate learning.

3   THE LOCI OF PLASTICITY

When we began our work on the chick passive-avoidance response, so ignorant were we of chick functional neuroanatomy that we did not know which areas of the brain might be involved in registering the effects of training. However, it seemed a reasonable assumption that both the experience of training and the memory consolidation process would involve enhanced neuronal activity. The accumulation of radioactively labeled 2-deoxyglucose (2-DG) is generally taken as a surrogate marker for neuronal—primarily synaptic—activity, and at an early stage in our research program we therefore compared 2-DG accumulation in autoradiographs derived from forebrains of MeA- and W-trained chicks. Two forebrain regions in particular, the intermediate medial hyperstriatum ventrale (IMHV, approximately homologous to mammalian striate cortex) and lobus parolfactorius (LPO, a basal ganglion region), showed increased 2-DG accumulation in MeA-trained chicks, and especially in the left IMHV (Rose and Csillag, 1985). That the IMHV should be a site of neural activity following training did not come as a great surprise to us, as it was already known to be a site implicated in imprinting (Horn, 1985); however, the LPO was unknown territory. That there should be lateralization of the sites of learning-related plasticity was also compatible with much other evidence concerning brain lateralization in avian species (Andrew, 1991; Rogers,1986). It seemed reasonable to assume that IMHV and LPO were good candidate sites at which to find evidence of neural and synaptic plasticity as a consequence of training on the passive-avoidance task.

3.1 Synaptic Transients: NMDA Receptors

Learning to suppress pecking at the bitter bead results in a flurry of synaptic activity. The IMHV is a region particularly richly populated with both NMDA-glutamate and muscarinic cholinergic receptors. Although some of the earliest experiments we made with the passive-avoidance protocol showed a transient enhancement of mAChR binding activity in the IMHV, peaking at about 30 min after training, recent interest has focused on the NMDA receptor. The initiation, though not maintenance, of LTP is known to depend on this class of glutamate receptor (Morris et al., 1986; Watkins and Collingridge, 1989), which has also been implicated in the mechanism of activity-dependent self-organization of synaptic connectivity in the kitten visual cortex (Constantine-Paton, 1990; Rauschecker, 1991). It therefore seemed logical to explore its role in the chick. NMDA receptor binding activity increases by 39% in the left IMHV of MeA-trained birds compared to W-trained controls 30 min after the training event (Stewart et al., 1992) but declines to control levels within 3 hr, suggesting that training results in a transient upregulation of receptor activity (either by increasing B_{max} or affecting Kd, but more likely the former). That the activity of the NMDA receptor is necessary for memory formation to occur is shown by the fact that if the noncompetitive NMDA antagonist MK801 is injected into the birds just before or just after training, there is amnesia for the task when the chicks are tested 3 or 24 hr subsequently (Burchuladze and Rose, 1992). Inhibitors of non-NMDA glutamate receptors, such as CNQX or NBQX, are without amnestic effect. It has of course been established for some time that antagonists of NMDA such as AP-5 will prevent retention of memory in hippocampal tasks in mammals, such as in rats learning a water maze (Morris et al., 1986).

The time of injection of the MK801 is important; if it is administered 1 or more hours after training there is no subsequent amnesia, implying that, as in the case of LTP, NMDA receptors are required for the initial phases of memory formation but not for later steps in the sequence, nor for recall of established memories. Furthermore, if chicks are injected with MK801 around the time of training, amnesia develops slowly; the birds show recall at 30 min, but are amnesic by 3 h. This means that NMDA receptors are not required for the short-term phases of memory formation; rather, they are part of the enabling procedures required for the development of long-term memory. The increase in NMDA receptor binding found at 30 min cannot then itself be responsible for "holding" the memory trace at that point in the sequence—further evidence that the synaptic mechanisms of short-term memory are distinct from those of long-term memory. Just which receptor processes are involved in the short-term phases is not clear from our data at present. Within the Hebbian paradigm, one must assume that the increased NMDA binding is a post-synaptic response to the contiguous arrival at neurons of the IMHV of inputs deriving from the visual processing of the image of the bead, motor feedback from the pecking activity, and registration of the aversive taste of the bead—

all plausible inputs considering what is known of the connectivity of the region (Bradley et al., 1985). Upregulating the NMDA receptor at any given synapse is a way of at least temporarily strengthening its input into the postsynaptic neuron.

3.2   Synaptic Transients: Retrograde Signals

As argued above, Hebbian mechanisms imply that at such a temporarily strengthened synapse, there is a retrograde signal to the presynaptic cell. A number of candidate molecules have been proposed for such a role; these include the recently identified diffusible signal molecule nitric oxide (Bredt and Snyder, 1992; Garthwaite, 1991). Nitric oxide is synthesized during arginine metabolism, and its synthesis is inhibited by the antimetabolite nitroarginine. Nitroarginine injected an hour before training results in profound and lasting amnesia for the bead in chicks tested as soon as 30 min after training, and, as would be predicted from the biochemistry, if arginine is injected together with the nitroarginine, amnesia is prevented (Holscher and Rose, 1992). Nitric oxide *could* therefore fit the bill as a retrograde signal in passive avoidance training, thereby "alerting" the presynaptic neuron to the need to increase its effectiveness vis-à-vis the postsynaptic neuron at a particular synapse or set of synapses. We have as yet no evidence in the chick of the possible involvement of other such candidate retrograde messengers as arachidonic acid (O'Dell et al., 1991).

3.3   Presynaptic Phosphorylation

What form might such an increase in effectiveness take? Plausible candidate mechanisms by which changes in synaptic efficacy might occur are known to include the reversible phosphorylation of membrane proteins, resulting in opening Ca^{2+} channels and triggering intracellular second messenger systems. A number of enzymes will phosphorylate membrane proteins, especially protein kinases A and C (PKC). Synaptic membrane and postsynaptic density fractions derived from chick forebrain contain several proteins that can be phosphorylated in vitro from ATP; one of particular interest is a specific *presynaptic* 52kD PKC substrate known variously as B50, GAP-43, and sometimes F1, depending on the laboratory concerned (Benowitz and Routtenberg, 1987; Bullock et al., 1990; Gispen and Routtenberg, 1986). In synaptic plasma membranes isolated from MeA-trained chicks 30 min after training, there was a specific decrease in the phosphorylation of B50 (a decrease in an in vitro phosphorylating system is generally assumed to imply a prior *increase* in phosphorylation in vivo) (Ali et al., 1988). This effect is believed to be mediated by a translocation of cytosolic PKC to the synaptic membrane, where it becomes bound to and phosphorylates proteins such as B50 (Akers et al., 1986; Linden and Routtenberg, 1989), and there is some evidence for such a translocation of PKC occurring in the left IMHV within 30 min of training (Burchuladze et al., 1990). Stronger evidence for the involvement of PKC-mediated processes comes from the evidence that inhibitors of PKC, such as melittin or H-7, injected at concentrations which prevent B50 phophorylation in vitro, will produce amnesia for the passive-avoidance response if injected at or just after the time of training. The specificity of this effect is striking; amnesia only occurs if the inhibitor is injected into the left but not the right IMHV (Burchuladze et al., 1990). As in the case of the NMDA inhibitors, amnesia is not apparent at 30 min, but has developed by 3 h, again indicating that the PKC-dependent processes are required for the development of long-term memory, rather than forming an aspect of the short-term store.

In the case of LTP, most attention has been paid to the postsynaptic effects of PKC inhibitors. Thus Malinow, Schulman, and Tsien (1989) have injected specific blocking agents such as PKC pseudosubstrates into the postsynaptic cell and shown that this blocks the induction, but not the expression of LTP, though their methods do not enable them to be sure that PKC-mediated phosphorylations are indeed inhibited by such injections. These results have been interpreted as showing that it is postsynaptic phosphorylation which is necessary for LTP to occur. This is not necessarily incompatible with our data. PKC has both presynaptic and postsynaptic substrates (for example, post-synaptically the 17kDa neurogranin). Malinow et al. have not shown that presynaptic PKC inhibition does not also prevent LTP, nor have we ruled out the possibility that there are other, postsynaptic proteins whose phosphorylation changes following training the chicks. The important feature of B50 in this context is that it is a specifically presynaptic reporter molecule for PKC-mediated phosphorylation, so at least some of the significant early synaptic events in memory formation must be presynaptic.

The molecular cascade of events initiated by PKC-mediated phosphorylations is substantive (Gispen and Routtenberg, 1986, 1991). Among them are the opening of synaptic membrane Ca^{2+} channels, and it is of interest that we have preliminary evidence both that there is an enhanced in vitro uptake of Ca^{2+} into tissue prisms derived from the IMHV of MeA-trained chicks, and that Ca^{2+} channel blockers such as nifedipine will also produce amnesia if injected prior to training. Altered calcium fluxes are certainly one way of providing the necessary intracellular signal by which synaptic events can potentially trigger nuclear activation, but there will certainly turn out to be complex pathways involved.

3.4 Synapse to Nucleus: Protein Oncogenes

The training-initiated events described so far are essentially transient, occurring within the minutes to an hour following training, and returning to base-line beyond this time. Some may be the neural correlates of short-term phases of memory which, in the chick, have been extensively pharmacologically dissected by Gibbs and Ng (1977), and by Rosenzweig, Bennett and their collaborators (1991). However, in most learning situations studied, training also results in the activation of the cell's general protein synthetic machinery. A general molecular biological mechanism in the switching on of protein synthesis involves the expression of a family of immediate early genes (IEGs) and transcription factors. Among the IEGs two in particular, originally identified as the protein oncogenes *c-fos* and *c-jun*, have been extensively studied in the context of neural plasticity (Chiarugi et al., 1989; Dragunow, et al., 1989; Kaczmarek, 1992). The genes are practically silent and unexpressed under quiescent conditions, but are activated by a wide variety of sensory stimuli, both noxious and nonaversive. NMDA upregulation, for instance, triggers IEG expression (Cole, et al., 1989). Like 2-DG, therefore, their expression serves as a marker of neural function, but whereas 2-DG signals an increase in neural activity, expression of the IEGs can be regarded as a mark of enhanced neural plasticity. IEG expression can be detected with appropriate probes either by Northern blotting, to identify the RNA, or by in situ hybridization, which enables the sites of enhanced expression to be identified; the gene product can also be mapped by immunocytochemistry. To sustantially simplify the IEG story, the genes are switched on by signals arriving at the neuronal nucleus, and their activation results in the expression, within about an hour, of their protein products *c-fos* and *c-jun*. These in turn act as signals for the expression of more conventional late genes, whose products may eventually serve to modify synaptic structure and function. Thus the IEGs are an essential link between synapse and nucleus, and their activation is a key step in the molecular cascade of memory formation.

Demonstrating that IEGs are expressed as a result of a training experience has not proved difficult; the problem is that because increased expression can result from so many aspects of the experience, it has been difficult to demonstrate unequivocally that an increase is associated with learning. As with many other treatments, from metrazole convulsions to light exposure, MeA training in the chick results in enhanced *c-fos* expression in IMHV, LPO, and other forebrain regions (Anokhin et al., 1991). To prove a learning-related effect, however, it was necessary to find a behavioral protocol in which the effects of learning could be distinguished from other aspects of the training experience. For this we have used an appetitive rather than an aversive pecking task, in which chicks learn, over a few trials, to distinguish food crumbs from similar looking but inedible pebbles glued to the floor of the training pen. There were three experimental groups of birds as well as a quiet control group, and the experiment took place over two days. All three groups had experience of the pebble floor on day 1, the first two groups without food, and the third with food. Thus only the third group learned the food discrimination on day 1. On day 2, all groups experienced the pebble floor again. Once again the first group was without food, and the third with food. This time, however, the second group also had food. Thus the first and third groups were repeating a previous experience, while the second group was learning something new. Behavioral activity was highest in the experienced chicks of the third group, but much the highest IEG expression occurred in the second, leaming group (Anokhin and Rose, 1991). The conclusion is that it is learning a piece of behavior, rather than merely repeating behavior already learned, which increases early gene expression. This increase is most marked in the IMHV.

3.5 Nucleus to Synapse: The Role of Glycoproteins

An increase in *c-fos* and *c-jun* expression in the IMHV is observable by 30 min after training on the passive-avoidance task; thus by this time some signal—perhaps Ca^{2+}-mediated—must have been transmitted from the activated synapse to the neuronal nucleus of either or both presynpatic and post-synaptic cells. But the activation of the IEGs is no more than an intermediate stage in the switching on of the late, structural genes that are responsible for the enhanced protein synthesis that occurs following training experiences such as passive avoidance. While the mechanism and role of the IEG expression are of intense interest to molecular biologists, neurobiologists are more likely to be concerned with the functional significance of the protein products of the late genes. Many early experiments in the field of memory studies, from as far back as the late 1960s, have reported prolonged increases in the incorporation of radioactively labeled amino acid precursors into protein following training (see, e.g., Matthies, 1986, 1989). Separating the labeled proteins from such experiments on gels reveals multiple bands showing enhanced labeling, but it has proved rather difficult to identify the specific proteins concerned. One protein in the chick IMHV that does show increases in incorporation of precursor and in absolute quantity as assayed immunochemically for up to 24 hr following training is the cytosolic microtubular protein tubulin (Mileusnic et al., 1980; Scholey et al., 1992). As microtubules are structural elements associated with both dendritic and anterograde and retrograde axonal transport, this may be of special relevance to the mechanism of longer-term synaptic remodeling. If those synapses that are to be remodeled as a result of training and memory formation are biochemically marked in some way—for instance, by transient changes in their phosphorylation state—the increased tubulin synthesis could be associated with the directed transport of relevant membrane constituents to these particular synapses so as to reconstruct them along the lines discussed below.

Such longer-term remodeling, however, must of necessity involve changes to the structure or geometry of synaptic and dendritic membranes. Key constituents of these membranes are glycoproteins, membrane-spanning molecules whose carbohydrate moiety extends into the synaptic cleft. Many receptors and ion channels are glycoproteins. Membrane glycoproteins, and especially the group of neural cell adhesion molecules (NCAMs) are key elements in cell-cell recognition and adhesion mechanisms. For many years there have been suggestions that they might play a key role in neural plasticity, most recently formulated as a general theory by Edelman (1989). A good precursor marker for cerebral glycoprotein synthesis is fucose, and increased fucose incorporation into synaptic membrane glycoproteins in the hours following training has been reported both in brightness discrimination tasks in rats (Matthies, 1986) and in passive avoidance in chicks (see Rose, 1989). A striking feature of the Matthies group's results was that there appeared to be two waves of glycoprotein synthesis, one around the time of training and one several hours subsequently (Pohle et al., 1979).

More recently we have identifed a number of presynaptic and postsynaptic membrane glycoproteins—memory-associated glycoproteins (MAGs)—in IMHV and LPO which show enhanced incorporation between 1 and 24 hr after training. At 24 hr in the LPO these include a presynaptic 50kDa and postsynaptic 33, 100–120, and 150–180kDa species (Bullock et al., 1992). It is of relevance that there are both 120 and 180kDa forms of NCAM; another interesting glycoprotein is the low-molecular-weight ependymin, which has been proposed as having a role in memory consolidation processes (e.g., Piront alld Schmidt,1988). In the chick the increased glycoprotein synthesis involves both *de novo* protein synthesis and subsequent glycosylation of the proteins by way of the fucokinase-fucosyl transferase enzyme pathway, and in parallel with the increased glycoprolein synthesis the activity of the rate-limiting fucokinase enzyme increases (Lossner and Rose, 1983). The fucose analog 2-deoxygalactose (2-dgal) competes with galactose for incorporation into nascent glycoprotein chains and, once incorporated, inhibits terminal fucosylation of the chains. Injected around the time of training into chicks (or rats trained on a brightness discrimination task), it produces amnesia in animals tested 24 hr subsequently, suggesting that fucoglycoprotein synthesis is necessary for long-term memory (Rose and Jork, 1987). Labeled 2-dgal is itself, as would be expected, incorporated into the MAG fractions.

It is our assumption that the presynaptic and postsynaptic MAGs are involved in some way in altering synaptic connectivity. Hence the similarity of their molecular weights with those of the NCAMs is striking. Regan and coworkers (Doyle et al., 1992; Doyle and Regan, 1993) have recently tested the effect of antibodies to NCAM on memory in rats trained on a one-trial step down passive-avoidance task. The antibody was without effect on recall in animals injected around the time of training, but if injected 6 hr after training resulted in amnesia in animals tested 48 hr later. Doyle and Regan interpret this effect as implying that the synaptic plasticity of memory formation involves what they term a "neurodevelopmental replay" in which there is transient overproduction of synapses followed by selection and stabilization in which an embryonic (highly sialylated) form of NCAM is converted into the mature, 180kDa, low sialylated form, a process with which the NCAM antibodies presumably interferes.

We were struck by the correspondence of the time window at which Doyle and Regan found anti-NCAM to be amnestic with that of the second wave of glycoprotein synthesis observed by Matthies and his colleagues. We therefore tested the amnestic effect of 2-dgal injected at various times after training in the chick, and observed that it too showed two time windows of amnesia. 2-dgal injected either within the first 1–2 hr after training, or 5–8 hr after training (but not at intermediate or later times) results in amnesia in chicks tested at 24 hr. In accord with the claims of Doyle and Regan, anti-NCAM injected at the second time window, but not the first, is also amnestic for passive avoidance in the chicks (Scholey et al., 1993). Antibodies to NCAM immunoprecipitate a macromolecular fraction that incorporates labeled 2-dgal, so it is reasonable to assume that one of the MAGs is indeed NCAM.

The existence of this second time window of biochemical plasticity, however, does not match any hitherto known phase of memory formation. A clue as to its implications however, is provided by the observations that (1) chicks trained to peck at even a dry bead retain a memory of it for a few hours and this memory is itself dependent on glycoprotein synthesis (Barber et al., 1989) and (2) if the chicks are trained on a weakly aversive stimulus, such as quinine, rather than the strongly aversive MeA, their avoidance response on test declines over a period of 6–9 hr, and under these circumstances there is no enhancement of glycoprotein synthesis over that in the W-trained chicks (Bourne et al., 1991). My interpretation of these data is that weak and rapidly decaying memories evoke only the first wave of glycoprotein synthesis; to produce a longer-lasting memory requires the second wave, and as will become clearer from the argument of the next sections, under these conditions Hebbian mechanisms in their simple form no longer apply.

4 BIOCHEMISTRY BECOMES STRUCTURE

Such issues can be delayed until the implications of enhanced synaptic membrane glycoprotein synthesis for synaptic structure are considered. If memory formation affects synaptic connectivity it might be expected that changes in synaptic number or morphology could be detected by light or electron microscopy. Such changes have indeed been found in *Aplysia* (Bailey and Chen, 1991) and in the rat (Greenough et al., 1990). In the chick, passive-avoidance training results in dramatic presynaptic and postsynaptic structural changes, observable at both light and electron microscope level. Twenty-four hours after training, there is a 60% increase in the spine density on dendrites of multipolar projection neurons of the left IMHV (Patel and Stewart, 1988). Synapses can be on the cell body, on the dendritic shafts, or on the dendritic spines. Theoretical calculations show that spine synapses are likely to be more powerful than shaft synapses in their effect on the postsynaptic cell, so whether the increase is as a result of the formation of entirely new synapses or the reorganization of dendrites so as to convert existing shaft synapses to spine ones, a change in connectivity at the structural level clearly occurs as a result of the training experience—indeed, as a consequence of memory formation (Patel et al., 1989). Presumably the enhanced synaptic membrane glycoprotein synthesis that occurs over the same time period is the biochemical correlate of this reconstuction.

Related but more complex presynaptic changes can be observed in both left IMHV and LPO by morphometric electron microscopy (reviewed by Stewart, 1991). By 24 hr after training there are striking increases in the numbers of synaptic vesicles per synapse in the left IMHV, and in the overall synaptic density (numbers of synapses per unit volume of tissue) in both left and right LPO. How such changes in connectivity can result in a changed expression of behavior that is the consequence of memory formation for this training task is not known. Nor do we know for how long these changes persist. The earliest time at which Stewart and colleagues have detected structural changes is 1 hr post training, but these (changes in synapse number in the right IMHV) are transient. It is pertinent that Scheich and collaborators (e.g., Wallhauser and Scheich, 1987) have found a *decrease* in dendritic spine density (in a region of the chick brain close to but distinct from IMHV) in the several days following exposure of chicks to an acoustic imprinting stimulus. One interpretation of the two sets of data, from Stewart and from Scheich, is that memory formation results in an initial efflorescence of dendritic spines and new synapses, but that in the days that follow there is a period of pruning of redundant connections in the manner proposed by Changeux and Danchin (1976), leaving only those which are necessary to retain the essential features of the memory. The dynamic state of synapses even in the adult and in the absence of specific training stimuli has been beautifully demonstrated by Purves (1988).

5 STRUCTURE BECOMES FUNCTION

Does a change in synaptic structure imply a change in functional connectivity? The appropriate measure of such a change would of course be electrophysiological, as in the context of LTP. But unlike the hippocampus, the wiring diagrams of the chick IMHV and LPO are unknown, although Bradley, Burns, and Webb (1991) have shown that trains of pulses injected into IMHV slices *in vitro* can result in LTP-like responses in the slice. However, extracellular recording from the IMHV or LPO of the anesthetized chick in the hours following training does show a remarkable, severalfold increase in the incidence of bursts of high frequency neuronal firing (Gigg et al., 1993; Mason and Rose, 1987). The physiological meaning of such bursts is unclear, but that it has to do with memory formation, rather than merely the experience of the bitter taste of the MeA bead is clear, for it is abolished by treatments that render the chicks amnesic (Mason and Rose, 1988).

The simple interpretation of the results presented so far would be that memory formation does indeed involve synaptic plasticity, and that an ensemble of synapses in the left IMHV, and another in the left and right LPO, respond to a significant learning experience by a cascade of molecular events that, beginning with synaptic transients, culminates in the *de novo* synthesis of macromolecules which, inserted into presynaptic and postsynaptic membranes, alter the number and strength of the synapses, affecting their signaling properties so as to form neural "representations" of the experience. It is on the basis of these representations that the bird's behavior is changed, and an initial "peck" response to a bead stimulus is transformed into a "no peck" one.

That the story is more complex, however, became apparent when, in the late 1950s, we began a series of lesion studies to confirm that the left IMHV was indeed necessary for memory of the avoidance response. The results of these experiments (reviewed in Rose, 1991) were initially paradoxical, for they showed that whereas pretraining lesions of the left IMHV resulted in chicks that could learn, but not remember, the passive-avoidance response, lesions made an hour or more post training were no longer amnestic. Conversely, pretraining lesions of the LPO were not amnestic, whereas bilateral post-training lesions were. On the basis of a series of double dissociation experiments we were able to interpret these results as suggesting that while an initial memory for the avoidance was made and stored in the left IMHV, there was subsequently a "flow" of memory from left to right IMHV and thence (probably via the archistriatum) to left and right LPO. Nor are these the only structures involved; the hippocampus, too, residual structure though it is in chicks by comparison with mammals, has a part to play (Sandi et al., 1992). This flow takes place in the hours following training on the passive-avoidance task, and it can be tracked rather elegantly by analyzing the time course of the bursting activity of the neurons, which, initially observed in both left and right IMHV, peaks specifically in the right about 6–7 hr after the time of training, and in both left and right LPO at 4–7 hr after trainig (Gigg et al., 1992). Perhaps coincidentally, the 6–7 hr time point is also that of the second wave of posttraining glycoprotein synthesis, and it is tempting to assume that it is functionally related to the "stamping in" of a memory trace in the LPO.

6 SYNAPSES AND SYSTEMS

This is not quite the end of the story, however. For if posttraining lesions of the left IMHV are not amnestic, and therefore the chick does not require this structure to recall the avoidance of a bitter bead, why should there nonetheless be lasting synaptic changes in that region as a result of training? Simple Hebbian models of memory formation cannot accommodate this paradox, and an explanation requires a broader neurobiological and behavioral understanding. When the chick pecks and learns to avoid the bead, it cannot know which aspect of the experience is the significant one; the bead is of a particular size, color, and shape and presented in a particular manner, and until the bird is able to refine its experience and test its own hypotheses about which aspect of the bead makes it unpleasant, it must clearly classify and store all possible relevant information about the bead in its context. Valloltigara, Zanforlin, and Compostella (1990) have indeed shown that chicks use a hierarchy of discriminators of color, size, and shape in learning particular tasks.

This suggested a simple resolution to the paradox of synaptic plasticity in the IMHV. Suppose that, after the initial registration of the bitter bead in the left IMHV, it is classified on the basis of these varied discriminators and the information concerning this classification is then distributed through the brain (for an analogy with human memory, think of trying to recall the name of an acquaintance; one may try to link it to the visual image of a face, or run through the alphabet until one hits a likely surname, or recall the context in which the person was last seen. Each strategy implies a different brain process). In the chick, the IMHV may retain the color information, the LPO that for shape and size, and so forth. If this were the case, a chick whose IMHV had been lesioned post training on a chrome bead would avoid it later because aspects of the representation would have moved ito the LPO, and the bead would be recognized on the basis of these other characteristics. If the chick is trained on a bitter yellow bead and then offered a choice between a blue and a yellow, it will avoid yellow and peck blue. If the left IMHV remembers the bead in terms of color, however, posttraining IMHV lesions will prevent this yellow-blue discrimination, and the chick will now avoid both beads, as the memory in the LPO will simply be that beads of a parlicular shape and size, irrespective of color, taste bitter. When we made such an experiment, this was indeed what we found; chicks trained to avoid a yellow bead and then given left IMHV lesions subsequently avoid both yellow and blue (Patterson and Rose, 1992).

It follows that the neural representations necessary for even such simple memories as avoiding pecking at a bitter bead are not confined to a single set of synapses in a defined brain locale, but, as long-term memory is formed, become widely distributed across several brain regions. In each region, there will be synaptic plasticity to encode the information within an appropriate ensemble of neurons, but the mechanism of such encoding will no longer be Hebbian, and it ceases to be possible to ask where in the brain a particular memory resides; rather it has become a distributed property of the system. The pruning of connections that occurs during development and following training is part of the process of refining that distribution and dirninishing its redundancy.

Tulving has made this point most clearly in a recent interview:

There is nothing wrong *in principle* with the idea that the information that is necessary for remembering something is recorded in a particular site in the brain... [however]... the concept of the engram has mesmerized brain scientists into acting as if there was nothing more to the problem of memory and the brain than the engram and its characteristics, including its location in the overall structure.... The engram is an unfinished thought about memory, at best only one-half the story of memory.... A biological memory system differs from a mere physical information-storage device by virtue of the system's inherent capability of using the information in the service of its own survival.... The Library of the Congress, a piece of videotape or a Cray supercomputer ... could not care less about their own survival. So anyone who is interested in memory, but looks only at the storage side of things, is essentially ignoring the fundamental distinction between dead and living storage systems, that is, ignoring the essence of *biological* memory. (Tulving, 1991)

In this interview, Tulving goes on to argue that the cognitive psychology does better than neurobiology in its understanding of memory by its recognition that "memory storage" is not the problem; while synaptic studies may reveal the processes of *learning*, the "problem of memory" is that of the retrieval of memories.

What, though, of a synaptic memory trace? Tulving offers the most radical challenge yet to Hebbian models in his suggestion that although there may be what he calls physical—that is changes in the brain in association with learning, a permanent engram as such does not exist as a durable "physical" change, but only comes into existence when activated (he calls it "ecphorised") by the act of remembering. He concludes his interview with a parody of a once better known phrase: "Students of memory of the scientific world, unite in the study of the myriad aspects of the essence of biological memory, unite in the study of the interaction between the processes of storage and recall."

Tulving's argument hinges on just what is meant by "physical." For sure, the biochemical and physiological phenomena discussed in this chapter are transient in the sense that the increases in protein synthesis, neural bursting activity and so forth do not persist beyond a few hours after the learning experience. But those few hours have permanently altered the brain, if only by shifting the number and position of a few dendritic spines on a few neurons in particular brain regions. The spatial map of cells and their connections in the brain—certainly as much of a physical change, in Tulving's sense, as is the imposing of a magnetic trace on a cassette tape—has been lastingly altered. In the limited sense that the music on the tape only exists when the cassette is subsequently played, the engram only exists when it is "ecphorised"—and the memory is retrieved. The task for neurobiology remains that of understanding how even a distributed change in synaptic weightings in many brain areas translates, in experimental animals, into changes in observable behavior, and in humans into the richly interconnected memories that last a lifetime and in a sense constitute us as individuals.

ACKNOWLEDGMENTS

The work described in this chapter has involved many people over the years; special thanks to Mlke Stewart, my morphological co-worker, and to the many colleagues of the Brain and Behaviour Research Group. Major funding for this work has come from the UK MRC, SERC, Royal Society, Wellcome Trust, and the Open University.

REFERENCES

Akers, R. F. Lovinger, D. M., Colley, D., Linden, D., and Routtenberg, A. (1986) Translocation of protein kinase C activity after LTP may mediate hippocampal synaptic plasticity. *Science* 231:587–589.

Ali, S. M., Bullock, S., and Rose, S. P. R. (1988) Phosphorylation of synaptic proteins in chick forebrain; changes with development and passive avoidance training. *J. Neurochem.* 50:1579–1587.

Andrew, R. J. (ed.) (1991) *Behavioural and Neural Plasticity: The Use of the Domestic Chick as a Model.* Oxford Universily Press, Oxford.

Anokhin, K. V., and Rose, S. P. R. (l991) Learning-induced increase of immediate early gene messenger RNA in the chick forebrain. *Eur. J. Neurosci.* 3:162–167.

Anokhin, K. V., Mileusnic, R., Shamakina, I., and Rose, S. P. R. (1991) Effects of early experience on *c-fos* gene expression in the chick forebrain. *Brain Res.* 544:101–107.

Bailey, C. H., and Chen, M. (l990) Morphological alterations at identified sensory neuron synapses during long-term sensitisation in *Aplysia*. In *The Biology of Memory*, E. Lindenlaub and L. R. Squire (ed.) pp. 135–154. Schattauer Verlag, Stuttgart.

Barber, A. J., Gilbert, D. B., and Rose, S. P. R. (1989) Glycoprotein synthesis is necessary for memory of sickness-induced learning in chicks. *Eur. J. Neurosci.* 1:673–677.

Benowitz, L. I., and Routtenberg, A. (1987) A membrane phosphoprotein associated with neuronal development, axonal regeneration, phospholipid metabolism and synaptic plasticity. *Trends Neurosci.* 10:527–532.

Bourne, R. C., Davies, D. C., Stewart, M. G., Csillag, A., and Cooper, M. (1991) Cerebral glycoprotein synthesis and long-term memory formation in the chick (*Gallus domesticus*) following passive avoidance training depends on the nature of the aversive stimulus. *Eur. J. Neurosci.* 3:243–248.

Bradley, P., Davies, D. C., and Horn, G., (1985) Connections of the hyperstriatum ventrale of the domestic chick. *J. Anat.* 140:577–589.

Bradley, P. M., Burns, B. D., and Webb, A. C., (1991) Potentiation of synaptic responses in slices from the chick forebrain. *Proc. Roy. Soc. Lond.* B 243:19–24.

Bredt, D. S., and Snyder, S. H. (1992) Nitric oxide, a novel neuronal messenger. *Neuron* 8:3–11.

Bullock, S., De Graan, P. N. E., Oestreicher, A. B., Gispen, W.-H., and Rose, S. P. R. (1990) Identification of a 52kDa chick brain membrane protein showing changed phosphorylation after passive avoidance training as B-50 (GAP 43). *Neurosci. Res. Comm.* 6:181–186.

Bullock, S., Rose, S. P. R., and Zamani, R. (1992) Characterisation and regional localisation of pre- and postsynaptic glycoproteins of the chick forebrain showing changed fucose incorporation following passive avoidance training. *J. Neurochem.* 58:2145–2154.

Burchuladze, R., and Rose, S. P. R. (1992) Memory formation in day old chicks requires NMDA but not non-NMDA glutamate receptors. *Eur. J. Neurosci.* 4:533–538.

Burchuladze, R., Potter, J., and Rose, S. P. R. (1990) Memory formation in the chick depends on membrane-bound protein kinase C. *Brain Res.* 535:131–138.

Changeux, J.-P., and Danchin, A (1976) Selective stabilisation of developing synapses as a mechanism for the specification of neuronal networks. *Nature* 264:705–712.

Constantine-Paton, M. (1990) NMDA receptor as a mediator of activity-dependent synaptogenesis in the developing brain. *Cold Spring Harbor Symp. Quant. Biol.* 55:431–443.

Cherkin, A. (1969) Kinetics of memory consolidation. Role of amnestic treatment parameters. *Proc. Natl. Acad. Sci. USA* 63:1094–1101.

Chiarugi, V. P., Ruggiero, M., and Coradetti, R. (1989) Oncogenes, protein kinase C, neuronal differentiation and memory. *Neurochem. Int.* 14:1–9.

Cole, A. J., Saffen, D. W., Baraban, J. M., and Worley, P. F. (1989) Rapid increase of an immediate early gene messenger RNA in hippocampal neurons by synaptic NMDA receptor activation. *Nature* 340:474–476.

Crick, F. H. C., (1984) Memory and molecular turnover. *Nature* 312:101–104.

Davis, H. P., and Squire, L. R. (1984) Protein synthesis and memory: A review. *Psychol. Bull.* 96:518–559.

Doyle, E., and Regan, C. M. (1993) *J. Neurochem.*, in press.

Doyle, E., Nolan, P., Bell, R., and Regan, C. M. (1992) Neurodevelopmental events underlying information acquisition and storage. *Network* 3:89–94.

Dragunow, M., Currie, R. W., Faull, R. L. M., Robertson, H. A., and Jansen, K. (1989) Immediate-early genes, kindling and long-term potentiation. *Neurosci. Biobehav. Rev.* 13:301–313.

Dudai, Y. (1989) *The Neurobiology of Memory.* Oxford University Press, Oxford.

Edelman, G. M. (1984) Cell surface modulation and marker multplicity in neural patterning. *Trends Neurosci.* 7:78—84.

Edelman, G. M. (1989) *The Remembered Present*. Basic Books, New York.

Garthwaite, J. (1991) Glutamate, nitric oxide and cell-cell signalling in the nervous system. *Trends Neurosci.* 14:60—67.

Gibbs, M. E., and Ng, K. T. (1977) Psychobiology of memory: Towards a model of memory formation. *Biobehav. Rev.* 1:113—136.

Gigg, J., Patterson, T. A., and Rose, S. P. R. (1993) Memory-specific elevation in focal bursting in the lobus parolfactorius of the day-old chick. *Behav. Neurosci.*, in press.

Gispen, W.-H., and Routtenberg, A. (eds) (1986) *Phosphoproteins in Neuronal Function. Prog. Brain Res.*, 89, Elsevier, Amsterdam.

Gispen, W.-H. and Routtenberg, A. (eds) (1991) *Protein Kinase C and its Brain Substrates. Prog. Brain Res.*, 69, Elsevier, Amsterdam.

Goelet, P., Castelluci, V. F., Schacher, S., and Kandel, E. R. (1986) The long and short of long-term memory—a molecular framework. *Nature* 322:419—423.

Greenough, W. T., Withers, G. S., and Wallace, C. S. (1990) Morphological changes in the nervous system arising from experience: What is the evidence that they are involved in learning and memory? In *The Biology of Memory*, L. R. Squire and E. Lindenlaub (eds) pp. 159—186. Schattauer Verlag, Stuttgart.

Hebb, D. O. (1949) *The Organization of Behavior*. Wiley, New York.

Holscher, C., and Rose, S. P. R. (1992) An inhibitor of nitric oxide synthesis prevents memory formation in the chick. *Neurosci Lett.* 145:165—167.

Horn, G. (1985) *Memory, Imprinting and the Brain*. Oxford University Press, Oxford,

Horn, G. (1991) In *Neural and Behavioral Plasticity: The Use of the Domestic Chick as a Model*. R. J. Andrew (ed.), pp. 219—261. Oxford University Press, Oxford.

Kaczmarek, L. (1992) Expression of c-fos and other genes encoding transcription factors in long-term potentiation *Behav. Neural Biol.* 57:263—266.

Linden, D. J. and Routtenberg, A. (1989) The role of protein kinase C in long-term potentiation: A testable model. *Brain Res. Rev.* 14:279—296.

Lossner, B., and Rose, S. P. R. (1983) Passive avoidance training increases fucokinase activity in the right forebrain base of day-old chicks. *J. Neurochem.* 41:1357—1363.

Lynch, G. S., and Baudry, M. (1984) The biochemistry of memory: A new and specific hypothesis. *Science* 224:1057—1063.

Malinow, R., Schulman, H., and Tsien, R. W. (1989) Inhibition of postsynaptic PKC or CamKII blocks induction but not expression of LTP. *Science* 245:862—866.

Mason, R. J., and Rose, S. P. R. (1987) Lasting changes in spontaneous multi-unit activity in the chick brain following passive avoidance training. *Neuroscience* 21:931—944.

Mason, R. J. and Rose, S. P. R. (1988) Passive avoidance learning produces focal elevation of bursting activity in the chick brain: amnesia abolishes the increase. *Behav. Neural Biol.* 49:280—292.

Matthies, H. J. (ed.) (1986) *Learning and Memory: Mechanisms of Information Storage in the Nervous System*. Pergamon Press, Oxford.

Matthies, H. J. (1989) In search of cellular mechanisms of memory. *Prog. Neurobiol.* 32:277—349.

McGaugh, J. L. (1964) Time-dependent processes in memory storage. *Science* 153:1351—1358.

Mileusnic, R., Rose, S. P. R., and Tillson, P. (1980) Passive avoidance learning results in region-specific changes in concentration of and incorporation into colchicine-binding proteins in the chick forebrain *J. Neurochem.* 34:1007–1015.

Morris, R. G. M., Andersen, E., Lynch, G. S., and Baudry, M. (1986) Selective impairment of learning and blockade of long-term potentiation by an NMDA receptor antagonist. *Nature* 319:774–776.

O. Dell, T. J., Hawkins, R. D., Kandel, E. R., and Arancio, O. (1991) Tests of the roles of two diffusible substances in long-term potentiation: evidence for nitrix oxide as a possible early retrograde messenger. *Proc. Natl. Acad. Sci USA* 88:11285–11289.

Patel, S. N., and Stewart, M. G. (1988) Changes in the number and structure of dendritic spines, 25 hr after passive avoidance training in the domestic chick, *Gallus domesticus. Brain Res.* 449:34–46.

Patel, S. N., Rose, S. P. R., and Stewart, M. G. (1989) Training-induced spine density changes are specifically related to memory formation processes in the chick, *Gallus domesticus. Brain Res.* 463:168–173.

Patterson, T. A., and Rose, S. P. R. (1992) Memory in the chick: Multiple cues; distinct brain locations *Behav. Neurosci.* 106:465–470.

Piront, M.-L., and Schmidt, R. (1988) Inhibition of long-term memory formation by anti-ependymin antisera after active shock-avoidance learning in goldfish. *Brain Res.* 442:53–62.

Pohle, W. M., Ruthrich, H. L., Popov, N., and Matthies, H. J. (1979) Fucose incorporation into rat hippocampus structures after acquisition of a brightness discrimination. *Acta Biol. Med. Germ.* 38:53–63.

Purves, D. (1988) *Body and Brain: A Trophic Theory of Neural Connections.* Harvard University Press, Cambridge.

Rauschecker, J. (1991) Mechanism of visual plasticity: Hebb synapses, NMDA receptors, and beyond. *Physiol. Rev.* 71:587–615.

Rogers, L. J. (1986) Lateralisation of learning in chicks. *Adv. Study Behav.* 16:147–189.

Rose, S. P. R. (1981) What should a biochemistry of learning and memory be about? *Neuroscience* 6:811–821.

Rose, S. P. R. (1989) Glycoprotein synthesis and post-synaptic remodelling in long-term memory. *Neurochemistry Int.* 14:299–307.

Rose, S. P. R. (1991) How chicks make memories: The cellular cascade from c-fos to dendritic remodelling. *Trends Neurosci.* 14:390–397.

Rose, S. P. R. (1992) *The Making of Memory.* Bantam Press, London.

Rose, S. P. R., and Csillag, A. (1985) Passive avoidance training results in lasting changes in deoxyglucose metabolism in left hemisphere regions of chick brain. *Behav. Neural Biol.* 44:315–324.

Rose, S. P. R., and Jork, R. (1987) Long-term memory formation in chicks is blocked by 2-deoxygalactose, a fucose analogue. *Behav. Neural Biol.* 48:246–268.

Rosenzweig, M. R., Bennett, E. L., Martinez, J. L., Beniston, D., Colombo, P. J., Lee, D. W., Patterson, T. A., Schulteis, G., and Serano, P. A. (1991) Stages of memory formation in the chick: Findings and problems. In *Behavioural and Neural Plasticity: The Use of the Domestic Chick as a Model,* R. J. Andrew (ed.), pp. 394–418. Oxford University Press, Oxford.

Sandi, C., Rose, S. P. R., and Patterson, T. A. (1992) Unilateral hippocampal lesions prevent recall of a passive avoidance task in day-old chick. *Neurosci. Lett.* 141:255–258.

Scholey, A., Bullock, S., and Rose, S. P. R. (1992) Passive avoidance learning in the young chick results in time- and locus-specific elevations of α-tubulin immunoreactivity. *Neurochem. Int.* 21:343–350.

Scholey, A. B., Rose, S. P. R., Zamani, M. R., Beck, F., and Schachner, M. (1993) A role for the neural cell adhesion molecule in a late, consolidarity phase of glycoprotein synthesis six hours following passive avoidance training in the young chick. *Neuroscience*, in press.

Singer, W. (1987) Developmental plasticity—self-organization or learning? In *Imprinting and Cortical Plasticity*, J. P. Rauschecker and P. Marler (eds.) pp. 171–176. Wiley, New York.

Singer, W. (1990) Search for coherence: A basic principle of cortical self-organisation. *Conc. Neurosci.* 1:1–26.

Stewart, M. G. (1991) Changes in dendritic and synaptic structures in chick forebrain consequent on passive avoidance learning In *Behavioural and Neural Plasticity: The Use of the Domestic Chick as a Model*, R. J. Andrew (ed.), pp. 305–328. Oxford University Press, Oxford.

Stewart, M. G., Bourne, R. C., and Steel, R. J. (1992) Quantitative autoradiographic demonstration of changes in binding in NMDA-sensitive ^{3}H glutamate and ^{3}H-MK801, but not ^{3}H-AMPA receptors in chick forebrain 30 minutes after passive avoidance training. *Eur. J Neurosci.* 4:936–943.

Tanzi, E. (1909) *A Textbook of Mental Diseases*, translated by W. F. Robertson and T. C. Mackenzie, p. 174. Rebman, London.

Thompson, R. F. (1992) Memory. *Curr. Opin. Neurobiol.* 2:203–208.

Tulving, E. (1991) Interview. *J. Cog. Neurosci.* 3:89, 94.

Vallortigara, G., Zanforlin, M., and Compostella, S. (1990) Perceptual organisation in animal learning: Cues or objects? *Ethology* 85:89–102.

Wallhauser, E., and Scheich, H. (1987) Auditory imprinting leads to differential 2-deoxyglucose uptake and dendritic spine loss in the chick rostral forebrain. *Devel. Brain Res.* 31:29–44.

Watkins, J. C., and Collingridge, G. L. (eds.) (1989) *The NMDA Receptor.* IRL Press, Oxford.

11 Synaptic Plasticity and Memory Storage

Richard F. Thompson, Judith K. Thompson,
Jeansok J. Kim, David J. Krupa,
Alan F. Nordholm, and Chong Chen

Whenever a mammal engages in adaptive learning, a number of brain systems become involved. Thus, when an animal learns a discrete behavioral response to deal with a strongly aversive stimulus, the animal rapidly learns a conditioned fear response, which is amygdala-dependent, neurons in the hippocampus exhibit a rapidly acquired learning-induced increase in activity, and the cerebellum becomes critically involved. While it is true that different brain systems play critical roles in different aspects or forms of learning and memory, it is also true that all memory systems become engaged in virtually all learning situations and play roles in modifying and modulating adaptive behavior. Thus, multiple brain sites may learn different things about a learning situation and these "memories" can interact. Integrated, adaptive behavior is the product of an ensemble of engrams (Lavond et al., 1993). Wagner and associates have developed elegant theoretical analyses (SOP; AESOP) showing how various memory systems can interact to yield adaptive behavior (Wagner and Brandon, 1989; Wagner and Donegan, 1989).

In this chapter we will briefly review brain substrates of several prototypic forms of learning and memory: classical conditioning of fear and of discrete adaptive responses; instrumental learning of passive and active avoidance and of spatial- and context-dependent tasks; and visual short-term and long-term object memory. Our focus will be on localization of memory traces and putative mechanisms of memory storage, particularly long-term potentiation (LTP) and long-term depression (LTD). The key brain structures to be considered are the amygdala, the cerebellum, the hippocampus-cerebral cortex, and their associated circuitries. The amygdala is critical for conditioned fear and active and passive avoidance (and the reward aspect of visual object memory in primates); the cerebellum is critical for discrete response learning. The hippocampus–cerebral cortex is critical for long trace classical conditioning, spatial- and context-dependenttasks in rodents, and for visual short-term and long-term object memory in monkeys. But all these brain systems are involved to varying degrees in virtually all learning situations.

With the recent resurgence of interest in "cognitive" science, there has been a tendency on the part of some to view humans as somehow unique, rather than as the product of biological evolution, and to view aspects of learning and memory that are not "mediated by consciousness" (definable only in humans) as being somehow noncognitive and therefore not important. With the apparent exception of language, phenomena of learning and memory appear to have basic similarities in all mammals. Classical or Pavlovian conditioning, viewed in the context of evolution, reflects the basic causal nature of associative learning, learning about inevitable temporal sequences of events in the world. Associative learning requires that a neutral warning stimulus (conditioned stimulus; CS) must occur before the stimulus that has biological consequences (unconditioned stimulus; US) in order for learning to occur. Further, the degree of learning that develops depends on the time between the onsets of the two stimuli. More remarkable, the *form* of the functional relationship between the onset times of the two stimuli is essentially the same for all kinds of associative learning (Rescorla, 1988b).

In general terms, associative learning is a process by which an organism benefits from experience so that its future behavior is better adapted to its environment. In more specific terms, it is the way organisms, including humans, learn about causal relationships in the world. It results from exposure to relations among events in the environment. To quote Rescorla, "Such learning is a primary means by which the organism represents the structure of its world" (1988b, p. 152). Viewed in this way, Pavlovian conditioning (associative learning) is a basic aspect of complex, cognitive learning. For both modern Pavlovian and cognitive views of learning and memory, the individual learns a representation of the causal structure of the world and adjusts this representation through experience to bring it into tune with the real causal structure of the world, striving to reduce any discrepancies or errors between its internal representation and external reality (see Rescorla, 1988a, b; Thompson and Gluck, 1991). This general view encompasses virtually all aspects of learning and memory.

1 AVERSIVE LEARNING, THE AMYGDALA, AND LONG-TERM POTENTIATION

1.1 Conditioned Fear

Initially neutral stimuli such as tones, light, or experimental chambers, when paired with aversive electric shock, can rapidly become CSs that are capable of eliciting a number of fear conditioned responses (CRs). Several lines of evidence point to the amygdala as a critical neural substrate for this type of emotional learning (see Davis, 1992; Kapp et al., 1991; Lavond et al., 1993; LeDoux, 1991 for detailed reviews and references). Various modalities of sensory information project to the amygdala through its basal and lateral nuclei (Amaral, 1987). These nuclei are reciprocally connected with the central nucleus via intra-amygdaloid projections. The central nucleus appears to be the major amygdaloid output structure that projects to various autonomic and somatomotor pathways involved in fear expression.

Amygdala lesions, particular of the central nucleus, reduce or abolish various conditioned fear-related behaviors in a number of mammalian species. Acquisition and retention of learned fear responses such as increase in blood pressure (Iwata et al., 1986a), changes in heart rate (Kapp et al., 1979), fear-potentiated startle (Hitchcock and Davls, 1986), analgesia (Helmstetter, 1992), and defensive freezing (Iwata et al., 1986a) are all attenuated by the lesion. In addition to acquired fear responses, amygdala lesions also impair innate or unconditioned fear responses. Amygdala lesions reduce reactivity to the footshock US and block shock sensitization of startle (Hitchcock et al., 1989) . Since amygdalectomy impairs both the conditioned and unconditioned fear responses, this indicates that the amygdala receives both CS and US information.

In two-process theories of learning (Prokasy, 1972; Rescorla and Solomon, 1967), fear conditioning results in "diffuse" or "nonspecific" conditioned fear responses. (The second process involves learning of particular skeletal muscle responses such as eyeblink or limb flexion that are specifically adaptive to deal with the particular US.) It has been suggested that CS activates a "central fear motivational state" (e.g., Bolles and Fanselow, 1980). The fact that amygdala lesions affect CRs in a range of response systems lends strong support for this notion.

Selective lesions of structures afferent to the amygdala can affect conditioning to specific sensory stimuli. For instance, lesioning of the medial geniculate nucleus of the thalamus, which sends auditory information directly to the lateral amygdaloid nucleus, blocks the formation of tone-footshock, but not light-footshock, association as measured by conditioned freezing and blood pressure responses and the fear-potentiated startle response to an auditory stimulus (Campeau and Davis, 1991; LeDoux et al., 1990). Similarly, hippocampal lesions affect context-footshock association but not tone-footshock association (Kim and Fanselow, 1992; Phillips and LeDoux, 1992).

On the efferent side, lesions confined to hypothalamic and brainstem areas to which the central amygdaloid nucleus projects affect specific conditioned fear response (Hitchcock et al., 1989; Iwata et al., 1986b). In a representative set of studies, LeDoux and his colleagues showed that lesions of the lateral hypothalamus and ventral region of the periaqueductal gray matter abolished blood pressure and freezing CRs, respectively (LeDoux et al., 1988). However, the lateral hypothalamus lesion did not affect freezing, and the periaqueductal gray lesions did not alter blood pressure. Thus, the lateral hypothalamus and the ventral periaqueductal gray matter appear to be efferent mediators for specific fear responses. This double dissociation of CSs and CRs, as a result of lesions made in structures that are afferent and efferent to the amygdala, further indicates that the amygdala is a critical mediator of fear learning.

Consistent with lesion data, electrophysiological studies reveal that neurons in the central nucleus of the amygdala respond to both conditioned and unconditioned fear stimuli (Pascoe and Kapp, 1985a,b), and undergo plastic changes during fear conditioning (Applegate et al., 1982). Moreover, the unit activity in the amygdala correlates with the conditioned fear response. Also, electrical or chemical stimulation of specific regions in the amygdala (e.g., the central nucleus) elicits fear responses that tend to mimic CRs (Iwata et al., 1987; Rosen and Davis, 1990).

Recent studies suggest that the *N*-methyl-D-aspartate (NMDA) class of excitatory amino acid receptors play an important role in fear conditioning. Administration of DL-2-amino-5-phosphonovaleric acid (APV), a selective NMDA antagonist, into the amygdala completely blocks the acquisition of the fear-potentiated startle response to a light or tone stimulus (Campeau et al., 1992; Miserendino et al., 1990). A similar effect was observed when APV was microinfused into the basolateral nucleus (a region rich in NMDA receptors), but not the central nucleus (a region sparse in NMDA receptors), of the amygdala using contextual fear conditioning and freezing (Fanselow et al., 1991). The drug APV, however, does not impair the performance of previously acquired fear responses such as freezing and startle (Kim et al., 1991; Miserendino et al., 1990). Moreover, APV blocks fear conditioning only when administered prior to the time that the CS-US association occurs, but not immediately following the CS-US association (Kim et al., 1991). These findings suggest that NMDA receptors in the amygdala may be specifically involved in the fear learning process.

The dependence of fear learning on NMDA receptors in the basolateral amygdaloid nucleus raises the possibility that a process like LTP may be involved. Since APV affects fear conditioning and LTP in similar manners, that is, blocks acquisition/induction but not performance/expression, LTP has been proposed as a possible synaptic mechanism that mediates fear learning (Kim et al., 1991, 1992; Miserendino et al., 1990). Recently, Clugnet and LeDoux (1990) demonstrated an LTP-like phenomenon in the auditory CS pathway from the thalamus (the medial division of the medial geniculate nucleus) to the lateral amygdala. This auditory projection to the amygdala is also known to be glutaminergic (Farb et al., 1989). LTP has also been demonstrated in the basolateral amygdala region using a brain slice preparation (Chapman et al., 1990), although Chapman and Bellavance (1992) have recently questioned the extent to which such plasticity in the amygdala can be selectively blocked by APV.

1.2   Instrumental Aversive Learning: Passive and Active Avoidance

A wide range of drugs and other treatments can facilitate or impair memory performance in passive and active avoidance paradigms. In brief, in passive or inhibitory avoidance, the animal (typically rat or mouse) is placed in a lighted compartment, and when it enters a darkened compartment the animal is shocked. On the next trial the amount of time it avoids entering the darkened compartment is an index of memory. The opposite is the case for active avoidance, where the animal is shocked in a distinctive compartment or with occurrence of a discrete CS (e.g., tone) and must move to another compartment to avoid shock. We focus here on these aversive learning paradigms, but most treatments that facilitate or impair memory performance of such tasks have similar effects on reward learning (see Gold, 1992; McGaugh, 1989, 1992, for detailed reviews).

Among the most effective memory facilitating drugs when given systemically are hormones such as epinephrine (or adrenaline), opioid antagonists (e.g., naloxone and naltrexone), GABA antagonists (e.g., picrotoxin and bicuculline), and glucose. Memory-impairing agents include beta-adrenergic antagonists (e.g., propranolol), opioid agonists (e.g., morphine and β-endorphin), GABA agonists (e.g., muscimol), and electroconvulsive shock.

Epinephrine, which is the adrenal medullary hormone *par excellence* released in response to stress, is among the most effective substances for memory facilitation. In the real world we and other mammals tend to remember best those experiences that occur at times of arousal and moderate stress. Epinephrine and other memory facilitating drugs show the same inverted U effect on memory as a function of drug dose that holds in general between performance and arousal.

Because epinephrine does not readily cross the blood-brain barrier, it appears that epinephrine's effect on modulating memory performance may not be acting directly on the brain. Systemic injection of doses of epinephrine that yield maximal memory facilitation are much too low to enter the brain to any appreciable degree. So how could it act on memory storage? It appears that the memory-modulating effects of epinephrine involve, via stimulating peripheral adrenergic receptors on visceral afferents, the release of central norepinephrine (NE) within the amygdaloid complex (McGaugh, 1989). Consistent with this view, memory-enhancing effects of peripherally administered epinephrine can be blocked by intra-amygdala infusions of NE antagonists (Liang et al., 1986).

Unlike epinephrine, the opioid and GABAergic drugs readily pass the blood-brain barrier. The effects of these agents on memory appear to be based on direct central effects since methylated agents (e.g., naltrexone methyl bromide) that do not readily pass the blood-brain barrier have no effect on memory. Infusions of very small doses of these drugs directly into the amygdala also produce similar memory facilitation (and impairment) to systemically injected drugs (Gallagher and Kapp, 1978; Liang et al., 1986) . McGaugh (1992) hypothesizes that the key system is a central NE projection to the amygdala and that GABAergic and opioid influences regulate the efficacy of NE transmissions in the amygdala. In a recent study, Kim and McGaugh (1992) showed that infusion of APV into the amygdala impaired memory performance much as do, for instance, NE antagonists, thus raising the possibility that an LTP-like process in the amygdala may underlie memory enhancement. However, they suggested that this effect might be independent of NE facilitation effects in the amygdala.

The amygdala hypothesis can account for both the facilitating and impairing effects of hormones and drugs on memory storage. However, it does not tell us where the memories themselves, (e.g., for passive and active avoidance) are actually stored. Liang et al. (1982) showed that if animals were trained in passive avoidance and the amygdala was lesioned immediately thereafter, memory performance was abolished. However, if the lesion was made a week after the learning experience, memory was not impaired. In current work (Parent et al., 1992) it was shown that with sufficient over-training, amygdala lesions made at the end of training did not impair memory performance in passive avoidance. All these data support the notion that an initial memory trace is formed in the amygdala and is necessary for subsequent storage elsewhere. With sufficient overtraining or time following training, the amygdala trace is no longer necessary.

These results appear to differ from those in classical conditioning of fear. At least in the conditioned potentiation of startle paradigm, overtraining does not protect against amygdala abolition (Kim and Davis, 1992). This may reflect a difference between classical and instrumental learning. On the other hand, a very surprising result in conditioned potentiation of startle is the fact that once animals have been overtrained and amygdala lesions have abolished retention of the learned fear, the animals readily relearn the conditioned potentiation of startle task (Kim and Davis, 1992). Collectively, these results suggest that fear memory traces are initially formed in the amygdala and subsequently transferred to other loci, or reestablished in other loci, in the brain. If LTP is indeed the synaptic mechanism of memory storage in the amygdala, then it is a time-limited storage process that in many situations serves to facilitate more permanent storage of memories elsewhere in the brain. Very similar results are reported by Rose (see chapter 10) for passive-avoidance learning (of a bitter-tasting bead) in a day-old chicks. A region of the forebrain homologous to mammalian cortex (IMHV) appears necessary for initial acquisition but is not necessary for longer-term retention.

2 SPACE, PLACE, TRACE, AND OLFACTORY LEARNING: THE HIPPOCAMPUS AND LONG-TERM POTENTIATION

The clearest evidence to date implicating LTP in memory storage comes from studies on spatial and context memory, olfactory memory in rodents, trace conditioning in rabbits, and passive-avoidance learning in chicks (see chapter 10). The pioneering studies on "place" neurons in the hippocampus by O'Keefe, Nadel, Ranck and others (e.g., Kubie and Ranck, 1983; McNaughton et al., 1983; O'Keefe and Dostrovsky, 1971; O'Keefe and Nadel, 1978; Olton et al., 1978) led to the notion that the hippocampus plays a key role in spatial memory, a notion reinforced by many hippocampal lesion studies. Two tasks in particular, David Olton's radial arm maze and Richard Morris' water maze, have become the *sine qua non* assays for hippocampal damage in rodents (Morris et al., 1982; Olton and Samuelson, 1976).

The key evidence implicating LTP in hippocampal spatial memory comes from the work of Morris and associates (Morris et al., 1986, 1989, 1990). In brief, infusion of APV in the hippocampus or lateral ventricle markedly impairs memory for location of the hidden platform in the water maze. Further, there is a substantial correlation between impairment in the task and impairment in the induction of LTP (Morris et al., 1990).

In conditioned fear, measured by freezing behavior, lesions of the hippocampus made directly after training abolish the learned fear to context (distinctive cage) but not to tone (as noted earlier, tone-fear memory is abolished by amygdala lesions). However, if the lesion is made a week or more after training it does not impair fear-context memory (Kim and Fanselow, 1992). Importantly, infusion of APV in the hippocampus at the time of context-fear training prevents learning of context-fear but not tone-fear (Young et al., 1992). The transient nature of the necessary role of the hippocampus in context-fear memory is reminiscent of the transient role of the amygdala in instrumental fear memory (see above).

As Baudry and Lynch note (see chapter 5), the most effective parameters for inducing hippocampal LTP are brief, high-frequency trains given at the theta frequency, a 5−7 Hz rhythm prominent in much of the olfactory and limbic systems. It is also the rate at which rats sniff in bouts when exploring an environment. Recent work indicates that the hippocampus plays a critical role in olfactory learning and memory (see Eichenbaum et al., 1992; Lynch, 1986). Staubli et al. (1984) showed that rats were able to form learning sets for successive odor discriminations and that lesions of entorhinal cortex (major olfactory input to hippocampus is from the lateral entorhinal cortex) did not impair this ability if intertrial intervals were less than 3 min. However, the animals were profoundly impaired with longer intertrial intervals. Further, when animals were trained on a particular odor discrimination, rested for an hour, and then retrained on the same odors with their significance reversed, normal animals were slow to learn (earlier learning interfered) but lesioned animals immediately acquired the correct (formerly incorrect) odor.

In an intriguing series of studies, Eichenbaum and associates (see Eichenbaum et al., 1992) compared normal and fornix-lesioned rats on simultaneous vs. successive olfactory discrimination tasks. The lesioned animals were impaired relative to controls on the simultaneous discrimination but were in fact superior to controls in successive discriminations. They interpret this last and seemingly paradoxical result in terms of a "relational representation" hypothesis of hippocampal function. Hippocampal unit recordings indicated that (1) unit activity was typically time-locked to ongoing sniffing and theta rhythm, and (2) some units responded selectively to appropriate odor cues in both simultaneous and successive discriminations (Eichenbaum et al., 1989; Otto et al., 1991). Further, the patterns of firing of hippocampal units seem to correspond to the most effective patterns of stimulation for inducing LTP (see above). Collectively, the data on olfactory learning argue strongly that the hippocampal system is critically involved in some (relational ?) aspects of olfactory memory but that this involvement may be time limited (see Eichenbaum et al., 1992; Lynch, 1986).

When rabbits are trained in the conditioned eyeblink response, pyramidal neurons in the hippocampus rapidly develop an increase in discharge frequency that precedes and predicts the occurrence and form of the learned behavioral CR (Berger et al., 1976, 1980, 1983; Berger and Thompson, 1978; Hoehler and Thompson, 1980), a learning-induced pattern of response that in many ways resembles the learning-induced neuronal model in the cerebellar interpositus nucleus (see below). Although lesions of the hippocampus do not impair learning of the basic behavioral CR in the standard delay paradigm, they massively impair learning in long-trace interval training and in more complex discrimination procedures (Berger and Orr, 1983; Moyer et al., 1990; Solomon et al., 1986). Virtually identical results hold for humans with medial temporal lobe (hippocampal) anterograde amnesia—no impairment in learning the basic CR but marked impairment in more complex discrimination paradigms with eyeblink conditioning (Daum et al., 1991; Weiskranz and Warrington, 1979).

Several lines of evidence converge in support of the notion that LTP plays a key role in these hippocampal dependent aspects of eyeblink conditioning:

1. The granule cell monosynaptic population spike response in the dentate gyrus to single-pulse stimulation of the perforant path (pulse given in the intertrial interval) increases across days of training in close correlation with the development of learning (unpaired control animals show no changes) (Weisz et al., 1984).

2. Induction of LTP (perforant path to dentate gyrus) markedly facilitates discrimination reversal learning (Berger, 1984).

3. Induction of LTP in vivo (anesthetized rat) (but not low-frequency stimulation) causes a marked increase in AMPA but not NMDA binding in hippocampal cell membranes (see chapter 5; Tocco et al., 1992).

4. Eyeblink conditioning (but not unpaired control training) in both delay and trace paradigms causes a very similar (to 3) increase in AMPA but not NMDA binding in hippocampal cell membranes (Annala et al., 1992; Tocco et al., 1991). Interestingly, learning induced increases in hippocampal pyramidal neuron response tends to decrease as animals are given extensive over-training, suggesting that the role of the hippocampus may be time limited (Sears and Steinmetz, 1990).

3   AVERSIVE LEARNING OF DISCRETE RESPONSES: THE CEREBELLUM AND LONG-TERM DEPRESSION

Evidence to date argues strongly that the cerebellum and its associated brainstem circuitry is essential (necessary and sufficient) for both learning and memory of classical conditioning of the eyeblink response and, to the extent tested, other discrete skeletal muscle responses, learned with an aversive US. We review this evidence briefly (see Lavond et al., 1993; Steinmetz et al., 1992; Thompson, 1990 for detailed reviews and references), then focus on current evidence that the memory traces for this form of learning are stored in the cerebellum, and examine the possible role of long-term depression (LTD) as a mechanism of memory storage in cerebellar cortex.

In overview, the evidence summarized immediately below supports the following circuit hypotheses: the CS pathway includes the pontine nuclei and mossy fiber projections to the cerebellum; the US pathway includes the inferior olive and its climbing fiber projections to the cerebellum; and the CR pathway includes the efferent projection from the cerebellar interpositus nucleus (via the superior cerebellar peduncle) to the red nucleus and rubral projections to premotor and motor nuclei.

We initially reported that lesions of the cerebellum ipsilateral to the trained eye abolished the eyeblink CR completely and selectively, that is, the CR was *completely* abolished but the lesion had no effect on the UR. The lesions did not prevent learning in the contralateral eye. If the lesion was made before training, animals were completely unable to learn any CRs with the eye ipsilateral to the lesion. In other studies we and others obtained the same results with lesions of the superior cerebellar peduncle, the efferent pathway from interpositus to red nucleus. We then completed a study of effects of electrolytic lesions of the interpositus nucleus ipsilateral to the trained eye. Results demonstrated that if the lesions completely destroyed the critical region of the anterior interpositus nucleus the CR was abolished, with no effect on the UR. Since electrolytic lesions of the interpositus cause retrograde degeneration in the inferior olive, we made kainic acid lesions of the critical region of the interpositus, with identical results, namely, complete and selective abolition of the CR. Yeo and associates (1985) replicated our interpositus lesion result, using light and white noise CSs and a periorbital shock US, thus extending the generality of the findings (we used tone CS and corneal air-puff US). Reversible inactivation by microinfusion of nanomolar amounts of neurotransmitter antagonists in the critical region of the interpositus in already trained animals completely and reversibly abolished the CR, with no effect at all on the UR, in a dose-dependent fashion. This effect was extremely localized. We have periodically trained and retrained electrolytic interpositus-lesioned animals for periods up to 8 months; no CRs ever develop on the side of the lesion.

Recordings from the anterior interpositus nucleus during eyeblink conditioning revealed populations of cells that discharged when the conditioning stimuli were presented, and, more important, populations of cells that also discharged as a result of training just prior to execution of the classically conditioned response. These cells fired in a pattern that was similar to the learned behavioral response, that is, they formed an amplitude-time course "model" of the learned response that preceded and predicted the occurrence of the behavioral CR within trials and over the trials of training.

Electrical stimulation of the pontine nuclei serves as a "supernormal" CS, yielding more rapid learning than does a tone or light CS. With a pontine-stimulation CS, lesion of the middle cerebellar peduncle abolishes the CR, ruling out the possibility that the pontine CS is activating noncerebellar pathways, for example, by stimulation of fibers of passage or antidromic activation of sensory afferents. Stimulation of the middle cerebellar peduncle itself is an effective CS, and lesion of the interpositus nucleus abolishes the CR established with a pontine- or middle peduncle-stimulation CS. Localized lesions of the pontine nuclei can abolish the CR to a tone CS but not a light CS (i.e., can be selective for CS modality). Finally, when animals are trained using electrical stimulation of the pontine nuclei as a CS (corneal air-puff US), some animals show immediate and complete transfer of the behavioral eyeblink CR and the learning-induced neuronal model of the behavioral CR in the interpositus nucleus to a tone CS, arguing that the pontine stimulus and tone must activate a large number of memory trace elements (neurons) in common. All this evidence supports the hypothesis that the essential CS pathway includes projections from sensory relay nuclei to pontine nuclei and mossy fiber projections to the cerebellum.

Lesions of the face region of the dorsal accessory olive (DAO) prevent acquisition of the contralateral eyeblink CR if made before training and result in extinction and abolition of the CR in previously trained animals. Electrical microstimulation of this region of the DAO elicits eyeblink responses before training; indeed, virtually any phasic behavioral response can be so elicited, depending on the locus of the stimulating electrode. When DAO stimulation is used as a US, the exact response elicited by DAO stimulation is learned as a CR to a tone CS (Mauk et al., 1986). Control procedures demonstrated that the stimulus was activating climbing fibers to the cerebellum. Further, movements elicited from stimulation of the adjacent reticular formation could not be conditioned to a CS. Lesion of the interpositus nucleus abolished both the CR and UR elicited by DAO stimulation, thus ruling out the possibility that the UR is elicited by antidromic activation of reflex afferents (interpositus lesions effective in abolishing the CR have no effect on the reflex UR to the corneal air-puff US).

Neuronal unit activity recorded in the critical region of the DAO exhibits no responses at all to the tone CS and a clear evoked increase in unit activity to onset of the corneal air puff US prior to learning. Interestingly, this US-evoked neuronal activity decreases as animals learn and perform the CR but is still fully present on US alone trials. All of these results together support the hypothesis that the US pathway includes neurons of the DAO and their climbing fiber projection to the cerebellum. They also rule out the possibility that the memory trace is localized to the DAO—neurons that form the associative memory trace must receive inputs from both the CS (tone) and US (corneal air puff).

Electrical microstimulation of the critical region of the anterior interpositus nucleus evokes an eyeblink response in naive animals, and lesion of the superior cerebellar peduncle abolishes this response; the eyeblink circuit is hard-wired from interpositus nucleus to behavior. The region of the magnocellular red nucleus that receives projection from the critical region of the anterior interpositus also exhibits a learning-induced pattern of increased unit activity in eyeblink conditioning very similar to that shown by interpositus neurons. Lesions or reversible inactivation of this region of the red nucleus abolishes the eyeblink CR and has no effect on the reflex UR. Microstimulation of this region of the red nucleus in naive animals also elicits eyeblink responses. If the red nucleus is reversibly inactivated, the eyeblink CR is reversibly abolished but the learning-induced neuronal model of the CR in the interpositus nucleus is unaffected. In contrast, when the anterior interpositus nucleus is reversibly inactivated, both the behavioral CR and the learning-induced neuronal model of the CR in the magnocellular red nucleus are completely abolished. All this evidence supports the hypotheses that the eyeblink CR circuit is hard-wired from interpositus to behavior, that the memory trace is not in the red nucleus and is at or before the interpositus nucleus in the circuit.

3.1 Localization of the Cerebellar Memory Trace

Evidence cited above strongly supports a cerebellar locus of memory storage but does not prove it. Current studies using several methods of reversible inactivation appear to provide decisive evidence for this hypothesis. The logic is as follows: reversible inactivation of a structure in the essential memory trace circuit (defined above) will prevent expression of the CR. Hence, if naive animals are trained during inactivation of an essential structure, no CRs will be expressed during training. In postinactivation training, if animals exhibit no learning and then learn as if naive, the memory trace cannot have been formed prior to the inactivated structure in the essential circuit and must therefore be formed in the inactivated structure or beyond it in the essential circuit. If, on the other hand, asymptotic learning is exhibited from the beginning of postinactivation training, then the memory trace must be formed prior to the inactivated structure in the essential circuit.

Muscimol microinjection is in many ways an ideal method to use for reversible inactivation of brain structures. Following brief (2 min) infusion, muscimol inactivates soma-dendrites of neurons containing $GABA_A$ receptors (most neurons) by prolonged hyperpolarization for a period of several hours but does not inactivate fibers of passage (Olsen and Venter, 1986). Further, the exact effective distribution can be determined using ^{3}H-muscimol. Finally, repeated infusions of muscimol do not appear to have persisting effects on neuronal function (see below).

The effects of muscimol (and saline control) infusions in the cerebellum (anterior interpositus and cortex of lobule HVI) and muscimol infusions in the red nucleus (magnocellular division) during training in eyeblink conditioning of naive animals are shown in figure 11.1 (Krupa et al., 1993). Muscimol was infused 1 hr prior to training on each of 6 successive days. Following 3 days of no treatment, training was continued with no infusions. Results are striking. Neither the cerebellar nor red nucleus muscimol animals show any appreciable CRs during the 6 days of infusion training, whereas the saline control infusion animals learn to asymptote in the first 3 days. In postinfusion training the cerebellar muscimol animals show no signs of having learned and subsequently learn normally in a manner identical to animals naive to the training situation. In complete contrast, the red nucleus animals exhibit asymptotic learning from the very beginning of postinfusion training. Importantly, muscimol infusions in cerebellum and red nucleus have no effect on performance of the UR on US alone trials over the course of infusion training (every tenth trial throughout training was a US alone trial); hence muscimol infusions in the cerebellum effective in completely preventing learning have no effect at all on performance of the reflex response.

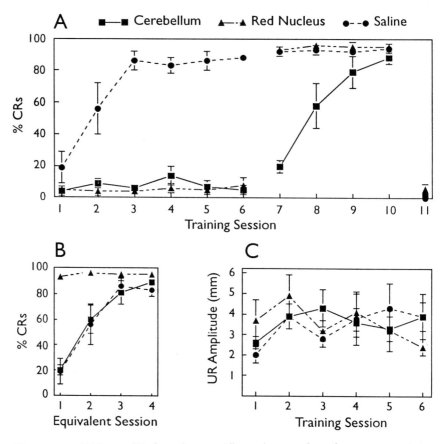

Figure 11.1 (A) Percent CRs for each group. All animals received an infusion prior to training on sessions 1–6. The cerebellar group (squarer; N = 6) received muscimol infusions into the ipsilateral lateral cerebellum, the red nucleus group (triangles; N = 6) received muscimol in the contralateral red nucleus, and the saline group (circles; N = 6) received 1 μl saline vehicle into the ipsilateral lateral cerebellum. No infusions were administered on days 7–10. All animals received muscimol infusions before session 11. Cerebellar muscimol infusions completely blocked any learning, whereas red nucleus infusions had no effect on learning but prevented expression of conditioned responses. (B) Percent CRs for equivalent sessions (sessions 1–4 of the saline group and sessions 7–10 of the cerebellar and red nucleus groups). (C) Unconditioned response (UR) amplitudes on airpuff only test-trials during the six sessions when infusions were administered. There were no significant differences between groups on these days. All data points are means ±SEM. Symbols are the same for all charts. (From Krupa et al., 1993)

Consequently, the memory trace must be formed and stored at or beyond the region of cerebellar inactivation and before the red nucleus. Since the CR pathway is a direct projection from interpositus nucleus to red nucleus (see above), we conclude that the memory trace must be formed and stored in the cerebellum.

Using a cold probe for reversible inactivation, Lavond and associates reported that training during cooling inactivation in the cerebellum (probe just dorsal to the anterior interpositus) completely prevented learning whereas training during cooling of the red nucleus did not prevent learning (Clark et al., 1992; Clark and Lavond, 1993). Cooling of each structure completely prevented expression of CRs during cooling training (5 days). In contrast, Welsh and Harvey (1991) claimed that infusion of lidocaine in the interpositus nucleus during training to a tone CS prevented expression of CRs during tone training (1 day) but did not prevent learning to tone as evidenced in post-inactivation training. However, their results are compromised by the fact that their animals had all previously been well-trained to a light CS and their control animals given saline during tone training showed marked transfer savings compared to naive animals.

To resolve this apparent discrepancy between results of cooling and lidocaine inactivation (note that in contrast to muscimol, both these methods inactivate axons as well as soma-dendrites), we used lidocaine infusions during training to a tone CS in naive animals (Nordholm et al., 1993). Lidocaine, incidentally, is more difficult to use than muscimol: it has a very short duration of action and must be infused continuously; because it does not bind to specific receptors, the effective distribution is difficult to determine. Results were strikingly clear. Naive animals given 3 or 6 days of tone CS training during continuous infusion of lidocaine just dorsal to the anterior interpositus, such that it inactivated the dorsal interpositus and cortex of lobule HVI (determined by infusion of ^{14}C-lidocaine), did not exhibit CRs during infusion training and did not learn at all—they subsequently learned as though naive to the training situation (directly comparable to saline control animals). A third group of naive animals were given lidocaine infusions during training in the white matter ventral to the anterior interpositus to inactivate the fibers of origin of the superior cerebellar peduncle, the efferent pathway from the interpositus. These animals showed no CRs during infusion training but exhibited virtually asymptotic learning from the beginning of postinfusion training. Importantly, the dorsal lidocaine infusion effective in completely preventing learning had no effect at all on performance of the UR on US-alone test trials over a wide range of US intensities. These lidocaine results completely confirm our muscimol results and Lavond's cold probe results—inactivation of the critical region of cerebellum (dorsal anterior interpositus nucleus and cortex of lobule HVI) completely prevents learning. Although it is possible that Welsh and Harvey's (1991) results were due to some of their cannulae being too ventral and hence inactivating the efferent pathway from the interpositus, it is more likely that their results are due to transfer of training—only a few trials where lidocaine was not completely effective would be needed to result in transfer of the already learned CR to the tone CS. The use of naive animals in our and Lavond's studies obviates this possibility.

More important, our lidocaine results demonstrate that the memory trace must be formed and stored at or beyond the dorsal region of inactivation and before the ventral region of inactivation in the cerebellum. Collectively, results of the reversible inactivation studies would seem to demonstrate conclusively that the essential memory trace for classical conditioning of the eyeblink response is formed and stored in the cerebellum.

3.2   Long-Term Depression and the Cerebellar Memory Trace

Although there is some disagreement about the extent to which lesions of cerebellar cortex impair or abolish the conditioned eyeblink response, there is general agreement that very large cortical lesions *markedly* impair the CR (Lavond et al., 1993; Yeo, 1991). At present, the most parsimonious hypothesis is that the essential memory trace involves processes of neuronal plasticity in cerebellar cortex and in the interpositus nucleus. Here we focus on cerebellar cortex and the hypothesis that LTD is the key underlying mechanism of synaptic plasticity.

As noted above, learning of the conditioned eyeblink response results in a marked increase in activity of neurons in the interpositus nucleus in the CS period that precedes and "models" the amplitude-time course of the behavioral CR. The simplest way this could occur would be for Purkinje neurons to decrease their activity in response to the CS so as to sculpt activity of interpositus neurons by decreasing inhibition (disinhibition) in a temporally patterned manner. The process of LTD, involving decreased excitability of parallel fiber synapses on appropriate Purkinje neurons, seems ideally suited to accomplish this. Recordings from Purkinje neurons in naive and trained animals provide evidence consistent with this hypothesis (Berthier and Moore, 1986; Donegan et al., 1985; Foy and Thompson, 1986; Krupa et al., 1990).

In brief, simple spike discharges (evoked by parallel fibers) recorded from Purkinje neurons in HVI and adjoining lobules exhibit the following patterns: before training, the majority of the Purkinje neurons that are influenced by the tone CS (many are not) show variable increases in tone-evoked discharge frequency (Foy and Thompson, 1986). In trained animals, the majority of Purkinje neurons that show CR-related activity exhibit decreases in discharge frequency in the CS period (but a significant minority show increases) (Foy et al., 1992). Gould, Miller, and Steinmetz (1991) provide an example where a single Purkinje neuron was held over training and the pattern shifted to a greater decrease in discharge frequency in the CS period over the course of learning. Interestingly, prior to training, US onset evokes complex spikes in Purkinje neurons influenced by the US but not in well-trained animals on trial where CRs occur (complex spikes are still evoked on US alone trials) (Krupa et al., 1991), an observation that led to the unit recording study in the inferior olive noted above.

Long-term depression has been amply demonstrated to occur in cerebellar cortex in vivo and in vitro (see chapter 6) and in other brain structures as well (see chapter 7). Several years ago we published an in vivo study that provides an analog to cerebellar LTD for eyeblink conditioning. In brief, electrical microstimulation of pontine nuclei or mossy fibers (middle cerebellar peduncle) served as a CS and microstimulation of the DAO—climbing fiber system that elicited movements served as the US. Animals learned whatever movement was elicited by DAO stimulation as a CR to the pontine CS in a normal manner and lesion of the interpositus abolished both the CR and the DAO elicited UR (Steinmetz et al., 1989). Temporal training parameters were analogous to those standard with peripheral stimuli (CS train onset preceded US train onset or single pulse by 250 ms). When one group of animals, trained with a single DAO pulse US, was given simultaneous presentations of CS and US after acquisition they exhibited extinction. This would seem to be inconsistent with LTD, particularly in most in vitro studies, where simultaneous or near-simultaneous stimulation of parallel fibers and climbing fiber is used.

We have recently explored this question in the in vitro cerebellar slice preparation, recording parallel fiber evoked field potentials (Chen and Thompson, 1992). In brief, we gave parallel fiber stimulation onset 250, 125, 0, or − 250 ms prior to onset of climbing fiber stimulation. A control parallel fiber pathway 300 μ away from the paired site was used to insure stability of the preparation. No GABA blocking agents were used. In overview, the 250 ms forward pairing condition gave the greatest amount of LTD, and backward pairing (climbing fiber stimulus 250 ms before parallel fiber stimulation) gave no LTD. Although simultaneous stimulation yielded much less LTD, with a sufficient number of stimulation trials simultaneous and all forward pairing conditions yielded LTD. Since all prior in vitro studies of LTD that used near-simultaneous stimulation also used GABA blocking agents, it may be that GABAergic interneuron processes play a critical role in temporal , properties of LTD (see also Schreurs and Alkon, 1992). Indeed, a recent mathematical/computational model of cerebellar cortex suggests a key role for the Golgi neurons in timing of eyeblink conditioning (Bartha and Thompson, 1992), as did Fujita earlier regarding adaptation of the vestibulo-ocular reflex (Fujita, 1982). In any event, these results at least suggest that the temporal properties of LTD and classical conditioning of discrete responses may not be inconsistent.

4 VISUAL MEMORY IN PRIMATES

We consider this large and important literature only briefly; it has been extensively reviewed (Dudai, 1989; Mishkin and Appenzeller, 1987; Squire, 1987). A good deal has been discovered about regions of cerebral cortex (and the hippocampus) that are necessary for various aspects of visual memory performance in monkeys. At least for long-term memory (e.g., of the shapes of visual objects), a region of temporal cortex (area TEO, see below) is often assumed to be the locus of storage, and there is some single-unit recording data consistent with this possibility (Miller et al., 1991; Sakai and Miyashita, 1991). Given the fact that long-term potentiation has now been demonstrated to occur in visual cortex (see chapters 7 and 8), such a locale and mechanism for long-term storage of visual information is an attractive possibility.

The visual system in the cerebral cortex of primates has been much elaborated over the visual regions in lower mammals; perhaps 20 different visual areas have been identified in the monkey and humans presumably have even more visual areas. These areas seem specialized for different aspects of visual function (e.g., V4 for color and V5 for movement). Humans with localized damage to one or another of these areas can show very specific kinds of defects in visual function, for example, inability to see color with all other aspects of visual perception normal, or inability to see movement with all other aspects of vision normal (Dowling, 1992).

There appear to be two major visual memory systems in the monkey brain. The details of these systems have been worked out mostly by Mishkin and associates, using the lesion method (Mishkin et al., 1983). One of these systems extends along the temporal lobe from the primary visual cortex through visual association areas to area TEO, to area VTE, and finally to hippocampus and amygdala. The other system projects from the visual areas to the parietal cortex. Monkeys were trained on visual discriminations where they must remember which of two objects seen over and over again is correct ("what") and in other tests they must learn the locations of objects in space ("where"). Lesions of the temporal area TEO markedly impair discrimination performance ("what" task) but not location performance ("where" task). Lesions in the parietal area have just the opposite effect, impairing "where" but not "what" tasks. Neurons in area TEO have very complex receptive fields for visual objects and neurons in the parietal association region appear to code the direction of intended reaching. So these two regions of cortex are necessary for these two types of visual memory tasks.

Are these the areas where "memories" for shape and location are stored? They are necessary for normal perception of shape and location but this may result from hard-wired circuits. Perhaps they are needed for seeing but not remembering. But on the other hand, if you can't see different shapes you can't remember that you have seen them before in a memory test. This question is very difficult to answer in evaluating effects of damage to visual areas on memory. Are the memories stored in the area or do the stimulus codings or "perceptions" necessary to form memories occur there but the memories are stored elsewhere? As of this writing, the issue is unresolved.

Lesions of area VTE and the hippocampus have quite different effects on visual performance then do lesions of area TEO In a now classic study, Mishkin (1978) used a short-term or working memory task—delayed nonmatching to sample. This is a task in which monkeys are presented with an object, which is then removed from vision. After a delay, two objects are presented and they are to select the noval object. He found that removal of both the hippocampus and the amygdala on both sides massively impaired this recent visual memory task, particularly with longer delay times. Similar results occur with lesions of cortical areas VTE. The monkey still remembers the principle that it was to choose the new object, but it cannot remember which was the old object. These monkeys can still see the difference between objects: they can be trained to choose one and not the other, and so it appears that their perceptions of objects are still normal. What has been lost is the ability to remember briefly what they have seen. Squire and associates more recently reported that monkeys with lesions limited to the hippocampus have this memory deficit, so the importance of the amygdala is at present not entirely clear (Zola-Morgan et al., 1989).

The short-term visual memory deficit Mishkin found in monkeys with limbic lesions seems rather different than human amnestic patients (e.g., H.M.) inability to place new experiences and facts into long-term memory (see Squire, 1987). Zola-Morgan and Squire (1990) devised a task that does seem to mimic some aspect of H.M.'s impairment. They trained monkeys to discriminate 100 pairs of objects, in which the animal had to learn which of two objects was rewarded for each pair, at different time periods prior to the time at which the hippocampus was surgically removed. Hence, objects learned earlier may involve long-term memory storage whereas objects learned recently may not. In a similar manner to the human amnestic patients, the monkeys with hippocampal damage remembered objects learned many weeks earlier better than recently learned objects. In fact, these monkeys remembered objects learned long ago prior to the surgery as well as did control monkeys. (H.M.'s memory for events prior to some months before his surgery were normal, whereas memory for events shortly before the surgery were entirely lost.) The strong implication is that in both monkeys and humans, the hippocampus is necessary for recent or "working" visual memory and for placing this information in long-term storage elsewhere in the brain (cerebral cortex?) but is not the locus of long-term storage.

5 OVERVIEW

The chapters in this volume address key contemporary issues in synaptic plasticity. It is perhaps useful here to provide a brief overview of the chapters in the larger context of putative mechanisms of memory storage.

Hockfield stresses the role of neuronal activity in development and developmental plasticity in the nervous system. She reminds us that the NMDA receptor, in addition to being critical for the induction of LTP, may play a key role in developmental plasticity and the regulation of such plasticity, that is, the end of the critical period in development. She adduces evidence that synaptic plasticity may be reduced by expression of the extracellular matrix, particularly the proteoglycan Cat-301, which can serve to stabilize synaptic structures. It seems that the NMDA receptor can regulate Cat-301 expression in motor neurons—activation causes expression, and blockade of NMDA receptors inhibits expression of Cat-301. From the perspective of memory storage the key issue is that bridges can exist between activation of the NMDA receptor that yields functional plasticity (LTP) and the regulation of gene expression that can yield long-lasting structural changes in synapses.

Steward focuses on one of the earliest and still most prominent hypothesis of memory storage, proposed initially by Tanzi and Ramón y Cajal: use promotes the formation of new synaptic connections and/or strengthens existing connections by long-lasting structural changes at synapses. He addresses the puzzling issue that if structural changes at synapses are due to changes in gene expression, namely, producing more, less, or different proteins, how does the neuron know to which synapses they go? Learning must involve changes in specific sets of synapses rather than changes in all synapses on a neuron (as do LTP and LTD). He explores three mechanisms (not mutually exclusive) for alterations in the postsynaptic structures of synapses—sorting of mRNA to dendrites and neuronal cell bodies, selective mRNA transport, and docking at synaptic sites.

Finch and McNeill utilize selective deafferentation of the hippocampus and striatum as models for neuronal changes that occur in aging and neurodegenerative disease. They focus on structural changes and changes in gene expression. From the point of view of mechanisms of memory storage, the key issue is that deafferentation can lead to massive structural changes in addition to simple degeneration, including the presumed formation of new synapses (e.g., sprouting, first discovered in hippocampus by Lynch and Cotman, and increases in gene expression). The adult nervous system is capable of extensive structural remodeling. These results amplify and extend to processes of aging occurrence of structural changes in neurons and synapses that occur with early experience (Greenough and Juraska, 1986) and are hypothesized by many to occur with specific memory storage.

Teyler and Grover focus on a relatively new aspect of LTP, the fact that a long-lasting form of potentiation resembling LTP can be induced in CA1 pyramidal neurons independent of activation of NMDA receptors. (NMDA independent potentiation had earlier been shown to occur in CA3 [Harris and Cotman, 1986].) The key variable is the frequency of tetanus—frequencies of 25–100 Hz appear to induce only NMDA-dependent LTP, but higher frequencies (> 150 Hz) induce both NMDA- and non-NMDA−dependent LTP. Calcium influx is necessary to induce both forms of LTP, the non-NMDA form apparently via voltage-dependent calcium channels. One functional difference between the two forms of LTP is time course; non-NMDA LTP is slower to develop and decline, requiring 10–20 min to peak expression. The implications of these two forms of LTP in the hippocampus for possible mechanisms of memory stortage are not clear. However, the differential effective tetanus frequencies for induction must surely have functional implications.

Baudry and Lynch provide a comprehensive overview of the current state of our understanding of biochemical mechanisms of LTP. There is general agreement that at least in the CA1 region of the hippocampus moderate-frequency tetanus (most effectively, theta-burst stimulation) induces LTP by activation of NMDA receptors (glutamate release from presynaptic terminals) and sufficient depolarization to release the Mg^{2+} block in the associated ion channel, leading to influx of Ca^{2+}. The authors stress a key issue that has plagued analysis of mechanisms of LTP: What forms or aspects of increased synaptic response are or are not LTP? For example, is the non-NMDA form of LTP induced by high-frequency stimulation (Teyler and Grover, chapter 4) "really" LTP? This question is not merely academic. The primary reason LTP (NMDA dependent in CA1) is viewed as a putative mechanism of memory storage is because it lasts for relatively long periods of time (weeks). However, since most current work on LTP-like phenomena is in slice, no evidence is available on duration. Indeed, as Baudry and Lynch note, there are very few in vivo studies of any form of increased synaptic response that have determined duration. All forms of increased synaptic response can result in increased transmission of information through the hippocampal circuitry; the key question is how long this increased transmission lasts. The authors present a convincing case (to this author, at least) that maintenance of LTP involves postsynaptic changes in AMPA receptors, but the authors do not rule out the possibility of presynaptic processes as well.

Ito provides a careful review of the possible intracellular biochemical mechanisms that may serve to underlie LTD. Ito first discovered LTD in cerebellar cortex, and this persisting form of decreased synaptic excitability has now been demonstrated in numerous studies in several brain structures (see chapter 7 by Artola and Singer). In brief, LTD in cerebellar cortex is a persisting decrease in the excitability of parallel fiber synapses on Purkinje neuron dendrites as a result of paired parallel fiber and climbing fiber activation. There is general agreement that both induction and expression are postsynaptic processes, that the expression is due to decreased sensitivity of AMPA receptors, that induction involves activation of the quis-metabotropic receptors (adult Purkinje neurons do not have NMDA receptors) and that the other key event in induction is influx of Ca^{2+}. LTD in cerebellar cortex is clearly associative in that paired activation of both parallel fibers and mossy fibers is required. Ito overviews the possible role of cerebellar LTD in motor learning and raises the interesting possibility that the cerebellum (and LTD) may also play a key role in complex cognitive processes (see also discussion above in this chapter).

Artola and Singer provide a very comprehensive review of the mechanisms of LTD in cerebellar cortex, neocortex, and hippocampus. They stress that two types of use-dependent LTD exist, heterosynaptic and homosynaptic. Heterosynaptic depression has been studied in hippocampus and in neocortex. In brief, it is expressed as reduced excitability on nonactivated synapses as a result of strong tetanic activation of other synapses on the same neuron, a condition that yields LTP at the stimulated synapses (both are often seen together). As in LTP, calcium influx is a necessary condition for heterosynaptic LTD. From a functional point of view, the concomitant development of LTP and heterosynaptic LTD could perhaps serve to enhance signal-to-noise for the relevant (tetanized) input. Homosynaptic depression was discovered by Ito in cerebellar cortex (see above) and has since been demonstrated to occur in hippocampus and neocortex as well. In these last two structures, LTD can be established by repeated stimulation of one excitatory input alone. Interestingly, in cerebellar cortex, repetitive stimulation of parallel fibers alone can induce an LTP-like increase in excitability (Sakurai, 1987, 1990) . On the other hand, evidence to date suggests that LTD in cerebellar cortex and neocortex share many common features: Ca^{2+} entry, a critical level of depolarization and activation of quis-metabotropic receptors are necessary for induction of LTD in both structures, and hyperpolarization can prevent LTD in both. Finally, activation of NMDA receptors is not necessary to induce LTD in either structure. In CA1, at least, homosynaptic LTD is induced by low-frequency stimulation and LTP by higher-frequency stimulation of the same afferent fibers. Artola and Singer's review presents a convincing case that LTP and LTD are robust phenomena in three major brain systems implicated in learning and memory: hippocampus, neocortex, and cerebellum.

Intrator, Bear, Cooper, and Paradiso present a very different approach to synaptic plasticity, a mathematical/computational model of the visual cortical network (initially developed several years ago by Cooper and associates). They use mean-field theory to represent the complexity of the network. The heart of the model is a theory of synaptic modifiability that expresses changes in synaptic efficacy as a function of input activity and quasi-local and time-averaged quasi-local variables. The theory makes predictions at two quite different levels, developmental plasticity of ensembles of neurons in visual cortex and processes of plasticity at synapses. At the former level, the theory can account remarkably well for a wide range of effects of various forms of visual deprivation during the critical period on the development of receptive field properties of neurons in visual cortex. At the synaptic level the theory predicted some years ago that synaptic depression (LTD) and synaptic potentiation (LTP) must develop at the same synapses as a function of input activity and quasi-local variables. Both of these processes have now, of course, been demonstrated to occur at the same synapses in visual and hippocampal cortex (see above and chapters 7 and 8 by Artola and Singer and Intrator et al.), a remarkable example of theoretical prescience. More generally, as we learn increasingly more about the details of neuronal circuits necessary for various apects of learning and memory and the associated processes of synaptic plasticity, it will be necessary to develop mathematical/computational models—the systems are far too complex to make meaningful quantitative predictions at a verbal-qualitative level of analysis.

Berger and associates present an elegant, coordinated theoretical and empirical analysis of the flow and transformations of information through the hippocampal system. In brief, nonlinear systems analysis applied to information processing in the hippocampus predicted unexpected aspects of information flow that were then verified empirically. Thus, instead of the traditionally assumed cascade relationship between the three subsystems of the hippocampus, excitatory input from the entorhinal cortex inltiates a two-stage feedforward excitation of pyramidal cells with the dentate gyrus providing feedforward excitation of CA3, and with both the dentate and CA3 providing feedforward excitation of CA1 . In addition, these authors prepared a mini slice of dentate gyrus that is open loop, to characterize the within-subsystem interactions. Interestingly, the input-output properties of granule cells within these mini slices were not distinguishable from those of whole slices, indicating that feedback from hilar interneurons were not substantial. In addition, the authors are developing a field theory model of the hippocampus that proves a continuous representation in space and time where the effects of molecular events on network dynamics can be described. These systems-level approaches share conceptual similarities with the work of Cooper and associates (see chapter 8) and would seem to be the way of the future to capture and analyze quantitatively the information processing properties of large ensembles of neurons.

Rose summarizes beautifully the result of the extensive series of studies on learning in the day-old chick, focusing on one-trial passive avoidance (having once pecked a bead coated with a bitter-tasting substance, they avoid similar appearing beads subsequently). (Results of these studies are similar in some ways to results of work on imprinting in day-old chicks [see Horn, 1991]). Rose and associates initially identified two regions of the brain that exhibited enhanced activity as a result of learning, as indexed by accumulation of radiolabeled 2-DG. One region was the intermediate medial hyperstriatum ventrale (IMHV, approximately homologous to mammalian visual cortex) and lobus perolfactorius (LPO, a part of the basal ganglia). Rose summarizes an extensive series of studies showing that NMDA activation of neurons in IMHV is necessary for learning and that a cascade of biochemical processes, including expression of immediate early genes, increased production of membrane glycoproteins and structural changes in synapses accompany the learning process, implying that alterations in gene expression are necessary for long-term storage. Lesion studies on the relative roles of IMHV and LPO indicate that the initial or short-term memory is formed in IMHV but that IMHV is not necessary for long-term memory; LPO and other regions are more critical for long-term storage. These results are strikingly analogous to the role of the amygdala in passive avoidance and the hippocampus in context-fear in aversive learning in mammals (see above, this chapter). Rose's chapter exemplifies very well the "model-system" approach to analyzing the neurobiological substrates of memory at all levels from behavior to gene expression. My only disappointment is that at the end of the chapter he surrenders to the cognitive psychologists and suggests that memories, even memories for bitter beads in day-old chicks, are widely distributed in the brain.

6 CONCLUSION

The chapters in this volume make clear that both LTP-and LTD-like processes occur in cerebral cortex, cerebellar cortex, and hippocampus, and an LTP-like process occurs in the amygdala. The blocking effects of APV in hippocampus on spatial memory, in amygdala on conditioned fear, and in IMHV on passive-avoidance learning in chicks certainly argue, at the least, that NMDA receptors in these structures play necessary roles in initial learning. The key issue remains whether LTP and LTD are in fact mechanisms of long-term memory storage in the mammalian brain.

Although hippocampal LTP is commonly viewed as a mechanism of long-term memory storage, from a systems-level viewpoint the hippocampus is not an island unto itself. It is a part of a larger circuit receiving input from cortical and subcortical sources and projecting to a variety of cortical and subcortical sites. The effect of LTP is to facilitate or enhance (and transform?) transmission of information that flows within and through the hippocampus and to its efferent targets and beyond. The nature of the information relayed through the hippocampus and the possible transformations effected by the hippo-campus are currently intense areas of investigation (see chapter 9 by Berger and associates).

As noted in this chapter, evidence from a variety of preparations suggests that the role of the hippocampus in memory storage is time-limited. Hippo-campal lesions made shortly after a learning experience markedly impair sub-sequent memory performance, whereas the same lesions made at a longer time after the experience do not, in visual object discrimination in monkeys, in context fear learning in rats, in olfactory discriminations in rats, in passive-avoidance learning in chicks (IMHV), and in declarative memory in humans. Furthermore, the hippocampus plays a key role in working memory (delayed nonmatching to sample) in monkeys. Similar results appear to obtain for the amygdala, at least in instrumental fear learning. Learning-induced increases in hippocampal unit activity in eyeblink conditioning (in rabbits) seem to de-crease with extensive over-training. If LTP is in fact a mechanism of memory storage in the hippocampus and amygdala (and IMHV in chicks), then perhaps it is a process that subserves time-limited storage, facilitating more permanent storage elsewhere in the brain.

Cerebellar storage of long-term memories for discrete response (e.g., eye-blink conditioning) does not appear to be time-limited—no matter how much time or how much training is given, effective lesions made before or after training completely and permanently prevent and abolish the learned response (Steinmetz et al., 1992). There is as yet no information regarding the duration of LTD. If LTD is time-limited and if LTD does subserve memory formation in cerebellar cortex, then perhaps both short-term and long-term storage storage processes occur in the cerebellum. One possible scenario would be that LTD in cerebellar cortex subserves "working" memory (e.g., for motor skills) and serves to induce the formation of long-term or permanent storage in cerebellar nuclei and/or in cerebellar cortex.

More generally, if LTP and LTD are time-limited processes in brain struc-tures, then perhaps they serve to enable more permanent structural changes in the brain. Several of the chapters in this volume focus on structural changes in synapses as the key aspect of synaptic plasticity that could subserve long-term memory storage.

We are still some distance from being able to demonstrate a strict causal chain from a process of LTP or LTD in a brain structure to the memory, that is, to the learned behavioral response. The hippocampal system is particularly difficult in this regard in that little is known about the readout from hippo-campus to behavior. At least in the amygdala (conditioned fear) and cerebel-lum (discrete responses) much of the readout circuitry is known. But as Baudry and Lynch (chapter 5) stress, very little information is available on the most elementary requirement for LTP and LTD as long-term memory mechanisms —how long do they persist in the intact, behaving animal? Equally important, only a few studies to date have addressed perhaps the most obvious require-ment of all—do learning experiences in fact result in the establishment of LTP-, or LTD-like processes in appropriate regions of the brain?

ACKNOWLEDGMENTS

Supported in part by grants from ONR (N00014-91-J0112), NSF (BNS-8117115), NIH (AG05142), and the McKnight Foundation to R.F.T.

REFERENCES

Amaral, D. G. (1987) Memory: Anatomical organization of candidate brain regions. In *Handbook of Physiology, Volume V: Higher Function of the Brain*, F. Plum (ed.), William and Wilkins, Baltimore.

Annala, A. J., Tocco, G., Baudry, M., and Thompson, R. F. (1992) Classical conditioning of eyeblink response in trace paradigm modifies AMPA and CNQX binding in the rabbit hippocampus. *Soc. Neurosci. Abstr.* 18:344.

Applegate C. D., Frysinger, R. C., Kapp, B. S., and Gallagher, M. (1982) Multiple unit activity recorded from the amygdala central nucleus during Pavlovian heart rate conditioning in the rabbit. *Brain Res.* 238:457−462.

Bartha, G. T., and Thompson, R. F. (1992) Cerebellar control of conditioned eyeblink timing. *Soc. Neurosci. Abstr.* 18:1206.

Berger, T. W. (1984) Long-term potentiation of hippocampal synatpic transmission affects rate of behavioral learning. *Science* 224:627−630.

Berger, T. W., and Orr, W. B. (1983) Hippocampectomy selectively disrupts discrimination reversal conditioning of the rabbit nictitating membrane response. *Behav. Brain Res.* 8:49−68.

Berger, T. W., and Thompson, R. F. (1978) Neuronal plasticity in the limbic system during classical conditioning of the rabbit nictitating membrane response. I. The hippocampus. *Brain Res.* 145:323−346.

Berger T. W., Alger, B., and Thompson, R. F. (1976) Neuronal substrate of classical conditioning the hippocampus. *Science* 192:483−485.

Berger, T. W., Laham, R. I., and Thompson, R. F. (1980) Hippocampal unit-behavior correlations during classical conditioning. *Brain Res.* 193:229−248.

Berger, T. W., Rinaldi, P. C., Weisz, D. J., and Thompson, R. F. (1983) Single-unit analysis of different hippocampal cell types during classical conditioning of rabbit nictitating membrane response. *J. Neurophysiol.* 50:1197−1219.

Berthier, N. E., and Moore, J. W. (1986). Cerebellar Purkinje cell activity related to the classically conditioned nictitating membrane response. *Exp. Brain Res.* 63:341−350.

Bolles, R. C., and Fanselow, M. S. (1980) A perceptual-defensive-recuperative model of fear and pain. *Behav. Brain Sci.* 3:291−323.

Campeau, S., and David, M. (1991) Lesions of the auditory thalamus block acquisition and expression of aversive conditioning to an auditory but not a visual stimulus measured with the fear potentiated startle paradigm. *Soc. Neurosci. Abstr.* 17:658.

Campeau, S., Miserendino, M. J. D., and Davis, M. (1992) Intra-amygdala infusion of the N-methyl-D-aspartate receptor antagonist AP5 blocks acquisition but not expression of fear-potentiated startle to an auditory conditioned stimulus. *Behav. Neurosci.* 106:569−574.

Chapman, P. F., and Bellavance, L. L. (1992) Induction of long-term potentiation in the basolateral amygdala does not depend on NMDA receptor activation. *Synapse* 11:310−318.

Chapman, P. F., Kairiss, E. W., Keenan, C. L., and Brown, T. H. (1990) Long-term synaptic potentiation in the amygdala. *Synapse* 6:271−278.

Chen, C., and Thompson, R. F. (1992) Associative long-term depression revealed by field potential recording in rat cerebellar slice. *Soc. Neurosci. Abstr.* 18:1215.

Clark, R. E., and Lavond, D. G. (1993) Reversible lesions of the red nucleus during acquisition and retention of a classically conditioned behavior in rabbits. *Behav. Neurosci.* 107:264–270.

Clark, R. E., Zhang, A. A., and Lavond, D. G. (1992) Reversible lesions of the cerebellar interpositus nucleus during acquisition and retention of a classically conditioned behavior. *Behav. Neurosci.* 106:879–888.

Clugnet, M. C., and LeDoux, J. E. (1990) Synaptic plasticity in fear conditioning circuits: Induction of LTP in the lateral nucleus of the amygdala by stimulation of the medial geniculate body. *J. Neurosci.* 10:2818–2824.

Daum, I., Channon, S., Pokey, C. E., and Gray, J. A. (1991) Classical conditioning after temporal lobe lesions in man: Impairment in conditional discrimination. *Behav. Neurosci.* 105:396–408.

Davis, M. (1992) The role of the amygdala in fear and anxiety. *Annu. Rev. Neurosci.* 15:353–375.

Donegan, N. H., Foy, M. R., and Thompson, R. F. (1985) Neuronal responses of the rabbit cerebellar cortex during performance of the classically conditioned eyelid response. *Soc. Neurosci. Abstr.* 11:835.

Dowling, J. (1992) *Neurons and Networks: An Introduction to Neuroscience.* The Belknap Press of Harvard University Press, Cambridge.

Dudai, Y. (1989) *The Neurobiology of Memory.* Oxford University Press, New York.

Eichenbaum, H., Wiener, S. I., Shapiro, M., and Cohen, N. J. (1989) The organization of spatial coding in the hippocampus: A study of neural ensemble activity. *J. Neurosci.* 2:2764–2775.

Eichenbaum, H., Otto, T., and Cohen, N. J. (1992) The hippocampus—what does it do? *Behav. Neural Biol.* 57:2–36.

Fanselow, M. S., Kim, J. J., and Landeira-Fernandez, J. (1991) Anatomically selective blockade of Pavlovian fear conditioning by application of an NMDA antagonist to the amygdala and periqaueductal gray. *Soc. Neurosci. Abstr.* 17:659.

Farb, C. F., LeDoux, J. E., and Milner, T. A. (1989) Glutamate is present in medial geniculate body neurons that project to lateral amygdala and in lateral amygdala presynaptic terminals. *Soc. Neurosci. Abstr.* 15:890.

Foy, M. R., and Thompson, R. F. (1986) Single unit analysis of Purkinje cell discharge in classically conditioned and untrained rabbits. *Soci. Neurosci. Abstr.* 12:518.

Foy, M. R., Krupa, D. J., Tracy, J., and Thompson, R. F. (1992) Analysis of single unit recordings from cerebellar cortex of classically conditioned rabbits. *Soc. Neurosci. Abstr.* 19:1215.

Fujita, M. (1982) Simulation of adaptive modification of the vestibular-ocular reflex with an adaptive filter model of th cerebellum. *Biol. Cybernet.* 45:207–214.

Gallagher, M. and Kapp, B. S. (1978) Manipulation of opiate activity in the amygdala alters memory processes. *Life Sci.* 23:1973–1978.

Gold, P. E. (1992) Modulation of memory processing: Enhancement of memory in rodents and humans. In pp. 402–414. *Neuropsychology of Memory* (2nd ed.), L. R. Squire and N. Butters (eds.), Guliford Press, New York.

Gould, T. J., Miller, D. P., and Steinmetz, J. E. (1991) Differences in acquisition and extinction of conditioning-related neuronal activity in rabbit cerebellar cortex and interpositus nucleus. *Soc. Neurosci. Abstr.* 17:323.

Greenough, W. T., and Juraska, J. M. (1986) *Developmental Neuropsychobiology.* Academic Press, Orlando.

Harris, E. W., and Cotman, C. W. (1986) Long-term potentiation of guinea pig mossy fiber responses is not blocked by *N*-methyl-D-aspartate receptor antagonists. *Neurosci. Lett.* 70:132–137.

Helmstetter, F. J. (1992) The amygdala is essential for the expression of conditional hypoalgesia. *Behav. Neurosci.* 106:518–528.

Hitchcock, J. M., and Davis, M. (1986) Lesions of the amygdala, but not of the cerebellum or red nucleus, block conditioned fear as measured with the potentiated startle paradigm. *Behav. Neurosci.* 100:11–22.

Hitchcock, J. M., Sananes, C. B., and Davis, M. (1989) Sensitization of the startle reflex by footshock: Blockade by lesions of the central nucleus of the amygdala or its efferent pathway to the brainstem. *Behav. Neurosci.* 103:509–518.

Hoehler, F. K., and Thompson, R. F. (1980) Effect of the interstimulus (CS-UCS) interval on hippocampal unit activity during classical conditioning of the nictitating membrane response of the rabbit (*Oryctolagus cuniculus*). *J. Comp. Physiol. Psychol.* 94:201–215.

Horn, G. (1991). In *Neural and behavioral plasticity: The use of the domestic chick as a model*, R. J. Andrew (ed.), pp. 219–261. Oxford University Press, Oxford.

Iwata, J., LeDoux, J. E., Meeley, M. P., Arneric, S., and Reis, D. J. (1986a) Intrinsic neurons in the amygdaloid field projected to by the medial geniculate body mediate emotional responses conditioned to acoustic stimuli. *Brain Res.* 383:195–214.

Iwata, J., LeDoux, J. E., and Reis, D. J. (1986b). Destruction of intrinsic neurons in the lateral hypothalamus disrupts cardiovascular but not behavioral conditioned emotional responses. *Brain Res.* 368:161–166.

Iwata, J., Chida, K., and LdDoux, J. E. (1987) Cardiovascular responses elicited by stimulation of neurons in the central amygdaloid nucleus in awake but not anesthetized rats resemble conditioned cardiovascular responses. *Brain Res.* 418:183–188.

Kapp, B. S., Frysinger, R., Gallagher, M., and Haselton, J. (1979) Amygdala central nucleus lesions: Effects on heart rate conditioning in the rabbit. *Physiol. Behav.* 23:1109–1117.

Kapp, B. S., Markgraf, C. G., Wilson, A., Pascoe, J. P., and Supple, W. F. (1991) Contributions of the amygdala and anatomically-related structures to the acquisition and expression of aversively conditioned responses. In *Current Topics in Animal Learning: Brain, Emotion and Cognition*, L. Dachowski & C. F. Flaherty (eds.). Lawrence Erlbaum: Hove.

Kim, J. J., and Fanselow, M. S. (1992) Modality-specific retrograde amnesia of fear. *Science* 256:675–677.

Kim, J. J., DeCola, J. P., Landeira-Fernandez, J., and Fanselow, M. S. (1991) *N*-methyl-D-aspartate receptor antagonist APV blocks acquisition but not expression of fear conditioning. *Behav. Neurosci.* 105:126–133.

Kim, J. J., Fanselow, M. S., DeCola, J. P., and Landeira-Fernandez, J. (1992) Selective impairment of long-term but not short-term conditional fear by the *N*-methyl-D-aspartate antagonist APV. *Behav. Neurosci.* 106:591–596.

Kim, M., and Davis, M. (1992) Electrolytic lesions of the amygdala block acquisition and expression of conditioned fear even with extensive training, but do not prevent reqcquisition, as assessed by fear-potential startle. *Soc. Neurosci. Abstr.* 18:652.5.

Kim, M., and McGaugh, J. L. (1992) Effects of intra-amygdala injections of NMDA receptor antagonists on acquisition and retention of inhibitory avoidance. *Brain Res.* 585:35–48.

Krupa, D. J., Weiss, C., Tracy, J., and Thompson, R. F. (1990) Single unit responses from the cerebellar cortex of naive rabbits. *Soc. Neurosci. Abstr.* 16:762.

Krupa, D. J., Weiss, C., and Thompson, R. F. (1991) Air puff evoked Purkinje cell complex spike activity is diminished during conditioned responses in eyeblink conditioned rabbits. *Soc. Neurosci.* 17:322.

Krupa, D. J., Thompson, J. K., and Thompson, R. F. (1993) Localization of a memory trace in the mammalian brain. *Science*, 260:989–991.

Kubie, J. L., and Ranck, J. B. (1983) Sensory-behavior correlation in individual hippocampus neurons in three situations: Space and context. In *Molecular, Cellular, and Behavioral Neurobiology of the Hippocampus*, W. Seifert (ed.). Academic Press, New York.

Lavond, D. G., Kim, J. J., and Thompson, R. F. (1993) Mammalian brain substrates of aversive classical conditioning. *Annu. Rev. Psychol.* 44:317–342.

LeDoux, J. E. (1991) Systems and synapses of emotional memory. In *Memory: Organization and Locus of Change*, L. R. Squire, N. M. Weinberger, G. Lynch, and J. L. McGaugh (eds.). Oxford University Press, Oxford.

LeDoux, J. E., Iwata, J., Cicchetti, P., and Reis, D. J. (1988) Different projections of the central amygdaloid nucleus mediate autonomic and behavioral correlates of conditioned fear. *J. Neurosci.* 8:2517–2529.

LeDoux, J. E., Farb, C., and Ruggiero, D. A. (1990) Topographic organization of neurons in the acoustic thalamus that project to the amygdala *J. Neurosci.* 10:1043–1054.

Liang, K. C., McGaugh, J. L., Martinez, J. L., Jensen, R. A., Jr., Vasquez, B. J., and Messing, R. B. (1982) Posttraining amygdaloid lesions impair retention of an inhibitory avoidance response. *Behav. Brain Res.* 4:237–249.

Liang, K. C., Juler, R., and McGaugh, J. L. (1986) Modulating effects of posttraining epinephrine on memory: Involvement of the amygdala noradrenergic system. *Brain Res.* 368:125–133.

Lynch, G. (1986) *Synapses, Circuits, and the Beginnings of Memory*. MIT Press, Cambridge.

Mauk, M. D., Steinmetz, J. E., and Thompson, R. F. (1986) Classical conditioning using stimulation of the inferior olive as the unconditioned stimulus. *Proc. Nat. Acad. Sci. USA* 83:5349–5353.

McGaugh, J. L. (1989) Involvement of hormonal and neuromodulatory systems in the regulation of memory storage. *Annu. Rev. Neurosci.* 12:255–287.

McGaugh, J. M. (1992) Affect, neuromodulatory systems and memory storage. In *Handbook of Emotion and Memory: Current Research and Theory*, S. A. Christoson (ed.), pp. 245–268. Lawrence Erlbaum, Hillsdale, N. J.

McNaughton, B. L., Barnes, C. A., and O'Keefe, J. (1983) The contribution of position, direction, and velocity to single unit activity in the hippocampus of freely-moving rats. *Exp. Brain Res.* 52:41–49.

Miller, E. K., Li, L., and Desimone, R. (1991) A neural mechanism for working and recognition memory in inferior temporal cortex. *Science* 254:1377–1379.

Miserendino, M. J. D., Sananes, C. B., Melia, K. R., and Davis, M. (1990) Blocking of acquisition but not expression of conditioned fear-potentiated startle by NMDA antagonists in the amygdala. *Nature* 319:716–718.

Mishkin, M. (1978) Memory in monkeys severely impaired by combined but not separate removal of amygdala and hippocampus. *Nature* 273:297–298.

Mishkin, M., and Appenzeller, T. (1987) The anatomy of memory. *Sci. Am.* 256:62–71.

Mishkin, M., Ungerledier, L. G., and Macko, K. A. (1983) Object vision and spatial vision: Two cortical pathways. *Trends Neurosci.* 6:414–417.

Morris, R. G. M., Garrud, P., Rawlins, J. N. P., and O'Keefe, J. (1982) Place navigation impaired in rats with hippocampal lesions. *Nature* 297:681–683.

Morris, R. G. M., Anderson, E., Lynch, G. S., and Baudry M. (1986) Selective impairment of learning and blockade of long-term potentiation by a N-methyl-D-aspartate receptor antagonist, AP5. *Nature* 319:774–776.

Morris, R. G. M., Halliwell, R. F., and Bowery, N. (1989) Synaptic plasticity and learning II: Do different kinds of plasticity underlie different kinds of learning? *Neuropsychologia* 27:41–59.

Morris, R. G. M., Davis, S., and Butcher, S. P. (1990) Hippocampal synatpic plasticity and NMDA receptors: A role in information storage? *Philos. Trans. R. Soc. Lond.* 329:187–204.

Moyer, J. R., Deyo, R. A., and Disterhoft, J. R. (1990) Hippocampectomy disrupts trace eye-blink conditioning in rabbits. *Behav. Neurosci.* 104:243–252.

Nordholm, A. F., Thompson, J. K., Dersarkissian, C., and Thompson, R. F. (1993). Lidocaine infusion in a critical region of cerebellum completely prevents learning of the conditioned eyeblink response. *Behav. Neurosci.*, in press.

O'Keefe, J., and Dostrovsky, J. (1971) The hippocampus as spatial map: Preliminary evidence from unit activity in the freely moving rat. *Brain Res.* 34:171–175.

O'Keefe, J., and Nadel, L. (1978) *The Hippocampus as a Cognitive Map.* Clarendon Press, London.

Olsen, R. W., and Venter, J. C. (1986) *Benzodiazepin/GABA Receptors and Chloride Channels: Structural and Functional Properties.* Alan R. Liss, New York.

Olton, D. S., and Samuelson, R. J. (1976) Remembrance of places passed: Spatial memory in rats. *J. Exp. Psychol. [Anim. Behav.]* 2:97–116.

Olton, D. S., Branch, M., and Best P. J. (1978) Spatial correlates of hippocampal unit activity. *Exp. Neurol.* 58:387–409.

Otto, T., Eichenbaum, H., Wiener, S. I., and Wible, C. G. (1991) Learning-related patterns of CA1 spike trains parallel stimulation parameters optimal for inducing hippocampal long-term potentiation. *Hippocampus* 1:181–192.

Parent, M. B., Tomaz, C., and McGaugh, J. L. (1992) Increased training in an aversively moti-vated task attenuates the memory-impairing effects of posttraining N-methyl-D-aspartate-in-duced amygdala lesions. *Behav. Neurosci.* 106:789–797.

Pascoe, J. P., and Kapp, B. S. (1985a) Electrophysiological characteristics of amygdaloid central nucleus neurons in the awake rabbit. *Brain Res. Bull.* 14:331–338.

Pascoe, J. P., and Kapp, B. S. (1985b) Electrophysiological characteristics of amygdaloid central nucleus neurons during Pavlovian fear conditioning in the rabbit. *Behav. Brain Res.* 16:117–133.

Phillips, R. G., and LeDoux, J. E. (1992) Differential contribution of amygdala and hippocampus to cued and contextual fear conditioning. *Behav. Neurosci.* 106:274–285.

Prokasy, W. F. (1972) Developments with the two-phase model applied to human eyelid conditioning. In *Classical Conditioning II. Current Research and Theory,* A. H. Black and W. F. Prokasy (eds.). Appleton-Century-Crofts, New York.

Rescorla, R. A. (1988a) Behavioral studies of Pavlovian conditioning. *Annua. Rev. Neurosci.* 11:329–352.

Rescorla, R. A. (1988b) Pavlovian conditioning: It's not what you think it is. *Am. Psychol.* 43:151–160.

Rescorla, R. A., and Solomon, R. L. (1967) Two process learning theory: Relationships between Pavlovian conditioning and instrumental learning. *Psychol. Rev.* 74:151–182.

Rosen, J. B., and Davis, M. (1990) Enhancement of electrically elicited startle by amygdaloid stimulation. *Physiol. Behav.* 48:343−349.

Sakai, K., and Miyashita, Y. (1991) Neural organization for the long-term memory of paired associates. *Nature* 354:152−155.

Sakurai, M. (1987) Synaptic modification of parallel fibre-Purkinje cell transmission in in vitro guinea-pig cerebellar slices. *J. Physiol.* 394:463−480.

Sakurai, M. (1990) Calcium is an intracellular mediator of the climbing fiber in induction of cerebellar long-term depression. *Proc. Nat. Acad. Sci. USA* 87:3383−3385.

Schreurs, B. G., and Alkon, D. L. (1992) Long-term depression and classical conditioning of the rabbit nictitating membrane response: An assessment using the rabit cerebellar slice. *Soc. Neurosci. Abstr.* 18:337.

Sears, L. L., and Steinmetz, J. E. (1990) Acquisition of classical conditioning-related activity in the hippocampus is affected by lesions of the cerebellar interpositus nucleus. *Behav. Neurosci.* 104:681−692.

Solomon, P. R., Vander Schaff, E. R., Thompson, R. F., and Weisz, D. J. (1986) Hippocampus and trace conditioning of the rabbit's classically conditioned nictitating membrane response. *Behav. Neurosci.* 100:729−744.

Squire, L. R. (1987) *Memory and Brain.* Oxford University Press, New York.

Staubli, U., Ivy, G., and Lynch, G. (1984) Hippocampal denervation causes rapid forgetting of olfactory information in rats. *Proc. Nat. Acad. Sci. USA* 81:5885−5887.

Steinmetz, J. E., Lavond, D. G., and Thompson, R. F. (1989) Classical conditioning in rabbits using pontine nucleus stimulation as a conditioned stimulus and inferior olive stimulation as an unconditioned stimulus. *Synapse* 3:225−232.

Steinmetz, J. E., Lavond, D. G., Ivkovich, D., Logan, C. G., and Thompson, R. F. (1992) Disruption of classical eyelid conditioning after cerebellar lesions: Damage to a memory trace system or a simple performance deficit? *J. Neurosci.* 12:4403−4426.

Thompson, R. F. (1990) Neural mechanisms of classical conditioning in mammals. *Philos. Trans. R. Soc. Lond. (Biol.)* 329:161−170.

Thompson, R. F., and Gluck, M. A. (1991) Brain substrates of basic associative learning and memory. In *Perspective on Cognitive Neuroscience*, H. J. Weingartner and R. F. Lister (eds.). Oxford University Press, New York.

Tocco, G., Devgan, K. K., Hauge, S. A., Weiss, C., Baudry, M., and Thompson, R. F. (1991) Classical conditioning selectively increases AMPA receptor binding in rabbit hippocampus. *Brain Res.* 559:331−336.

Tocco, G., Maren, S., Shors, T. J., Baudry, M., and Thompson, R. F. (1992) Long-term potentiation is associated with increased ^{3}H-AMPA binding in rat hippocampus. *Brain Res.* 573:228−234.

Wagner, A. R., and Brandon, S. E. (1989) Evolution of a structured connectionist model of Pavlovian conditioning ESOP). In *Contemporary Learning Theories: Pavlovian Conditioning and the Status of Traditional Learning Theory*, S. B. Klein and R. R. Mowrer (eds.). Lawrence Erlbaum, Hillsdale, N.J.

Wagner, A. R., and Donegan, N. H. (1989) Some relationships between a computational model (SOP) and a neural circuit for Pavlovian (rabbit eyeblink) conditioning. In *The Psychology of Learning and Motivation*, R. D. Hawkins and G. H. Bower (eds.). Academic Press, San Diego.

Weiskrantz, L., and Warrington, E. K. (1979) Conditioning in amnestic patients. *Neuropsychologia* 17:187−194.

Weisz, D. J., Clark, G. A., and Thompson, R. F. (1984) Increased responsivity of dentate granule cells during nictitating membrane response conditioning in rabbit. *Behav. Brain Res.* 12:145–154.

Welsh, J. P., and Harvey, J. A. (1991) Palovian conditioning in the rabbit during inactivation of the interpositus nucleus. *J. Physiol.* 444:459–480.

Yeo, C. H. (1991) Cerebellum and classical conditioning of motor responses. *Ann. N.Y. Acad. Sci.* 627:292–305.

Yeo, C. H., Hardiman, M. J., and Glickstein, M. (1985) Classical conditioning of the nictitating membrane response of the rabbit. I. Lesions of the cerebellar nuclei. *Exp. Brain Res.* 60:87–98.

Young, S. L., Fanselow, M. S., and Bohenek, D. L. (1992) The dorsal hippocampus and contextual fear conditioning. *Soc. Neurosci. Abstr.* 18:652–611.

Zola-Morgan, S., and Squire, L. R. (1990) The primate hippocampal formation: Evidence for a time-limited role in memory storage. *Science* 250:288–290.

Zola-Morgan, S., Squire, L. R., and Amaral, D. G. (1989) Lesions of the amygdala that separate adjacent cortical regions do not impair memory or exacerbate the impairment following lesions of the hippocampal formation. *J. Neurosci.* 9:1922–1936.

Index